FOSTERING SOCIAL JUSTICE
THROUGH QUALITATIVE INQUIRY

FOSTERING SOCIAL JUSTICE THROUGH QUALITATIVE INQUIRY

A METHODOLOGICAL GUIDE

Corey W. Johnson
Diana C. Parry

editors

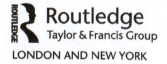

Routledge
Taylor & Francis Group

LONDON AND NEW YORK

First published 2015 by Left Coast press, Inc.

Published 2016 by Routledge
2 Park Square, Milton Park, Abingdon, Oxon OX14 4RN
711 Third Avenue, New York, NY 10017, USA

Routledge is an imprint of the Taylor & Francis Group, an informa business

Library of Congress Cataloging-in-Publication Data
Fostering social justice through qualitative inquiry : a methodological guide / Corey W. Johnson, Diana C. Parry, editors.
        pages cm
 Includes bibliographical references and index.
  ISBN 978-1-61132-374-0 (hardback) -- ISBN 978-1-61132-375-7
(paperback) -- ISBN 978-1-61132-736-6 (consumer ebook)
 1. Social justice--Research--Methodology. 2. Qualitative research--
Methodology. I. Johnson, Corey W., 1973- II. Parry, Diana C., 1973-
  HM671.F6787 2015
  303.3'72--dc23

                               2014047038

ISBN 978-1-61132-374-0 hardback
ISBN 978-1-61132-375-7 paperback

CONTENTS ||||||||||||||||||||||||||||||||||||||||||||||||||||||||||||||||||||||||||||||||||||||

Do people still read prefaces? We *hope* so, because this is a book about *hope*. In fact, it is a book written for the hopeful. We cannot lose sight of hope, especially when it is easy to be overwhelmed by the injustice of the world. Alongside the media's obsession with celebrity gossip, headlines tout missing planes and missing passengers, mass kidnappings, rapid climate change, military threats, national security breaches, political scandals, corporate ethics, and lingering racism, sexism, heterosexism, ableism, and classism. Yet, amid these stories of crisis and concern are stories that keep us optimistic. The two-time election of a black president in the United States, the US Supreme Court's 2013 decision to federally recognize same-sex marriage, the "Idle No More" protests that galvanized Canada's indigenous populations, and the international Occupy movement give us hope. Research has helped the goals of social justice move forward. Take, for example, the Center of Global and Health Development (http://www.bu.edu/cghd/), who are attempting to understand how human rights conditions influence the spread of HIV in women living in Vietnam and Ghana.

Given our hopeful outlook, we wanted to write a text to try to convince *all* scholars that they can make a difference using qualitative research to create a more socially just world. We believe that qualitative researchers are in a unique position to add value to this endeavor. We do not argue that quantitative researchers cannot contribute to positive social change, but our definition of social justice does not include goals of reductionism, generalizability, or resting on the white, male, capitalist, elite, hegemonic values on which positivist and postpositivist notions of science were built. In short, social justice research is about more than one's intent to *believe it can get*

7

better; it is bound up in questioning and dismantling power structures not encouraged or supported by other philosophical commitments. Social justice is built on a commitment and action to *make it better*!

As we set about to create this text, we were intentional in many aspects. We wanted to execute a particular vision for the book that lived somewhere between a dual-authored and edited contribution. As such, we wrote several of the early foundational chapters and the final one charting future directions. Then we set about identifying authors who would bring diversity to the text in terms of methodological expertise, disciplinary background, content area, length of time in the academy, rank, and social identity (race, age, gender, sexual identity, and class). Social workers, counseling psychologists, geographers, historians, and scholars of leisure studies, women's studies, and tourism, among others, can be found within. In addition to detailing epistemology, theory, common elements of qualitative research, and seven methodological strategies, we ground the discussions in important issues such as lesbian, gay, bisexual, transgender, and queer (LGBTQ) identity and faith reconciliation; resilience and sexual abuse for women in South Asian communities; people living homeless in public parks; women's health and body image; and gendered family memory keeping, to name a few. Finally, we have authors who understand social justice issues, having experienced injustice related to their own identities as women, people of color, non-heterosexual, and working class (or having lived poor). We did our best to ensure that our selections matched the spirit and intent of the text; of course, full representation always falls short, but we did try. Our efforts meant making difficult decisions, sometimes not inviting close colleagues or the "expert," and also involved some risks of working with others we did not know well. We believe these decisions paid off, and we are proud of their contributions.

Finally, we learned much about ourselves and the craft of qualitative research by working with our authors and each other on this book. We hope you find it a meaningful contribution to your endeavors to create "justice to come."

Acknowledgments

Throughout the process of writing this book, a number of people helped us along the way. Thus, we owe many a debt of gratitude. First and foremost, to our husbands, Troy and Yancey, thank you both for your support, patience, encouragement, and love. We dedicate this book to you. Claire and Charlotte, thanks for making your Mummy smile and laugh throughout the writing process. A special thank you to our contributing authors, whose inspiring chapters provide a pathway for social justice; it was our pleasure working with you. Thanks to Nuria Jaumot-Pascual and Brian Kumm for their attention to detail and impressive APA skills. To the anonymous reviewers, we appreciate your helpful feedback that undoubtedly resulted in a stronger book. We thank Stephanie Jones and Anneliese Singh (Corey's seven-year writing group) for their constant critique, review of drafts, and their encouragement to write an intellectual yet accessible book. Thanks to Bettie St. Pierre for encouraging thoughts about what comes next (postqualitative, posthumanistic inquiry) while thinking and writing about how to do what we do now, better. Thanks to Callie Spencer and Karen Paisley for creating a space for us to retreat, think, and write. We are grateful to Jobeth Allen: thanks for encouraging the writing of books. Last, but not least, thanks to Bill Stewart for always encouraging us to think of the values that underpin the process and end states of our research.

Corey W. Johnson and Diana Parry

Contextualizing Qualitative Research for Social Justice

Corey W. Johnson & Diana C. Parry

> Injustice anywhere is a threat to justice everywhere.
> —*Martin Luther King, Jr. (1963)*

Most of us come to a social justice paradigm because we have experienced injustice in our own lives and want to do something about it. For example, Diana was drawn to feminism as a result of the patriarchy she encountered in daily life as a woman. Meanwhile, Corey's attraction to social justice was grounded in the distinct differences he felt moving through the social world as a gay man and the stereotypes and homophobia that existed around who he could love. Regardless of how one comes to the work of social justice, there is much work to still be done. Many people think we have tackled the major social identity issues of injustice and solved these social ills. However, this "color-blind" approach to viewing the world is problematic. We bet you can look at your own classroom and/or campus and easily identify issues needing attention from social justice activists. In fact, as we wrote this text, active racism and homophobia were swelling to intolerant levels at Corey's home campus and people were taking to the streets, marching as Martin Luther King, Jr. did in his day. The local paper reported:

> Hundreds of University of Georgia students and community activists marched over the Sanford Drive bridge today to call attention to racism and homophobia on campus. Caroline Bailey, a UGA student and president of the university's Black Affairs Council, organized the march after someone posted "Why can't you dumb dirty niggers stop stinking up the place? Let UGA be RIGHT for good WHITE Christian

Corey W. Johnson & Diana C. Parry, editors, "Introduction: Contextualizing Qualitative Research for Social Justice" in *Fostering Social Justice Through Qualitative Research: A Methodological Guide*, pp. 11-22. © 2015 Left Coast Press, Inc. All rights reserved.

students," to the council's Facebook page. The message was posted anonymously using an account created in the name of a UGA student, but according to university police, someone else started the account with his name. Bailey said she was "very, very disheartened" that someone could post such a message 50 years after UGA began admitting black students. Activists [also] used the occasion to call attention to other issues [such as the state's] policy barring undocumented immigrants from attending UGA. (Aued, 2013)

Inequities and discrimination such as classism, racism, sexism, ageism, transphobia, and heterosexism create major social problems. To address such social problems, Paisley and Dustin (2010) argue that we need to "stop 'othering,' treating people who are at the margins… as if they [are] somehow inferior to us…. It is time to adopt a more caring and connected attitude toward the world around us" (p. v). Caring and connection are at the heart of a social justice research paradigm that aims to make the world a better place by enacting social change for marginalized and/or oppressed groups. Charmaz (2011) explains that social justice inquiry "attends to inequities and equality, barriers and access, poverty and privilege, individual rights and the collective good, and their implications for suffering" (p. 359). To achieve this aim, the processes and outcomes of scholarship must move beyond academic discourse to benefit communities or groups that are treated unfairly in the social world (Angrosino & Rosenberg, 2011; Lincoln, Lynham, & Guba, 2011). A social justice paradigm, therefore, is a moral, ethical, and political task that challenges traditional notions of universal truth, scientific neutrality, and researcher dispassion (Parry, Johnson, & Stewart, 2013.)

One of the underlying themes related to social justice inquiry is that the world is capable of being changed; that change can come from any direction, and especially from the bottom up. A social justice paradigm literally changes the way one thinks and views the world. Such a paradigm means that we are all capable of—and therefore responsible for—changing the world. Given this shared responsibility, it helps if the processes and outcomes of social justice research are made visible. With this goal in mind, the purpose of this textbook is fourfold: 1) to explain how using a social justice paradigm orients qualitative inquiry as a socially relevant, socially responsible, multidisciplinary, globally sensitive endeavor; 2) to document common features of social justice–oriented qualitative inquiry; 3) to detail and exemplify research methodologies frequently used in qualitative inquiry aimed to enact social justice; and finally 4) to create a proliferation of theories for social justice that speak to multiple and diverse global contexts.

The Evolution of Social Justice Research

> There must exist a paradigm, a practical model for social change that includes an understanding of ways to transform consciousness that are linked to efforts to transform structures. —*bell hooks (1995)*

Two decades ago, only a handful of scholars were explicitly concerned with connecting their research outcomes with issues of social justice (Denzin & Lincoln, 2011). These scholars conceptualized social justice as "the ability of social science to be put to policy objectives with the purpose of redressing a variety of historically reified oppressions in modern life: racism, economic injustice, the 'hidden injuries of class,' discrimination in the legal system, gender inequities, and the new oppressions resulting from the restructuring of the social welfare system" (Denzin & Lincoln, 2011, p. 715). Since then, a large array of scholars have taken up issues of social justice in both the *process* and *products* of their research. These scholars premise social justice on an epistemology that values emotions, personal relationships, an ethic of care, political praxis, and multivocality to purposefully reveal inequities in all facets of society (Charmaz, 2011; Denzin & Lincoln, 2011).

Epistemology questions what is the nature of knowledge? How do we come to know what we know? It will influence the way we think about what is Truth, truths, and/or the production of knowledge.

Today, scholars working within a social justice paradigm cover a wide range of topic areas including environmental issues, critical medical studies, critical management studies, animal rights, and a large field of literature on a broad range of topics connected to activist movements both contemporary and historic. This broad scope of social justice research is reflected in academic journals devoted to the topic (e.g., *Social Justice Research, Studies in Social Justice*) and in research centers (e.g., Southern Poverty Law Center, Canadian Centre for Social Justice) in various institutions across the globe.

Given that the purpose of this book is to outline social justice research methodologies, we will not address the historical evolution in great depth or detail. We are sensitive to the complexity that might be left out of the following overview, but would encourage you to follow up on the deep philosophical and historic roots of social justice offered through some of the readings cited throughout the text. We also acknowledge that social justice is very much a Western ideal, and that other philosophies exist to promote peace and tranquility.

However, our specific focus on social justice is inextricably linked to the shift toward a more critical approach to interpretation and representation of research (Denzin & Giardina, 2009). Indeed, the epistemological underpinnings of social justice have evolved through a variety of philosophical paradigms. According to Denzin and Lincoln (2011), the "narratives or stories scientists tell are accounts couched and framed within specific storytelling traditions, often defined as paradigms (e.g., positivism, postpositivism…)" (p. 6). To contextualize the social justice research paradigm used throughout this text, we turn next to the evolution of social justice that has informed current day understandings. Here we trace the history of social justice research, including positivism into (post)positivism, and then discuss the interpretive turn.

What Is (Post)Positivism?

Positivists believe by obtaining pure, truthful observations, they are able to offer causal explanations for social behavior and law-like generalizations (Schwandt, 2001). The purposes of research, from a positivist perspective, are for both prediction and control (Lincoln, Lynham, & Guba, 2011). From an ontological perspective, positivists believe in a single, identifiable reality wherein there is a truth to be measured and reported (Lincoln, Lynham, & Guba, 2011).

Ontology deals with the nature of reality; the study of reality and what constitutes the world (Schwandt, 2007). What does it mean to be?

Positivism, Crotty (2003) explained, "postulates the objective existence of meaningful reality. It considers such meaningful reality to be value-neutral, ahistorical, and cross-cultural. It believes that, if one goes about it in the right way, one can identify such reality with certitude" (p. 40). In short, through the use of proper methods positivists "discover truths" about which they have supreme confidence because of their belief that knowledge is accurate and certain.

Philosophers and social scientists have critiqued the assumptions and claims of positivism since its inception (Crotty, 2003; Phillips & Burbules, 2000). Without completely abandoning the need for objectivism, the critiques centered on degrees of objectivity, precision, and certitude, calling for more modest research claims or a "less arrogant form of positivism" (Crotty, 2003, p. 29). This more modest, less arrogant form of positivism is what we know as postpositivism. There is no singular unified approach to postpositivism, and there are many issues upon which postpositivists disagree (Phillips & Burbules, 2000). However, the one issue that postpositivists seem to agree upon is that knowledge is conjectural; human knowledge is not based on rock-solid foundations, but is challengeable and can change in light of new or further investigation (Phillips & Burbules, 2000). Postpositivists "admit that, no matter how faithfully the scientist adheres to scientific method, research outcomes are neither totally objective nor unquestionably certain" (Crotty, 2003, p. 40). As a result, methodologically, the best way to gather or seek out new knowledge is through a hypothetical deductive method (hypothesize, deduce, and generalize) (Guba & Lincoln, 2005); researchers aim for objectivity to ensure the results are not unduly influenced and can be used to generalize to the larger population. Throughout this process the goal is for the researcher to remain distant from research subjects (intentional use of the word) and processes (Crotty, 2003). In short, the goal of postpositivist research is to generate knowledge that helps better understand reality and generalize that reality to other populations.

What postpositivism does not do is appreciate the *process* of research as a component of social change, provide solutions, or suggest the type of change that needs to be created to address social problems. If solutions emerge from postpositivistic approaches, they are because researchers stepped out of their role as scientists and into roles as citizens, advocates, or practitioners. Postpositivists are not researchers who enact mechanisms of change or become advocates for the group or community under study (they aim to be distant and thus objective throughout the research process). Postpositivistic research is indifferent about the need for, and direction of, social justice: its philosophical commitments are directed at objective understanding, and those who practice it would be committed to the same.

To be clear, this is not a data-level discussion, but rather a philosophical one. There is nothing we have outlined that identifies postpositivism with the use of quantitative methods, data, or statistics (Phillips & Burbules, 2000). Labeling an approach as quantitative or qualitative is a data-level discussion that masks and/or ignores the philosophical commitments of the researchers. Discussions of the approach and outcome of research are philosophical in nature, not data driven. Indeed, researchers from across many disciplines increasingly are using qualitative approaches, but do so from a postpositivist paradigm.

Recently, however, a shift has occurred within qualitative research toward exploring conversational, multivocal, and critical representations of research. Rather than simplifying and reducing lived experiences, scholars seem to want to contextualize experiences and treat them as a complex phenomenon (Denzin & Lincoln, 2011). This shift in priorities has implications for both the processes and products of research, with a focus on social justice as part of the practice of research.

The Interpretive Turn

Interpretivism was born out of a need to escape the excess of scientific approaches to social science (Willis, 2007). While most research was still based in a postpositivist approach that focused on absolute truth, external reality, and the development of theory, interpretivists wanted to escape the boundaries of the scientific method and develop understanding in context (Willis, 2007). Rooted in the thinking of Immanuel Kant and Edmund Husserl, interpretivism, at its core, states that the nature of reality is socially constructed and that meaning making happens both in context and within the social process of a group (Prasad, 2005; Willis, 2007). Central to the interpretivist paradigm is the idea that the reality we know is socially constructed and that human interpretation is the starting point for increasing knowledge about the social world (Prasad, 2005). "Humans in groups, and using the tools and traditions of the group (including language), construct meaning and thus are able to share their understanding with other members of the group" (Willis, 2007, p. 97). This idea of social construction implies that the members of the group under study best understand the research being conducted; those who are not a part of the group will struggle to understand the reality constructed and the validity of the research (Angen, 2000).

The goal of interpretivist inquiry is not to locate an absolute truth, but instead highlight the socially constructed reality of a phenomenon or social group. "It is this inherent capacity for meaningful social construction that Interpretivists term as being subjective since it departs from the idea of a fixed external reality" (Prasad, 2005, p. 14). By moving beyond the scientific method side of research and accepting something other than an external reality, researchers will begin to see the knowledge available both to them and the groups they study.

One defining feature of interpretivist philosophies is that social phenomena are not accorded the same status as physical phenomena. Specifically, interpretivists believe that the phenomenon of inquiry and the aim of social scientific research differ from that of the physical world (Schwandt, 2001) and "hard" sciences. Instead, interpretivist philosophies believe that "what distinguishes human (social) action from the movement of physical objects is that the former is inherently meaningful" (Schwandt, 2001, p.191). Scientifically, the goal of intrepretivism is to understand human action (Rosenberg, 2012).

A second defining feature of interpretivist philosophy is that it requires interpretation. More specifically, for a researcher to claim an understanding means that she or he has interpreted human action and deemed it to be meaningful (Schwandt, 2001). Thus, in interpretivist research positionality and the subsequent interpretation play a key role in social scientific inquiry and its communication to outside audiences.

The third defining feature of interpretivism is that the subjectivity of human action is appreciated and viewed as a contribution to understanding. More specifically, to "say human action is meaningful is to claim either that it has a certain intentional content that indicates the kind of action it is" (Schwandt, 2001, p.191).

Intentional means pregiven lifeworlds exist prior to our awareness of them. Being and experience are already in the world and the uniting of the object and subject bring them to consciousness.

Thus, interprevisits believe that knowledge is developed through understanding the intentions of another. From the empathic identification perspective, this means trying to understand the intentions of human action from within the actor: the emic view. Because interpretivists focus on the intentions of another, inquiry is often limited to the individual or idiosyncratic.

Enacting a Social Justice Research Agenda

> We know too much, we understand too deeply, to go back now.
> (Lincoln & Denzin, 2011, p. 716)

Rather than framing success in research as understanding or identifying problems in the social world, social justice scholars are committed to the breakdown, challenge, and change of social structures and ideologies that perpetuate marginalization, discrimination, and oppression as an integral part of the research process from start to finish. Social justice is concerned with "how society's practices and institutions create and distribute society's benefits and burdens in terms of rights and disabilities, privileges and disadvantages, equal or unequal opportunities, power and dependency, wealth (which is the power to control the disposition of certain resources) and poverty" (Kalsem & Williams, 2010, p. 15). According to Freysinger, Shaw, Henderson, and Bialeschki (2013), social justice is "a vision of society where the distribution of resources is equitable and all members are physically and psychologically safe and secure. In this society, individuals are both self-determining and interdependent. Justice involves a sense of one's own agency and a sense of social responsibility towards others, and for society as a whole" (p. 553). Similarly, North (2006) argues social justice is about recognition for an individual's and/or group's struggle for personal and collective identity. Toward this end, Reid (2004) explains that social justice "concerns the degree to which a society contains and supports the conditions necessary for all individuals to exercise capacities, express experiences, and participate in determining actions. It requires not the melting away of difference, but the promotion and respect for group differences without oppression" (p. 2). Thus, while social justice refers most broadly to fairness and equality, it is also understood to represent a global struggle for human rights, recognition, and dignity (Kalsem & Williams, 2010). While the term *social justice* is dynamic and thus continues to evolve, our current conceptualization, and the one that underpins this book, tends to emphasize a transformative process that changes society by taking up issues of fairness connected to rights, allocation of resources, and power (Kalsem & Williams, 2010).

A social justice approach therefore requires a researcher to work *with*, as opposed to merely doing something *for*, a community or group (Angrosino & Rosenberg, 2011; Denzin, 1997). Merely working *for* a community or group (a value of postpositivism) implies a distant stance between the researcher and the researched with objectivism as a goal of the research process (Lincoln, Lynham, & Guba, 2011). In contrast, working *with* a community or group presumes that a researcher has a deep kinship (political and emotional) with research participants based upon membership or links to the community or group (Angrosino & Rosenberg, 2011). Within a social justice research agenda, participants are not distant objects of study, but rather neighbors, lovers, friends, family members, and/or allies. Knowledge is built from the lived experiences of people as opposed to distant or objective scholarly claims. The social justice researcher becomes an additional spokesperson or advocate for causes and issues, helps people articulate enduring and emergent problems, or brings together key stakeholders for community discussions/actions (Angrosino & Rosenberg, 2011). In myriad ways, social justice research reflects an emancipatory vision that works toward creating a different world for communities of concern (Charmaz, 2011).

Locating research within a social justice agenda reflects the philosophical commitment of scholars (Creswell, 2009). Ontologically, social justice scholars see human nature operating in a world that is rooted in power struggles that lead to "interactions of privilege and oppression that can be based on race or ethnicity, socioeconomic class, gender, mental or physical abilities, or sexual [identity]" (Lincoln, Lynham, & Guba, 2011, p. 102). This ontological premise has major implications for beliefs about acquiring and advancing knowledge: an epistemological stance (Schwandt, 2007). As you will note in the chapters that follow, social justice researchers ask questions such as:

- Whose knowledge?
- Where and how was that knowledge obtained, created, or legitimized?
- By whom?
- For whom?
- And for what purposes? (compare with Harding, 1991; Olesen, 2011).

Moreover, membership or connections with the group or community under investigation creates knowledge that is always subjective, within the goals of the collective. Although always suspect, knowledge is simultaneously emancipatory and full of possibility for marginalized or oppressed groups. Within a social justice framework, "research is judged by its authenticity, its fairness, and its ability to provoke transformations and changes in the public and private spheres of everyday life—transformations that speak to the conditions of oppression" (Denzin, 1997, p. 275). Toward this end, epistemology and, by implication, ontology, matter:

> Epistemology does matter. Standpoint matters. Each of these things—one philosophical, one embodied and sociocultural—gives meaning and inflection to both the beginning (the research question) and the ending (the findings) of any inquiry. To deny their influence is to miss most of the major debates of the last quarter-century of qualitative research and indeed, the social sciences more broadly. (Denzin & Lincoln, 2011, p. 716)

Since epistemology is such an important component of social justice research agendas, so is the way scholars seek to advance knowledge: through methodologies. Schwandt (2007) defines methodologies as "the principles of our inquiry and how inquiry should proceed" (p. 190). Dialogic approaches to gathering knowledge that both empower participants and support change fit well within the goals for social justice (Lincoln, Lynham, & Guba, 2011; Merriam, 1991). Social justice methodological strategies demand a friendly, connected relationship between the researcher and participants that enable transformation throughout the research process (not just as an end state). As scholars undertake inquiry, naming values and exploring positions for emancipation are crucial elements of a politics of hope (Denzin, 2000; Parry, Johnson, & Stewart, 2013). One's stance on ontological and epistemological issues generally drives theoretical and methodological principles that lead to research design and execution. As a result, we turn next to an overview of seven common theoretical orientations for social justice.

REFERENCES

Aued, B. (2013, November 8). UGA students protest racist Facebook post. *Flagpole*. Retrieved from http://flagpole.com/news/in-the-loop/uga-students-protest-racist-facebook-post

Angen, M. J. (2000). Evaluating interpretive inquiry: Validity debate and opening the dialogue. *Qualitative Health Research, 10*(3), 378–395.

Angrosino, M., & Rosenberg, J. (2011). Observations on observation: Continuities and challenges. In N. K. Denzin & Y. S. Lincoln (Eds.), *The Sage handbook of qualitative research (4th ed.)* (pp. 467–478). Thousand Oaks, CA: Sage.

Charmaz, K. (2011). Grounded theory methods in social justice research. In N. K. Denzin, & Y. E. Lincoln (Eds.), *The Sage handbook of qualitative research* (4th ed.) (pp. 359–380). Thousand Oaks, CA: Sage.

Creswell, J. W. (2009). *Research design: Qualitative, quantitative, and mixed methods approaches* (3rd ed.). Thousand Oaks, CA: Sage.

Crotty, M. (2003). *The foundations of social research*. Thousand Oaks, CA: Sage.

Denzin, N. K. (1997). *Reading the crisis: Interpretive ethnography*. Thousand Oaks, CA: Sage.

Denzin, N. K. (2000). Aesthetics and the practices of qualitative inquiry. *Qualitative Inquiry, 6*(2), 256–265.

Denzin, N. K., & Giardina, M. D. (Eds.). (2009). *Qualitative inquiry and social justice: Towards a politics of hope*. Walnut Creek, CA: Left Coast Press.

Denzin, N. K., & Lincoln, Y. S. (Eds.). (2011). *The Sage handbook of qualitative research* (4th ed.). Thousand Oaks, CA: Sage.

Freysinger, V., Shaw, S., Henderson, K., & Bialeschki, D. (Eds.). (2013). *Leisure, women and gender.* State College, PA: Venture.

Guba, E. G., & Lincoln, Y. S. (2005). Paradigmatic controversies, contradictions, and emerging confluences. In N. K. Denzin & Y. S. Lincoln (Eds.), *The Sage handbook of qualitative research* (3rd ed.) (pp. 191–216). Thousand Oaks, CA: Sage.

Harding, S. (1991). *Whose science? Whose knowledge?* Ithaca, NY: Cornell University Press.

hooks, b. (1995). *Art on my mind: Visual politics.* New York, NY: New Press.

Kalsem, K., & Williams, V. L. (2010). Social justice feminism. *UCLA Women's Law Journal, 18*(1), 131–193.

King, Jr., M. L. (1963). Letter from Birmingham jail. April, 16, 1963. Retrieved from http://www.uscrossier.org/pullias/wp-content/uploads/2012/06/king.pdf

Lincoln, Y. S., & Denzin, N. K. (2011). Toward a "refunctioned ethnography." In N. K. Denzin & Y. S. Lincoln (Eds.), *The Sage handbook of qualitative research* (4th ed.) (pp. 715–719). Thousand Oaks, CA: Sage.

Lincoln, Y. S., Lynham, S. A., & Guba, E. G. (2011). Paradigmatic controversies, contradictions, and emerging confluences, revisited. In N. K. Denzin & Y. S. Lincoln (Eds.), *The Sage handbook of qualitative research (4th ed.)* (pp. 97–128). Thousand Oaks, CA: Sage.

North, C. E. (2006). More than words? Delving into the substantive meaning(s) of "social justice" in education. *Review of Educational Research, 76*(4), 507–535.

Olesen, V. L. (2011). Feminist qualitative research in the millennium's first decade. In N. K. Denzin, & Y. S Lincoln (Eds.), *The Sage handbook of qualitative research* (4th ed.) (pp. 129–146). Thousand Oaks, CA: Sage.

Paisley, K., & Dustin, D. (Eds.) (2010). *Speaking up and speaking out: Working for social and environmental justice through parks, recreation and leisure.* Champaign, IL: Sagamore.

Parry, D. C., Johnson, C. W., & Stewart, W. (2013). Leisure research for social justice: A response to Henderson. *Leisure Sciences, 35*(1), 81–87.

Phillips, D. C., & Burbules, N. C. (2000). *Postpositivism and educational research.* Lanham, MD: Rowman & Littlefield Publishers.

Prasad, P. (2005). *Crafting qualitative research: Working in the postpositivist traditions.* Armonk, NY: M. E. Sharp, Inc.

Reid, C. (2004). Advancing women's social justice agenda: A feminist action research framework. *International Journal of Qualitative Methods, 3*(3), 1–15.

Rosenberg, A. (2012). *Philosophy of social science.* Boulder, CO: Westview Press.

Schwandt, T. S. (2001). *Dictionary of qualitative inquiry* (2nd ed). Thousand Oaks, CA: Sage.

Schwandt, T. S. (2007). *The Sage dictionary of qualitative inquiry* (3rd ed). Thousand Oaks, CA: Sage.

Willis, J. W. (2007). *Foundations of qualitative research: Interpretive and critical approaches*. Thousand Oaks, CA: Sage.

Theoretical Perspectives for Social Justice Inquiry

Diana C. Parry & Corey W. Johnson

How do we infuse theory with "justice to come"? (Derrida, 1994)

Once you have decided that a social justice paradigm is one that suits you, it is important to ground your work theoretically. Although by no means an exhaustive list or incompatible with each other, the following seven theoretical orientations represent the most common for qualitative research using a social justice approach. They include those that we have employed commonly in our own work and/or those taken up by our co-authors later in the text. These include Marxism, critical race theory, feminism, gay/lesbian theory, queer theory, poststructuralism, and postcolonialism. One word of caution: summarizing these theories in an introductory text such as this one is a tricky endeavor, for they are complex with their own cannons of literature, a variety of contributors, smaller theoretical trajectories within them, and debates on their deployment. We hope these summaries give you a place to start to delve into their complexity. Summarized key references for each approach are provided in an appendix at the back of the book; we hope you find these useful as you prepare to dig deeper.

Marxism

Although many still harbor post–Cold War perceptions about his ideas regarding communism, Karl Marx is widely recognized as a social activist. His success at blending philosophy, history, and economics suggest that he was an academic who was most interested in books and theories, yet his chief concern was ordinary people (Crotty, 1998). Arguing that change needs to start with social realities, Marxist philosophy is

Diana C. Parry & Corey W. Johnson, editors, "Theoretical Perspectives for Social Justice Inquiry" in *Fostering Social Justice Through Qualitative Research: A Methodological Guide,* pp. 23-41. © 2015 Left Coast Press, Inc. All rights reserved.

grounded in a belief that knowledge must come from those at the "bottom" (i.e., people who are marginalized and not in positions of power) as opposed to from the "top" down (i.e., those who oppress or exploit) to create change (Harding, 1991).

As a materialistic theory, physical realities of human existence serve as the "cause of change in beliefs, attitudes, values roles, institutions, and whole societies. In particular, it is facts about the modes of production, the means people employ to survive and perpetuate themselves, that dictate the rest of society" (Rosenberg, 2012). According to Marx, the crux of social problems lies in a class struggle or, as he conceived it, "a basic conflict between capital and labour, between the bourgeoisie and the proletariat" (Crotty, 1998, p. 118). These class struggles resulted in the proletariat (working class) having a more accurate perception on social reality than the dominant bourgeois. Indeed, Marx argued the bourgeois were incapable of truly understanding the functioning of society largely because they had constructed a system to suit their own needs (Harding, 1991). Such a privileged position prevented the bourgeois from understanding the lives of the proletariat. According to Marx, economic forces were the most important to address because those who hold financial power are able to shape the perceptions and viewpoints of those who do not (Crotty, 1998).

Others continued to develop Marx's philosophies after his death in 1883, although often with less emphasis on the force of economics and instead with more grounding in culture—also known as the "superstructure" of society—including legal and political forces (Crotty, 1998). Regardless of the shift in focus, the commitment to social justice remained clear; some would argue that Marxist insights are foundational for any form of critical research today (Kincheloe, McLaren, & Steinberg, 2011).

For example, Marxism is a powerful theoretical approach when used to explain the origins and continuation of racism (Kincheloe, McLaren, & Steinberg, 2011), and much of feminist theory, in particular feminist standpoint theory, is rooted in "Marxist historical materialism in that knowledge develops in a complicated and contradictory way from lived experiences and social historical context" (Naples, 2007, p. 580). Thus, contemporary Marxist scholars continue to embrace critical, historical, and economic theory to argue the real-world implications of race, gender, and class (Denzin & Lincoln, 2011). Empirical approaches and theoretical contributions are evaluated in terms of their emancipatory potential and often entail criteria such as dialogue and personal accountability (Denzin & Lincoln, 2011). A great illustration of the principles of Marxist theory put to work can be found in Jeff Rose's chapter on ethnography in this book (chapter 5), where he uses both Marxist theory and poststructuralism (described below) in his study of people living in public space.

Critical Race Theory

Critical Race Theory (CRT) proponents operate with the understanding that the civil rights movement addressed only overt racism—primarily the exclusion of black people—but the subtle racism that encompasses American society continues, supported by the legal system. CRT facilitates an investigation of race and power, especially in arenas that insist they are devoid of overt, formal racism. Striving for the seemingly simple idea of fair and equal treatment of all without investigating how power is distributed only results in a false sense of equality that CRT is dedicated to addressing. (Crenshaw, Gotanda, Peller, & Thomas, 1995)

CRT enables an exploration of the social systems at work on a deeper level than merely addressing discrimination based on skin color. Racial identity is not cloaked entirely in skin color, but also in culture, community, and politics (Crenshaw et al., 1995). However, the acknowledged social construction of race still results in unequal distribution of money, power, and education as we place people in undefined, unexplained, and unquestioned social categories. As a result, researchers may perpetuate hegemonic power structures because the reader must use stereotypes to assume what it means to be placed in each category. (Kivel, 2000)

CRT theorists believe that it is not possible to be neutral or objective when speaking of legal studies and race. CRT strives to bring race consciousness to the forefront, in contrast to the accepted model of color-blindness, in an effort to combat the limited understanding of how racism exists within hegemonic power structures in American society. Because legal studies and the law reinforce white privilege, CRT challenges the construction of race in both legal studies and American culture to understand how white privilege is maintained and how the subordination of minorities continues. CRT must not only generate understanding and knowledge, but also support change. (Crenshaw et al., 1995)

In an attempt to combat the unequal distribution of power surrounding race and the social construction of race, Hylton (2005) identified five main tenants used by CRT proponents. The first is that race and racism cannot be isolated from power structures and are always affected by outside influences. The second component calls into question the use of colorblind policies, meritocracy, and so-called objective, race-neutral policies.

> Meritocracy is an idea where people are judged on their individual abilities and not the social circumstances, relations, and/or access of resources available.

Third, CRT uses techniques of social justice to position the oppressed at the center of the discussion or research and not at the periphery. Fourth, topics that white researchers have examined and their resulting research are considered the truth in relation to races, resulting in a political viewpoint. Therefore, it becomes necessary to perform research from the viewpoint of the other. Finally, it is useful to employ CRT across disciplines; by applying information learned to other forms of social sciences, a transdisciplinary way of exploring race emerges. CRT belief holds that we live in an unequal society, with unequal distributions of power and resources. This distribution of power marginalizes minorities and their position in society (Hylton, 2005).

Glover (2007) outlines three interrelated principles that facilitate the social justice outcomes of CRT research. First, those who adopt CRT recognize and acknowledge that race is socially constructed. Race as a biological concept, posits Glover, has been refuted in the academic literature because there is greater genetic variation within racialized groups than between them (Haney Lopez, 2000). Despite this acknowledgement, critical race theorists assert that race continues to be a powerful social construct and as such, warrants attention. CRT therefore facilitates a focus on the myriad ways that race characterizes the lived experiences of people of color, which suggests it ought to be the starting point for much social justice inquiry (Glover, 2007).

The second principle of CRT is "skepticism of color-blindness and commitment to expose white privilege" (Glover, 2007, p. 196). As noted above, when colorblind policies are in effect, race is ignored or dismissed as a nonissue, and we fail to appreciate the significance of race in the lived experiences of people of color. Indeed, Glover (2007) argues that colorblind policies silence criticism about white privilege, which serves to thwart efforts to discuss the implications of institutional policies and practices that constrain people of color. With this in mind, one of the key goals of CRT is raising awareness regarding race and the implications of racism for people of color (Glover, 2007).

A racialized epistemology that privileges storytelling is the third principle of CRT (Glover, 2007). CRT appreciates that knowledge is not neutral. Instead, knowledge is often used as "a function of the ability of the powerful to impose their own views, to differentiate between knowledge and myth, reason and emotion, and objectivity and subjectivity" (Peller, 1995, p. 142). Certain types of knowledge, such as that produced from a postpositivist paradigm, are privileged within the social sciences. Parker and Lynn (2002) explain what is considered knowledge "often...become[s] shrouded in a language that fails to address important questions regarding the origins, uses, and abuses of social scientific inquiry and the importance of minority representation in this enterprise" (p. 13). The result is what Rappaport (2000) refers to as dominant cultural narratives that construct knowledge in a manner that reproduces the current social structures to the benefit of the majority group. Glover (2007) explains that CRT uses counter-stories as a way of intentionally resisting dominant cultural narratives. In his words,

> Counter-stories build a common culture of shared understandings among minority communities whose voices are missing from scientific discourse while simultaneously destroying stock stories, which are challenged through the effective depiction of injustice. Counter-stories, therefore, are used for their transformative possibilities". (p. 196)

Although he does not take up CRT specifically, Brett Lashua's chapter in this volume (chapter 6) does offer an illustration of counter-stories.

Feminism(s)

Feminism is a social and collective identity that represents a complex intersection of political and personal ideologies (Zucker & Bay-Cheng, 2010). Feminists see gender as a

> basic organizing principle that profoundly shapes/mediates the concrete conditions of our lives.... Through the questions that feminism poses and the absences it locates, feminism argues the centrality of gender in shaping our consciousness, skills, and institutions as well as in the distribution of power and privilege. (Lather, 1998, p. 571)

Feminists share a consciousness about women's distinct and shared disadvantages within patriarchal society. They see the political nature of everyday life (hence the slogan "the personal is political") and link these everyday experiences to larger social injustices (Rupp & Taylor, 1999). As a social, collective, and political identity, feminists are dedicated to calling attention to the existence, injustice, and negative impacts of sexism (hooks, 2000). Toward this end, feminists place "emphasis on the equal worth and rights of all people and [have a] collective orientation to social justice" (Zucker & Bay-Cheng, 2010, p. 1911).

Social justice from a feminist perspective involves envisioning and creating a society that is outside the bounds of patriarchy.

Patriarchy is a social system in which power rests with men and privileges them through greater access to institutional power, higher incomes, higher labor force participation, and greater access to all social and cultural resources among other beneficial arrangements (Hibbins, 2013; Kirkley, 2000).

With a focus on patriarchy, feminism is inclusive of everyone (women and men). To be clear, the patriarchy does not serve marginalized groups of men well (i.e., gay men, poor men, men with mental health challenges) (Hibbins, 2013). As Jaggar (1988) explains, feminism refers to all those who seek to end gendered injustice.

Feminists thus connect through a shared desire to challenge the social conditions of oppression that stem from the patriarchy. Beyond this unifying focus, however, there is a vast amount of difference across feminists based upon different conceptualizations of power as structuring, constraining, and regulating, as well as productive, affective, resistant, and relational. Feminists seek a new form of solidarity that unites folks across blurred, overlapping, and at times contradictory aspects of identities that results in multiple feminisms (Fixmer & Wood, 2005).

Indeed, there is growing interest within the feminist literature in thinking about gender identities, experiences, diversity, and interconnections. This approach moves us further away from "one size fits all" thinking and instead focuses on relationality and interconnections. Building on the concept of intersectionality that grew out of black feminist theorizing, recent scholars, such as Bhavani and Talcott (2012), have advocated for an interconnection that "connotes more movement and fluidity than lies in the metaphor of intersection, as well as offering a way of thinking about how not only race and gender, but also nation, sexuality, and wealth all interconnect, configure, and reshape each other" (p. 137). Interconnectivity demonstrates how a social justice lens can bring a "feminist consciousness that opens up intellectual and emotional spaces for all women to articulate their relations to one another and the wider society—spaces where the personal transforms into the political" (Hesse-Biber, 2012, p. 2).

Feminist scholarship recognizes women as the experts of their own experiences and the importance of women's lived experiences to unearthing subjugated knowledge (Hesse-Biber, 2012). Placing women (and other marginalized groups) at the center of inquiry, feminist scholarship asks "new" questions (Hesse-Biber, 2012) and disrupts traditional ways of knowing to create rich, layered, holistic, nuanced understandings of the systemic gendered nature of society.

When feminism is joined with social justice, it creates a focus that is "structural in its orientation, identifying issues that contribute to systemic subordination and developing theories and strategies for change" as linked to the patriarchy (Kalsem & Williams, 2010, p. 27). Social justice feminism seeks multiple ways to change the material conditions of women's (and other marginalized groups) everyday lives. There is a focus on formal and informal patterns of society in reproducing oppression and privileging dominant social groups (Reid, 2004). Perhaps most important, social justice feminism is driven by hope and desire for the type of society in which feminists wish to live (Kalsem & Williams, 2010).

Social justice feminism asks important questions of the past to approach the future with new paths forward. Social justice feminism produces frameworks that provide "more complete understandings of the factors that perpetuate social injustices while providing strategies for responding [to] such injustices through advocating collective action towards social change" (Reid, 2004, p. 10). Finally, social justice feminism heals as it brings people together to engage across various divides. Social justice feminism seeks to build confidence in women and other marginalized people so that they can speak up, be heard, and create change. In this way, social justice feminism is focused on sharing and caring about one another.

Whether it occurs at the micro and/or macro level, action is vital to feminist social justice research; it is through action that "we learn how the world works, what we can do, and who we are.... [W]e learn with mind and heart and this is how we become aware and emancipated" (Reid, 2004, p. 6). Tracy Penny Light's and Caitlin Mulcahy's chapters in this book (chapters 7 and 9, respectively) serve as excellent exemplars for how social justice is achieved through different forms of feminist research.

Lesbian, Gay, Bisexual, Transgender Theory

The terms "homosexuality" and "heterosexuality" emerged in the nineteenth century to describe behaviors of individuals—not their identities as individuals—who were homosexual or heterosexual (Katz, 1976). Weeks (1991) notes that "just as homosexuality was defined as a sexual condition peculiar to some people but not others… so the concept of heterosexuality was invented to describe 'normality,' a normality circumscribed by a founding belief in the sharp distinctions between the sexes and the assumption that gender identity (to be a man or a woman) and sexual identity were linked through the naturalness of heterosexual object choice" (p. 72).

With the growth of psychology in the twentieth century, a shift occurred from theorists who focused on biological determinism to those who examined behavior in terms of identity development and formation (compare Erik Erikson and Erving Goffman). Biology was only one characteristic that influenced one's behavior and identity development. For this newer generation of theorists, the individual had more agency in developing her/his identity than a biological determinist perspective would allow. Identities were now seen as the result of selection, "self actualization, and apparently choice" (Weeks, 1991, p. 74).

Since the 1940s, theorists have examined homosexuality by conflating behavior with identity. Researchers from across many disciplines—medicine, psychology, genetics, sociology, nursing, etc.—continue to spend a great deal of time trying to understand the "causes" of homosexuality. Their research does not examine the "causes" of heterosexuality, since the latter is thought to be the universally accepted standard for "normative" sexual identity. Yet, instead of formulating questions that focus on "why" individuals are "homosexual" or "heterosexual," a more interesting set of questions might focus on the origins of desire and the role of social, historical, and cultural forces in shaping one's desires. As Herdt and Boxer (1993) have suggested, "desires interact with cultural experiences and social learning to achieve particular set goals or end points. Desire is not a timeless universal…both form and content are historically, culturally and psychologically negotiated through life" (p. 179).

As theorists sought to understand the origins of homosexual identity, there also emerged people who, individually and collectively, began to self-identify as "homosexuals." With the advent of the civil rights movement beginning in the 1950s and the second wave of the women's movement in the 1960s, these social/historical movements gave rise to another movement: the movement for homosexual rights, which later became the lesbian/gay (L/G) rights movement. The lesbian/gay rights movement of the 1980s created a politics of identity and an identity politics that was based less on one's sexual practices and instead used this marker of identity as a rallying point to end discrimination and harassment of individuals who identified as lesbian and gay. Radical and queer political groups have tried to decenter the ideology of heterosexuality as the standard for "normative" sexual-identity formation. Theorists such as Shane Phelan (1997) have articulated the basis for such an argument. She argues, "once heterosexuality is revealed to be no more original than homosexuality, having no greater claim to being natural than the other, then much more energy must be expended to make heterosexuality compulsory, to appear natural, to become original" (p. 184). Parallel arguments about privileged sexual identities were made by people who identified as bisexual and, later, transgender, against their exclusion from lesbian and gay political movements. Eventually, in the 1980s and 1990s, resting on the belief that people with non-normative sexual identities should work together for social and political causes, the L/G movement became the lesbian, gay, bisexual, transgender (LGBT)[1] movement.

How is LGBT theory useful in a social justice paradigm? Given that estimates of between 4% and 5% of both Canadians and Americans identify as LGBT (Carlson, 2012; Gates 2011), we need to explore how they experience life similarly and/or differently than straight people. Of course the key word in the previous sentence is *identify*. This statistic does not account for the millions of individuals who either do not explicitly identify as LGBT or those who defy categories of sexual identity as well as those who are questioning their sexual identity and have yet to claim one. Regardless, individuals who self-identify as LGBT face significant stigmatism. Despite a civil rights movement that began more than 40 years ago and the removal of "homosexuality" as a pathological disorder from the *Diagnostic and Statistical Manual of Mental Disorders* (DSM) of the American Psychiatric Association in the early 1970s, prejudice and violence against people who express an LGBT identity remains. This is why a social justice approach is so important.

Using LGBT theory in a social justice paradigm means that first, it is important to acknowledge that sexual identity is only one marker of an individual's personal and social identity. The gender and sexual socialization processes that occur in society might influence what individuals come to "do" and "enjoy"; however, markers of identity such as sexuality do not inherently determine or lead people to engage in certain behaviors (Kivel & Klieber, 2000). Second, we need to focus on how society views and treats people as a result of their sexual-identity expression and how these views influence our assessment, planning, implementation, and evaluation of services.

As a result, when LGBT theory materializes in a social justice paradigm we are able to ask: What assumptions, based on stereotypes, do we make about people who identify as or who are perceived as being LGBT? What misinformation do we hold that might influence how we interact with and facilitate programs and services for people who are LGBT? How might myths and stereotypes influence policymaking and personnel decisions? We point you to Denise Levy's chapter on grounded theory methodology (chapter 3) to illustrate how she employs LGBT theory to assist in resolving the conflict of LGBT individuals reconciling their sexual identity with their religious faith for a social justice–oriented outcome.

Queer Theory

"Queer is decidedly promiscuous" (Barnett & Johnson, in press). In its pejorative heyday, the years before the late 1980s, the term *queer* served to denigrate perverts and/or men who fancied other men (Beemyn & Eliason, 1996; Eaklor, 2008; Marinucci, 2010). The first inkling of queer's reclamation came in the early 1990s, when AIDS Coalition to Unleash Power (ACT-UP) members formed Queer Nation, a direct-action organization aimed at abolishing homophobia and creating new visions of queers in America (Levy & Johnson, 2012). Efforts on both activist and scholarly fronts have similarly imagined queer as another way to think of, through, and against identity.

What is queer? Queer can be an identity, theory, or practice. In the most general sense, queer can be thought of as heteronormativity's antithesis, a defiantly nonnormative notion of human social relations that rejects sex and gender binaries, obfuscates essentialist identities, and celebrates the unwieldy—and remarkable—ways in which sex means much more than reproduction (Barnett & Johnson, 2013).

> Heteronormativity refers to a complex entanglement of gender and sexual ideologies that function to maintain the (often unquestioned or essentialized) systems that privilege heterosexuality.

As an affirming personal identity or way of understanding the world, queer takes many forms. One form is the refusal to adhere to, or identify with, essentialist categories such as woman/man, gay/straight, or feminine/masculine, and opting for queer instead. Identifying as queer, however, does not entail or suggest other identity categories are lurking inside; instead, queer serves as a decidedly ambiguous identity category. As an identity, queer is fluid, malleable, and transgresses boundaries as a way of establishing agency and unity. "Queer refuses to be locked into any permanent state of identification. In this way, queer-as-identity allows individuals to transcend or outright reject normative labels, or to carve out an identity that more accurately represents who they are and how they relate to others" (Barnett & Johnson, in press). In addition to adopting queer as a personal identity, many also claim it as a political identity. Queer's deliberate ambiguity provides a framework for building coalitions. Queer activists today rally around a diverse swath of social issues spanning race, class, gender, and sexual orientation, which makes it seemingly congruent with a paradigm on social justice (Barnett & Johnson, in press). However, the use of queer as an identity category is not without contestation. Because of its historically pejorative use, some do not understand or value the reclamation of the term (Eaklor, 2008).

As an academic endeavor, queer theory has its roots in feminist and poststructuralist frameworks. First coined by Teresa de Lauretis, queer theory "conveys a double-emphasis—on the conceptual and speculative work involved in discourse production, and on the necessary critical work of deconstructing our own discourses and their constructed silence" (1991, p. iv). In other words, queer theory's goal is to challenge and subvert dominant, heteronormative discourses and to consider the construction of nonnormative subjectivities. Queer theory functions to complicate existing academic frameworks and conceptions of social relations by deconstructing the dominant, heteronormative structures undergirding extant scholarship (Marinucci, 2010).

As an activist framework, queer functions as a verb: "to queer" is to "challenge the dominance of heterosexist discourses" (Beemyn & Eliason, 1996, p. 165) or is "a distorting, a making the solid unstable" (Corber & Valocchi, 2003, p. 25). To put it another way, "queering" complicates the taken-for-granted heteronormativity of everyday practices, spaces, and discourses. Queer activism takes many forms, from "queering spaces" (Barnett & Johnson, 2013) to resisting mainstream (read: assimilationist) gay and lesbian movements (Warner, 2000) and, at times, to being conflated with the social movements being led by LGBT people (Eaklor, 2008). Like the ambiguity of the term itself, queer activism or queer politics is many things at once. Gay rights and queer activists thus struggle alongside and against one another as they endeavor for related, but quite different, measures of success. Although most of Denise Levy's chapter employs LGBT theory, some tenets of queer theory become evident in her framework as she encounters people who both identify as both LGBT and queer (Levy & Johnson, 2012), which is also the case with some of the participants in Anneliese Singh's chapter on phenomenology (chapter 4).

Poststructural Theory

Often used interchangeably with postmodernism, we distinguish between postmodernism and poststructuralism for our purposes here.

> Finding its origins in modernist architecture and used more frequently in the humanities than the social sciences, Postmodernism is a critique of modernism that rejects both convention and academic tradition. Grounded in opposition to the enlightenment, it defies the free subjects, foundationalist thinking, reason as universal, and the investment in social and moral advancement (Crotty 1998; Schwandt, 2007).

We treat postmodernism as Schwandt (2007) does, as a totalizing term which serves as more of a diagnosis than a theory. Our focus here is on one theory that has grown out of that diagnosis: poststructuralism.

Most people assume that the inclusion of "post" in the term is based on its chronological development "after" other theories. However, instead, *post* refers to a position that calls for a critique or deconstruction, an afterthought, or a revisiting of that which already *exists*. It is a position that exists *after* to critique that which is *before* (Berbary & Johnson, 2013). According to Lather and St. Pierre (2007), *post* theories, such as poststructuralism and postcolonialism, are all connected by their general critique or troubling of humanist theoretical positions. Humanist positions such as positivism, feminism, gay and lesbian studies, and critical theory are typically a departure point for critique in poststructuralism. In particular, these critiques center on humanist reliance on equalizing binary structures, belief in "progress," desire for mass movements, defined "Truths," metanarratives, and positions of objectivity or constructionism, both of which value the object of knowing more than or equal to the subject's knowing (Berbary & Johnson, 2013; Crotty, 1998).

Although there is a lot of diversity among poststructuralist scholars, several central themes can be identified (Schwandt, 2007). First, post-structural scholars focus on the decentering of an individual and instead take into account the self-aware condition of being a subject. Second, poststructuralist theorists adopt pantextualism, or the notion that every-thing is a text. They view all texts as related, which leads to intertextuality. Third, from a poststructuralist perspective, meaning is never fixed, never determined or determinable, and therefore not representative. Last, post-structuralists use deconstruction as a strategy for reading texts to unmask the supposed "truth" or meaning of a text by undoing taken-for-grant-ed binaries (Schwandt, 2007). Therefore, poststructuralism is constantly re-deploying meanings, deconstructing social expectations, uncovering power relations, and troubling taken-for-granted truths. It provides us with the lens to question our existence, consider subversion of expecta-tion, construct space for multiplicity, and re-create oppressive discourses. Such a lens is particularly relevant to the re-theorization of subjectivity, the process through which one becomes a self, an identity, an "I" (Berbary & Johnson, 2013). In short, a poststructuralist perspective

> suspects all truth claims of masking and serving particular interests in local, cultural, and political struggles. But conventional methods of knowing and telling are not automatically rejected as false or archaic. Rather, those standard methods are opened to inquiry, new methods are introduced, and then they also are subject to critique.... No meth-od has a privileged status [and] does allow us to know "something" without claiming to know everything. Having a partial, local, historical knowledge is still knowing. (Richardson & St. Pierre, 2005, p. 961)

From a social justice perspective, the continuous re-theorization of subjectivity, specifically the reconsideration of the humanist subject, has been of great importance in efforts toward social justice because it has helped people without power deconstruct their social positions as sub-ordinates to those with power. While the mere idea that all people can be "represented" is an essentialist claim in need of questioning, there is also the general critique of the traditional concept that some people always rep-resent the lesser half of the binary. Both Tracy Penny Light (chapter 7) and Jeff Rose (chapter 5) employ some of the tenants of poststructural theory in their chapters on historical inquiry and ethnography later in the text.

Postcolonialism

Postcolonialism brings to the fore a critical analysis of the impacts of imperialism, colonialism, and neocolonialism (Kincheloe, McLaren, & Steinberg, 2011). It stems from colonial domination in which conquering European nations wanted to establish their intellectual and moral superiority over the people they intended to rule (Ashcroft, Griffiths, & Tiffin, 2002; McLeod, 2000; Muldoon, Qiu, Yudina, & Grimwood, 2013). The result was a colonial discourse that established Europeans as superior and dominant to those who originally inhabited the land. Muldoon et al. (2013) report Canadian residential schools as one prominent example insofar as they were intended to "civilize" Aboriginal children (Blackburn, 2012; Elias et al., 2012). To accomplish this, schools separated the children from their families and prevented them from speaking their languages, all in an effort to "kill the Indian in the child" (TRCC, 2012).

Young (2001) argues that postcolonial theory provides a critical lens for the examination of the discourses of colonialism and the ways in which they construct power. Postcolonial theorists question the role and impact of colonialism, including its role in normalizing assumptions about who is the "other" (Muldoon et al., 2013). In this way, postcolonial theory serves as a corrective mechanism to the ways in which colonialism continues to shape current-day interactions with one another. Kincheloe, McLaren, and Steinberg (2011) explain that postcolonialists ensure their research moves "beyond the objectifying and imperialist gaze associated with the Western anthropological tradition (which fixes the image of the so-called informant from the colonizing perspective of the knowing subject)" (p. 171). To do so, postcolonialists take up issues of power and knowledge while paying attention to both local and global contexts (Hesse-Biber & Brooks, 2007). Of particular interest to postcolonial theorists are methodologies that "create an equitable research field and disallow a proclamation to correctness, validity, truth, and the tacit axis of Western power through traditional research" (Kincheloe, McLaren, & Steinberg, 2011, p. 173). Such methodologies demand a decolonizing of self and "other" (Kim, Millen, Irwin, & Gershman, 2000). Toward this end, postcolonial thought is concerned with the "invidious effects of 'othering' (invidious, oppressive definitions of the people with whom research is done)" (Olesen, 2011, p. 130). Much of this theory informs Bryan Grimwood's chapter on participatory action research (chapter 8) and Anneliese Singh's chapter on phenomenology (chapter 4).

Conclusion

Until the great mass of the people shall be filled with the sense of responsibility for each other's welfare, social justice can never be attained. —*Helen Keller*

In this introduction we have given a brief overview of theories that characterize social science research and then oriented the reader to those focused on social justice. In the next chapter, we detail the common features found most frequently in qualitative research and examine the degree to which a social justice paradigm creates researchers who "understand the world and the way it is shaped in order for them to transform it" (Kincheloe, McLaren, & Steinberg, 2011, p. 171).

NOTE

1. We are intentionally leaving out the "Q" typically found in the acronym LGBTQ because the implications for queer theory are different than those discussed here. Queer is taken up separately. We also acknowledge that the acronym can also take on many other "sexual minority" groups such as intersex, questioning, and asexuals. However, the root of the theoretical literature initially grew out of LGBT.

REFERENCES

Ashcroft, B., Griffiths, G., & Tiffin, H. (2002). *The empire writes back: Theory and practice in post-colonial literatures.* London, New York: Routledge.

Barnett, J., & Johnson, C. W. (in press). Queer. In Sherwood Thompson (Ed.), *The encyclopedia of diversity and social justice.* New York: Routledge.

Barnett, J., & Johnson, C. W. (2013). We are all royalty. *Journal Of Leisure Research, 45*(5), 677–694.

Beemyn, B., & Eliason, M. J. (Eds.). (1996). *Queer studies: A lesbian, gay, bisexual and transgender anthology.* New York: New York University Press.

Berbary, L., & Johnson, C. W. (2012). The American sorority girl recast: An ethnographic screenplay of leisure in context. *Leisure/Loisir, 36*(3-4), 243–268.

Bhavnani, K. K., & Talcott, M. (2012). Interconnections and configurations: Toward a global feminist ethnography. In S. N. Hesse-Biber (Ed.), *Handbook of feminist research: Theory and praxis* (pp. 135–153). Thousand Oaks, CA: Sage.

Blackburn, C. (2012). Culture loss and crumbling skulls: The problematic of injury in residential school litigation. *Polar: Political & Legal Anthropology Review, 35*(2), 289–307.

Carlson, K. B. (2012, July). The true north LGBT: New poll reveals landscape of gay Canada. *The National Post.* Retrieved from http://

news.nationalpost.com/2012/07/06/the-true-north-lgbt-new-poll-reveals-landscape-of-gay-canada/

Corber, J., & Valocchi, S. (2003). *Queer studies: An interdisciplinary reader*. Malden, MA: Blackwell Publishing.

Crenshaw, K., Gotanda, N., Peller, G., & Thomas, K. (Eds.). (1995). *Critical race theory: The key writings that formed the movement*. New York: New Press.

Crotty, M. (1998). *The foundations of social research: Meaning and perspective in the research process*. London, Thousand Oaks, CA: Sage.

de Lauretis, T. (1991). *Queer theory: Lesbian and gay sexualities*. Bloomington, IN: Indiana University Press.

Denzin, N. K., & Lincoln, Y. S. (Eds.). (2011). *The Sage handbook of qualitative research* (4th ed.). Thousand Oaks, CA: Sage.

Derrida, J. (1994). *Spectres of Marx*. New York: Routledge.

Eaklor, V. (2008). *Queer America: A GLBT history of the 20th century*. Westport, CT: Greenwood Press.

Elias, B., Mignone, J., Hall, M., Hong, S. P., Hart, L., & Sareen, J. (2012). Trauma and suicide behaviour histories among a Canadian indigenous population: An empirical exploration of the potential role of Canada's residential school system. *Social Science & Medicine, 74*(10), 1560–1569.

Fixmer, N., & Wood, J. T. (2005). The personal is *still* political: Embodied politics in third wave politics. *Women's Studies in Communication, 28*(2), 235–257.

Gates, G. J., (2011). *How many people are lesbian, gay, bisexual and transgender?* Los Angeles: The Williams Institute.

Glover, T. D. (2007). Ugly on the diamonds: An examination of white privilege in youth baseball. *Leisure Sciences, 29*(2), 195–208.

Haney Lopez, I. F. (2000). The social construction of race. In R. Delgado, & J. Stefancic (Eds.), *Critical race theory: The cutting edge* (pp. 191–203). Philadelphia, PA: Temple University Press.

Harding, S. (1991). *Whose science? Whose knowledge?* Ithaca, NY: Cornell University Press.

Herdt, G. H., & Boxer, A. (1993). *Children of horizons: How gay and lesbian teens are leading a new way out of the closet*. Boston: Beacon Press.

Hesse-Biber, S. N. (Ed.). (2012). *Handbook of feminist research: Theory and praxis*. Thousand Oaks, CA: Sage.

Hesse-Biber, S. N., & Brooks, A. (2007). Core feminist insights and strategies on authority, representations, truths, reflexivity, and ethics across the research process. In S. N. Hesse-Biber (Ed.), *Handbook of feminist research: Theory and praxis* (pp. 419–424.). Thousand Oaks, CA: Sage.

Hibbins, R. (2013). Reconstructing masculinities, migration, and transnational leisure spaces. In V. Freysinger, S. Shaw, K. Henderson, & D. Bialeschki (Eds.), *Leisure, women and gender* (pp. 451–463). State College, PA: Venture.

hooks, b. (2000). *Feminist theory: From margin to center*. Boston: South End Press.

Hylton, K. (2005). "Race," sport and leisure: Lessons from critical race theory. *Leisure Studies, 24*(1), 81–98.

Jaggar, A. M. (1988). *Feminist politics and human nature*. Totowa, NJ: Rowan and Littlefield.

Kalsem, K., & Williams, V. L. (2010). Social justice feminism. *UCLA Women's Law Journal, 18*(1), 131–193.

Katz, F. E. (1976). *Structuralism in sociology: An approach to knowledge*. Albany, NY: State University of New York Press.

Kim, J. Y., Millen, J. V., Irwin, A., & Gershman, J. (Eds.). (2000). *Dying for growth: Global inequality and the health of the poor*. Monroe, ME: Common Courage Press.

Kincheloe, J. L., McLaren, P., & Steinberg, S. R. (2011). Critical pedagogy, and qualitative research: Moving to the bricolage. In N. K. Denzin, & Y. S. Lincoln (Eds.), *The Sage handbook of qualitative research* (4th ed.) (pp. 163–178). Thousand Oaks, CA: Sage.

Kirkley, D. L. (2000). Is motherhood good for women? A feminist exploration. *Journal of Obstetric, Gynecologic, & Neonatal Nursing, 29*(5), 459–464.

Kivel, B. D. (2000). Leisure experience and identity: What difference does difference make? *Journal of Leisure Research, 32*(1), 79–81.

Kivel, B. D., & Kleiber, D. A. (2000). Leisure in the identity formation of lesbian/gay youth: Personal, but not social. *Leisure Sciences, 22*(4), 215–232.

Lather, P. (1998). Feminist perspectives on empowering research methodologies. *Women's Studies International Forum, 11*(6), 569–581.

Lather, P., & St. Pierre, E. A. (2007). Chart 1. Postpositivist new paradigm inquiry (revised June 2005). In P. Lather, *Getting lost: Feminist efforts toward a double(d) science* (p. 164). SUNY Series in the Philosophy of the Social Sciences. Albany, NY: State University of New York Press.

Levy, D. L., & Johnson, C. W. (2012). What does the Q mean? Including queer voices in qualitative research. *Qualitative Social Work: Research And Practice, 11*(2), 130–140.

Marinucci, M. (2010). *Feminism is queer: The intimate connection between queer and feminist theory*. London, New York: Zed Books.

McLeod, J. (2000). *Beginning postcolonialism*. Manchester, UK: Manchester University Press.

Muldoon, M., Qiu, J., Yudina, O., & Grimwood, B. S. R. (2013). *A post-colonial reading of responsibility in tourism*. Paper presented at the International Critical Tourism Studies Conference V, Sarajevo, Bosnia & Herzegovina, June 25–28.

Naples, N. A. (2007). Feminist methodology and its discontents. In W. Outhwaite & S. P. Turner (Eds.), *The Sage handbook of social science methodology* (pp. 547–564). Los Angeles, London: Sage.

Olesen, V. L. (2011). Feminist qualitative research in the millennium's first decade. In N. K. Denzin, & Y. S Lincoln (Eds.), *The Sage handbook of qualitative research* (4th ed.) (pp. 129–146). Thousand Oaks, CA: Sage.

Parker, L., & Lynn, M. (2002). What's race got to do with it? Critical race theory's conflicts with and connections to qualitative research methodology and epistemology. *Qualitative Inquiry, 8*(1), 7–22.

Peller, G. (1995). Race-consciousness. In K. Crenshaw, N. Gotanda, G. Peller, & K. Thomas (Eds.), *Critical race theory: The key writings that formed the movement* (pp. 127–159). New York, NY: The New Press.

Phelan, S. (Ed.). (1997). *Playing with fire: Queer politics, queer theories*. New York, NY: Routledge.

Rappaport, J. (2000). Community narratives: Tales of terror and joy. *American Journal of Community Psychology, 28*, 1–24.

Reid, C. (2004). Advancing women's social justice agenda: A feminist action research framework. *International Journal of Qualitative Methods, 3*(3), 1–15.

Richardson, L., & St. Pierre, E. A. (2005). *Writing: A method of inquiry*. In N. K. Denzin, & Y. S. Lincoln (Eds.), *The Sage handbook of qualitative research* (3rd ed.), (pp. 959–978). Thousand Oaks, CA: Sage.

Rosenberg, A. (2012). *Philosophy of social science*. Boulder, CO: Westview Press.

Rupp, L. J., & Taylor, V. (1999). Forging feminist identity in an international movement: A collective identity approach to Twentieth-Century Feminism. *Journal of Women in Culture and Society, 24*(2), 363–386.

Schwandt, T. S. (2007). *The Sage dictionary of qualitative inquiry* (3rd ed). Thousand Oaks, CA: Sage.

Truth and Reconciliation Commission of Canada (TRCC). (2012). *They came for the children. Canada, aboriginal peoples, and residential schools*. Winnipeg, Manitoba, Canada: TRCC.

Warner, M. (2000). *The trouble with normal: Sex, politics, and the ethics of queer life*. Cambridge, MA: Harvard University Press.

Weeks, J. (1991). *Against nature: Essays on history, sexuality and identity*. London, UK: Rivers Oram Press.

Young, R. (2001). *Postcolonialism: An historical introduction*. Oxford, UK: Blackwell Publishers.

Zucker, A. N., & Bay-Cheng, L. Y. (2010). Minding the gap between feminist identity and attitudes: The behavioural and ideological divide between feminists and non-labellers. *Journal of Personality, 78*(6), 1895–1924.

Common Features of Qualitative Inquiry

Corey W. Johnson & Diana C. Parry

> Social justice in the twenty-first century will be considerably tougher than it has been in the last half of the twentieth.... [W]e have to think much harder about the questions of scope, about what the universe of social justice should be in a world in which economic, social and political boundaries no longer neatly coincide. (Miller, 1999, p. 265)

In the first few chapter we discuss the paradigmatic orientation of social justice research and briefly explain some of the frequent theories employed for its purposes. Here, we provide a glance into the more pragmatic aspects of research, namely, the common features of qualitative inquiry. First, we offer recommendations on how to identify a problem, formulate the purpose of the study, and construct questions that provide adequate and appropriate scope. Second, we discuss the importance of reflexivity, including researcher subjectivity. Third, we briefly describe the common methodological strategies used in qualitative research for social justice, and refer to the subsequent chapters in this volume for a deeper exploration of these strategies of inquiry and their implications for social justice. Following these brief descriptions, we explore issues of early interactions with other data collection and analysis strategies, attending to issues of trustworthiness and challenges of representation. Our goal is to offer a broad overview of the project of qualitative inquiry for social justice so that researchers are equipped to more deeply examine the history, disciplinary roots, subtleties, strengths, and weaknesses of the methodologies in

Corey W. Johnson and Diana C. Parry, editors, "Common Features of Qualitative Inquiry" in *Fostering Social Justice Through Qualitative Research: A Methodological Guide*, pp. 43-70. © 2015 Left Coast Press, Inc. All rights reserved.

the seven chapters that follow. Although we advocate and describe these commonalities or traditions, we are mindful of their critiques (St. Pierre, in press) and address some of these concerns in our final chapter (chapter 10) on paradigm proliferation.

Initial Design Considerations

One of the most fundamental moments in designing a qualitative research study is the identification of a social justice issue to be explored, its characterization in a larger social context and within research literature, its articulation for the purpose of the study, and developing appropriate research questions to achieve the study goals.

Problem Statements and Reviewing the Literature

After identifying a social justice issue, narrow the scope to something that can be accomplished in a reasonable undertaking. This is often a major challenge, especially for novice researchers. Ask these questions: What is your beef and what do you want to do about it? In other words, what is your goal for social justice? Two things can help: 1) understanding everyday discussions about an issue (media reports, water-cooler conversations, Facebook threads, etc.) and 2) a thorough review of the academic literature to identify gaps and/or locations where the research might make a significant and meaningful contribution. There are a variety of resources on writing literature reviews and debates about their utility in qualitative research. Regardless, researchers need to be well informed and articulate about how the proposed studies fit into the larger landscape of scholarship in and around the particular social justice issue; literature reviews and problem statements help achieve these means.

Purpose Statements and Research Questions

Unlike a problem statement that outlines the entire scope of the issue and situates the study within the current literature, a purpose statement is a concise (one or two sentences) articulation of the goal of the study with four or five pivotal pieces: the issue being addressed, the theoretical orientation, the methodological tradition being used, the participants, and the context (cultural and/or historical). Corey Johnson recently conducted a study with drag performers (Barnett & Johnson, 2013); his purpose statement read, "This feminist project adopts a genderqueer lens and the methodological approach of narrative inquiry to better understand the complex lives of enduring drag performers" (p. 680).

Building on a purpose statement, well-designed qualitative research studies usually have two to four research questions appropriate for supporting the purpose and that can feasibly be addressed with the data that are generated through the collection method(s). Qualitative research questions tend to use descriptive or critical verbs; however, the choice of language will often be dictated by theoretical and methodological choices, so it is a matter of working back and forth between scholarly interests, the influence of the theory, and the strengths and limitations of the methodology. Take a look at Corey's research questions for the previously discussed study of drag performers and see how feminist theory and narrative inquiry show up in the questions.

1) What are the important stories and events that have shaped the performers drag identity?

2) What are the daily struggles and joys of being a serious drag performer?

3) What is interesting or meaningful about managing a multiple-gendered identity?

4) What are the relationships between drag performers and the queer community (activism, friendships, politics, space), and how does this challenge/reinforce gender norms?

Diana Parry's research questions from her study on women's consumption of sexually explicit material also reflect her theoretical orientation and are consistent with her interview method. Once some of these crucial design elements are in place, it is likely time for the researcher to begin a thorough and ongoing interrogation of his or her own reflexivity and subjective positioning in relation to the chosen social justice issue.

Researcher Subjectivity and Reflexivity

Often characterized as researcher bias in positivistic accounts, subjectivity is the personal view of an individual and, more broadly, the lived experience of that individual in historical, physical, and political contexts (Schwandt, 2007). It also includes the important aspects of reflexivity and emotions that occur in and around a qualitative research project.

Self-awareness of researcher subjectivity is paramount when endeavoring to understand the complexity of social issues. In reviewing one's subjectivities, scholars are able to appreciate their connection to the research and more fully understand how personal life story and narrative leads to engagement with a particular research endeavor and shapes relationships with the individuals participating in the study. Attending to subjectivities in social justice research can also reveal additional theoretical influences, researcher assumptions, issues of marginalization, oppression, and privilege. deMarrais and Tisdale (2002) explain, "Researcher subjectivity is a conscious attempt on the part of qualitative researchers to distance themselves from the positivistic, objectivist orientations of traditional research and, in effect, is the recognition of the engagement of the emotional life of the researcher with the research" (p. 120).

So how does one go about creating a subjectivities statement? Although the primary directives may or may not be clear and are likely to shift over the course of the study (perhaps several times) before research is complete, it must start somewhere. But where to begin? Obviously, a subjectivity statement begins with the researcher, but when? The approach will undoubtedly be influenced by the personal experiences the scholar brings to the particular issue under study, so we believe it should start there. But what is relevant? How much does one share with the reader about the complexities of your subjectivity? For example, Corey might provide a reader with the following, somewhat expected or typical list: *white, male, middle class, college educated?* He could also add to the list *bad driver, meat eater, liberal, tall,* and *queer.* Does that tell a reader what they need to know? Depends on the study, right?

The subjectivities we reveal might not necessarily be clear in the beginning of our project. But since qualitative research is as much a process as a product, we can only begin to imagine or speculate what subjectivities may become important. We suggest taking Peshkin's (1988) advice and realize that

> [s]ubjectivity is not a badge of honor; something earned like a merit badge and paraded around on special occasions for all to see. Whatever the substance of one's persuasions at a given point, one's subjectivity is like a garment that cannot be removed. It is insistently present in both the research and non-research aspects of our life. (p. 1)

Although we encourage everyone to attend to their subjectivities prior to undertaking research, scholars should also engage in ongoing critical reflection throughout the process. This practice is called *reflexivity.* Reflexivity documents the personal experiences, ideas, mistakes, dilemmas, epiphanies, reactions, and thinking connected with a qualitative study. Reflexivity can be captured in researcher journals, memos, field notes, blogs, and in other's reactions to the work. For example, when undertaking ethnography on a country-western gay bar, Corey marked an important shift in his own subjectivity, captured in his reflexive research journal. He wrote:

> The personal is truly political and it is amazing to me how my personal life will ultimately impact my study. This study was planned as a man, involved in a committed relationship, which presented its own struggles in relation to studying a gay bar. However, now I am going to be a single man studying a gay bar and that seems to present a new set of challenges. There seem to be a new set of ethical dilemmas as a result of my "availability" in the bar. When coupled I had a ready and convenient excuse for battling come-ons and pickups. However now that excuse is unavailable to me. How will I respond to those men who I am attracted to in the site? How will my availability as a researcher be compromised? Will this change impact my focus?

Although reflexivity creates an opportunity to capture the subjective experiences of the researcher, it also provides an opportunity to interrogate the theoretical and methodological tensions encountered in the work, to justify and rationalize the decisions made, and lay the groundwork for interpreting the data. For example, when studying women's experiences with roller derby, Diana encountered a tension among some of the participants who were questioning the inclusion of transgender players. This tension forced Diana to consider the feminist implications of this tension as well as methodological consequences. She wrote the following in her journal:

> An interesting turn of events during my interview today. Melanie [pseudonym] raised the issue of transgender players on her team and other teams. When I asked how she felt about transgender players she was less than positive. Her concerns were twofold. One, physical safety. She feels there is a difference being hit by a transgender player who is large and broad. Two, emotional safety. She argues (my research supports this) that many women seek out derby in response to bad relationships with men. They purposively seek out a safe space in an all-woman environment and Melanie feels transgender players change the emotional safety that the sport offers. This issue is inherently feminist as it raises the question, what does it mean to be a woman? Who is a woman and what makes a woman (Biology? Identity?)? I will follow this line of questioning up in future interviews and see if there is a transgender person who would be willing to be interviewed. I also need to delve into the feminist literature in this area and look at previous examples of all women spaces that engaged in these debates (ex. Lilith Fair).

Common Methodologies

There are many different qualitative research methodologies. A methodology is a philosophically situated plan of inquiry, orienting the choice of particular data collection and data analysis methods and linking them to the desired aims of the research. Many methodologies are tied to disciplinary tradition. Indeed, there are too many to name in one text. However, in our work with social justice issues, we have identified seven well-known methodological approaches common to the social sciences: grounded theory, phenomenology, ethnography, case study, historic inquiry, participatory action research, and evocative inquiry. Each one is detailed in the chapters that follow, but we briefly describe them here.

Grounded Theory

Grounded theory is a type of qualitative research methodology that generates and/or discovers theory (Creswell, 2014) usually using semistructured interviews as the form of data collection and constant comparison as the form of data analysis. Grounded theory was developed in the field of sociology, particularly from Anselm Glaser and Barney Strauss's 1960s research on dying (Charmaz, 2006). As opposed to deductive analytic methods, which start with a hypothesis or theory, Glaser and Strauss proposed the use of inductive analytic methods. This analysis uses the data to inform the development of theory without any preconceived hypotheses (Ezzy, 2002). Simply stated, "grounded theory methods consist of systematic, yet flexible guidelines for collecting and analyzing qualitative data to construct theories 'grounded' in the data themselves" (Charmaz, 2006, p. 2). These grounded theories are interpretive rather than predictive, meaning that they call "for the imaginative understanding of the studied phenomenon. This type of theory assumes emergent, multiple realities" (Charmaz, 2006, p. 126).

Phenomenology

Phenomenology is an evolving philosophy and methodology useful for the study of social life. Though Husserl codified modern phenomenology between the first and second World Wars, it garnered more reputable authority in the 1970s when a methodological realization of the philosophy was established (Groenwald, 2004). Phenomenology is first and foremost a philosophy (Moran, 2002; Sokolowski, 2000). As with any philosophical approach, phenomenology is grounded in and informed by core tenets and assumptions as it addresses broader and more metaphysical questions and assertions. Posited as an onto-logical and epistemological orientation (Dahlberg, Dahlberg, & Nyström, 2008; Heidegger, 2002; Vagle, 2010, 2014), phenomenology adherents typically employ repeated interviews with participants in an attempt to "get behind" taken-for-granted perspectives of lived experiences to reveal glimpses, both tentative and fleeting, of phenomena as they are lived, not theorized. The goal is to approach a phenomenon openly, allowing for individuals' lived experiences and their expression of those experiences to provide context, insight, and substance. This understanding is always coming-to-be, never finalized, and contextual yet salient (Vagle, 2010, 2014). A result is a discursive representation of the phenomenon through interpretive and descriptive reporting.

Ethnography

Ethnography is a methodology that typically employs the data-collection methods of participation observation, ethnographic interviewing, and artifact analysis as a researcher lives in and across a culturally bound "field." Historically associated with cultural anthropologists, ethnography has also expanded well into the world of both social and natural scientists (Bernard, 2006). As Goodall (2000) indicates, ethnography is "a way of working, a way of entering the world every day, which privileges asking questions about others in cultural contexts constructed and understood by a self whose presence is very much in the text" (p. 21). And with a social justice focus, it also accounts for the "meeting of multiple sides in an encounter with and among the Other(s), one in which there is negotiation and dialogue toward substantial and viable meanings that make a difference in the Other's world" (Madison, 2012, p. 9). Thus, the role of the researcher in social justice ethnographies is not merely to engage somewhere along the participant observation spectrum, but to become advocates, supporters, and champions of a culture, in defiance of oppressions within a culture, or oppressions toward the entire culture more generally.

Case Study

Case study research is useful for those interested in the contextual conditions that might affect the phenomenon being studied (Yin, 2009). Yin (2009) indicates that "case study as a research strategy comprises an all-encompassing method—covering the logic of design, data collection techniques, and specific approaches to data analysis" (p.

18). Stake (1998) argues a somewhat contradictory stance, saying, "case study is not a methodological choice, but a choice of the object to be studied" (p. 86). Regardless of this difference, both agree on the value of investigating individual cases. Stake (1998) operationalizes several forms of case study research and argues that to maximize learning, the case is expected to be something that functions, that operates; the study is the observation of operations. There is something to be described and interpreted. Case studies emphasize objective description and personal interpretation, a respect and curiosity for culturally different perceptions of phenomena, and empathic representation of local settings.

Historic Inquiry

Historic inquiry includes methodologies such as narrative inquiry, genealogy, and archeology. Narrative inquiry has the inherent potential to position participant's subjectivities in cultural and historical contexts; illuminate examples of agency and cultural contestation; reveal human transformation; and promote advocacy through connection with the reader. These approaches can also empower participants by emphasizing their shared humanity through personal stories of joy, sorrows, struggles, and activities of daily living (Costa & Matzner, 2007).

Narrative inquiry puts the participant in the center of the research process as the "expert" of their own life story, which sharply contrasts to traditional methods of the researcher taking full control, considering themselves as the "experts" to guide and interpret the participants' stories (Riessman, 2008). Through the use of mostly unstructured interviewing techniques, researchers allow participants to share their stories in the way the participants feel is most appropriate and relevant, providing an opportunity to be heard in ways that might otherwise be dismissed or redirected (Riessman, 2008). It is this opportunity that makes narrative research a potential tool for mobilizing positive change and emancipation for those who find themselves on the margins (Mattingly & Lawlor, 2000; Riessman, 2008). Furthermore, the narrative platform allows the participant to create and become "part of a written document—a testimony of what occurred at a particular moment of history" (Stuhlmiller, 2001, p. 75). This sense of empowerment is especially salient in cases where the participant feels like their voice and/or story was originally silenced or ignored and may be even more significant for participants who additionally find themselves in the social margins for other stigmatized characteristics (Mattingly & Lawlor, 2000).

Foucault used archaeology early in his career because it supported a historiography that did not rest on the primacy of the consciousness of individuals. However, archaeology's critical force was restricted to the comparison of the different discursive formations of different periods and could say nothing of causes of the transition from one way of thinking to another (Gutting, [2003] 2012). As a result, Foucault (1995) developed and used the method known as *genealogy* to analyze a history of the present to reveal how accepted truths have become natural. History is used in this method "as a way of diagnosing the present" (Kendall & Wickham, 1999, p. 4) and helps us understand the discourse around institutions and, in this case, the relationship between welfare, work, and leisure. Foucault believed many of our historical advances came about by accident (Kendall & Wickham, 1999); he used the method of genealogy to explore these historical accidents, also known as *contingencies*, in an effort to reveal systems of power active in society.

Participatory Action Research

Participatory action research (PAR) elevates participants' stories by including them in the process of data collection, analysis, and subsequent action planning and change implementation (McIntyre, 2006; Tuck, 2009). PAR operates from an epistemology that assumes research for and about the participants necessitates a degree of involvement beyond that of informant. To attain a more comprehensive understanding of the social issues affecting their lives, PAR involves participants as partners in research and action (Tuck, 2009). In addition to providing an insider's perspective, PAR methodology seeks to empower participants by fostering the critical self-awareness necessary for individual and systemic transformation (McIntyre, 2006). Central to this tradition is Freire's (1970) concept of conscientization, in which popular education enables socially dispossessed peoples to come to critical consciousness and challenge the oppressive status quo. Such an approach is particularly beneficial for marginalized populations whose voices are seldom represented in the scholarship.

Expressive Inquiry

We use expressive inquiry to describe the methodologies of autoethnography and arts-based inquiry. At its core, autoethnography is a systematic examination of the self. The emergence of autoethnography as a method of inquiry moves researchers' "use of self-observation as part of the situation studied to self-introspection or self-ethnography as a legitimate focus of study in and of itself" (Ellis, 1991, p. 30). Autoethnography also challenges traditional forms of empirical science and engages and celebrates a variety of representational forms (Wall, 2006). Similarly, arts-based inquiry is firmly rooted aesthetic power of the arts; it privileges imagination, novelty, and unpredictability above replicability, which also stands in opposition to much of our modernist scientific inquiries (Wang, 2001). Arts-based inquiry reconceptualizes artmaking as an interactive, reflexive practice of problem finding, transforming previous knowledge and misunderstandings through the manipulation of material and symbolic tools and the reconstruction of social and cultural meanings (Barone & Eisner, 2006; Johnston, 2009).

Beginning Interactions with Participants

Regardless of the methodology one chooses, there are likely to be interactions with others in a variety of stakeholder roles. In this section we focus on targeting data sources, connecting with gatekeepers and key informants, securing informed consent, and ethical decision-making in qualitative inquiry.

Targeting Data Sources

Targeting data sources (how researchers access the field of inquiry and/or identify participants) might be one of the most underestimated challenges faced by novice social justice scholars. "You must consider how you enter the terrain of your subjects in ways that are appropriate, ethical, and effective" (Madison, 2012, p. 24). Of course, a good research design, as discussed in the previous section, is the first step in preparation for beginning interactions. In addition, most institutions of higher education, government agencies, and research centers require approval of that design prior to inquiring into the lives of human subjects. So the first step should be to secure written permission from an institutional and/or ethics review board.

That permission usually requires researchers to have also defined the boundaries of their intended field of inquiry and/or the basic criteria (often referred to as *sampling*) of the intended participants. Both the research questions and methodological strategy should be used to determine these parameters. For example, when Corey examined masculinity in a country-western gay bar using ethnography, he not only studied the bound space (Johnson, 2005) of a specific bar, but also the social networks of gay men who frequented the bar as they traveled outside that space (Johnson, 2008). Meanwhile, his narrative inquiry of drag performers (Barnett & Johnson, 2013) had nothing to do with a specific bound space or social network of people, but instead he selected to examine drag performers from across North America who had eight or more years of experience performing and were "famous" in their hometown. Each of these data-targeting decisions were grounded in the research questions, influenced by the methodology, and approved by human subjects review.

So, once the parameters for data generation are set, it is important to identify leaders and/or organizations that might help facilitate access or connection to the field or population and effectively broker admission. These facilitators are frequently referred to as *gatekeepers*. Gatekeepers can provide access and also direct researchers to and away from important information. For example, when Diana embarked on her study of women's experiences playing roller derby, she met first with one of the original organizers of the local league. First, she provided that person with a lay summary of who she was (a researcher at a local university); what she wanted to study and why (women's experiences—both positive and negative—with roller derby to understand how women resist and simultaneously reproduce gendered ideologies in the sport); how she planned to use the data she collected (for academic and advocacy purposes); who she wanted to interact with (interviews with team members); the risks and benefits of the proposed interactions (bringing to the fore negative aspects of women's involvement with roller derby and learning how women resist gendered ideologies through the sport); how she planned to protect participant's confidentiality (use of pseudonyms); how much time their involvement would take (an interview of one to two hours plus reviewing their transcript and group analysis of the data); and how she planned to document interactions (digital recording of interviews plus researcher notes) (Madison, 2012).

As an outsider to a population, community, or organization, you should remember that access usually takes more time and energy than you might initially anticipate. For example, Diana met repeatedly with the organizer for the roller derby league. In part, Diana had to convince the organizer that was she was not going to sensationalize and/or exploit women involved in roller derby. Even after successfully convincing the organizer of the aims and purpose of her study, Diana had to wait for approval from the team's board of directors before starting her interviews. They decided to take the issue to the league for a group vote since all players would be invited to participate. Because Diana approached the team during their off season (thinking they would be less busy and have more time to participate in an interview), they were not meeting frequently. As a result, Diana had to wait weeks before she heard her study had been approved. All told, the process took a few months. Insiders may have easier access, but relationships may be more complex and require the negotiation of previously established relationships. Keep in mind that each scenario will be different and context specific. Regardless of insider/outsider status, once a scholar gains "access," they will need to build rapport with key informants or those who have access to the information needed. DeWalt & DeWalt (2011) indicated that rapport with key informants is an ongoing relationship "when both the 'informant' and researcher come to the point when each is committed to help the other achieve his or her goal" (p. 47).

Once access to key informant(s) is obtained, and as dictated by the human subjects approval, scholars will need to seek informed consent. Informed consent is the participants' right to know they are being researched, the purpose and questions of the research, the risks and benefits of participation, and how they can withdraw participation and/or contact others if they want more information or feel violated during the process (Schwandt, 2007). Sometimes informed consent is verbally communicated; sometimes it is secured via a written consent form. Regardless, informed consent is a fundamental requirement of ethical behavior in qualitative research for social justice. Of course, this is often complicated by some methodological strategies and therefore should be handled in consideration of researcher ethics. For her research, Diana has always used informed, written consent. Diana likes to explain the informed consent process and send the forms electronically when she contacts participants to remind them of an upcoming interview. Diana still brings hard copies of the forms to the actual interview, but sending them as an email attachment prior to the meeting gives participants time to read the forms and think of any questions. She hopes this process avoids participants feeling as though the forms were "sprung" on them and opens up a dialogue about consent in an informed, sensitive manner. This is particularly important when dealing with marginalized groups.

Ethical Considerations

Ethics play a huge role in social justice research because they are the rudiments of what is right and what is wrong. Philosophical by nature, ethics beg us to consider what is good and how to be virtuous, generate goodwill, determine norms of human behavior, and privilege justice over injustice (Madison, 2012). Clearly, ethics—philosophically and pragmatically—are of the utmost importance to the social justice scholar given our propensity for advocacy. Madison elaborates:

Advocacy and ethics require that the "I" of my personal responsibility to [research] be explicitly stated to address what is for me the fundamental question: "what do I do now?" The challenge of having "something to do," of defining "a distance between what is and what ought to be," requires a turning inward toward self-reflection and my own positionality.… Advocacy and ethics are interconnected, responding to the question: "what should I do with what I have witnessed [or learned]?" (p. 97)

Many professional associations associated with human services (social work, counseling, nursing, etc.) and research disciplines (anthropology, sociology, psychology, etc.) will have their code of ethics for practice laid out clearly. They include things such as transparency, informed consent, anonymity or confidentiality, practical competency, creating no harm, respecting human dignity, working for mutual benefit, not knowingly deceiving or falsifying data, offering appropriate renumeration and reciprocity, and ethical representation and publication (DeWalt & DeWalt, 2011; Madison, 2012). Both the philosophical and pragmatic questions of ethics should remain a central feature of the social justice researcher from start to finish.

Although we have both encountered a myriad of ethical dilemmas in our collective thirty-plus years of conducting qualitative research hoping for social justice, Corey's biggest was balancing participant incentives with issues of protecting confidentiality. If he offered the monetary incentives to the LGBT youth in one of his projects (grant-funded), the University of Georgia required participants provide their Social Security number (SSN). This meant the university staff might be able to trace the SSN to an individual student. This was of particular concern, given that a number of the young people were not out of the closet and that some of their parents did live in Athens (GA) and/or work for the university. Eventually, Corey was able to convince the institutional review board and accounts payable at the university that the amount was not enough to concern themselves for tax purposes; however, it delayed the project by more than five months.

Data-Gathering Decisions

Interviewing

The qualitative interview is one tool used in an attempt to capture the multitude of views and perspectives of participants in our complex social world. The qualitative interview is a purposeful conversation that takes place to gather descriptions of an interviewee's reality.

Thus, qualitative interviewing becomes much more than a typical communicative interaction as it requires careful questioning and listening in relation to the interviewer's interest. Interviews in qualitative research are typically designed in one of three ways: unstructured, semistructured, or as focus groups. Although there are entire texts devoted to the practice of qualitative interviewing (Roulston, 2010), we discuss some key features here.

Structured Interviews

Also referred to as the *closed interview*, the structured interview is usually reserved for the quantitative researcher, though qualitative researchers can make use of this question strategy. Closed questions are simple and elicit either "yes" or "no" (Do you like strawberries?), "agree" or "disagree" (Strawberry ice cream is the only flavor we should keep in the fridge) answers, offer a limited range of answer possibilities (Do you prefer chocolate, vanilla, or strawberry ice cream?), or denote selection among predetermined varieties (What is your favorite flavor of ice cream?). As we indicated earlier, the closed question can be useful in qualitative research, but is usually when paired with more open-ended questions. In fact, the closed questions can provide comfirmability quite quickly; however, we should be prudent in our use of them (Kvale & Brinkman, 2009; Roulston, 2010).

Semistructured Interviews

Likely the most prominent data-gathering method of qualitative research is the semistructured interview. Most of Diana's research uses a specific type of semistructured interview called *active interviews*, which are conversational and capitalize upon a dynamic interplay between the researcher and respondents. Active interviews build upon mutual disclosure and sharing of information (Dupuis, 1999).

Thus, the active interview creates a space where participants and Diana can share their own narratives and explain their own experiences. For example, in her study with mothers who used a social networking site called Momstown.ca, Diana and her research assistant Caitlin (see chapter 9) were able to draw upon their experiences as mothers and also Momstown members to conduct active interviews. These interviews yielded rich data that would not have been possible without a forum in which they were able to share their experiences of motherhood and Momstown throughout the interviews.

Focus Groups

Focus groups identify a number of people (usually between five and ten) who have common or varying experiences with a topic and bring them together with a facilitator to discuss the matter. What is notable about the focus group is that the interactional style is intended to use groupthink to generate data: multiplicities of perspectives, confirmability, dissention, new ways of thinking, notable silences, and diversity of experience.

Focus groups are used in a variety of settings for a variety of purposes; however, when used for research, they are often used either in conjunction with other methods and/or for comfirmability of tentative findings (i.e., member checking).

For example, in the second phase of her research with the participants of Gilda's Club, a place for people whose lives have been touched by cancer, Diana used a series of intimate focus groups with participants to solicit feedback on her interpretation of findings and to gain additional insights. Although focus groups are often used to confirm the accuracy of interpretation, our experiences have taught us they are an excellent source of additional data. Therefore, Diana hosted focus groups that were open to both participants from the interviews and new members who wanted to attend. Each focus group included five to six participants and was held at Gilda's Club. Starting with a general overview of the purpose and methods of the study, the bulk of the focus group reviewed the findings of the study to provoke dialogue and additional insights regarding the role of Gilda's Club in the members' lives.

Although often used in a confirmatory way, focus groups can also be used as the primary data-generation method, which characterizes most of Corey's work with LGBTQ youth in high school (Johnson, Singh, & Gonzales, 2014). His research team recruited participants from university LGBT resource centers and LGBT youth-serving agencies throughout the state of Georgia. Three separate focus groups delineated the project: one for gay/bisexual men, one for lesbian/bisexual women, and one for self-identified transgender, queer, or questioning youth. As such, they recruited four to five students for each focus group, secured consent, provided incentives, and then engaged participants in writing about one positive and one negative memory that affected their sexual identity development or their gender identity development during their time in high school.

After the stories were written, they were collected and then redistributed as a package to be read in totality by all participants prior to the next focus group session. A research facilitator invited the participants to express opinions and ideas about each story, look for similarities and differences in each story, and identify generalizations and overarching themes regarding sexual and/or gender identity. In addition, the researchers focused the discussion around certain questions: How do we define sexual identity? How do we define gender? How have school experiences influenced our understandings of these terms? How do these stories (discussed one at a time) influence our attitudes and understandings of sexual identity and gender in schools? In this case, the stories and focus groups complement each other in data generation.

Before using focus groups, there needs to be consideration about the group interactions, facilitation of group dynamics, and mediating conflict and/or emotional trauma. As Roulston (2010) suggests,

> a well-conducted focus group looks deceptively easy—however, managing talk in a way that will generate data that will serve the researcher's purposes may not always go smoothly. With careful and thoughtful planning…researchers can use focus groups to generate useful data for analysis. (p. 49)

Unstructured Interviews

Often used interchangeably with ethnographic interviewing, unstructured interviews are usually a reciprocal discussion between the interviewer and the interviewee in "real-world" conversation. According to Spradley (1980), ethnography is a "series of friendly conversations into which the researcher slowly introduces new elements to assist informants to respond as informants" (p. 58). During Corey's participant observations (discussed below), he had the opportunity to engage in many ethnographic interviews with a variety of participants. Using ethnographic, unstructured interviews allowed him to keep the culture of the site central to his conversations, and to directly follow up on his observations. For example, one night after watching the dance floor for several hours, he approached Jack, a bartender, and asked him to explain the two-step.

During unstructured interviews Corey used three kinds of questions to assist in the task of gathering cultural data: descriptive questions, structural questions, and contrast questions. Descriptive questions offered him the opportunity to learn the culture's language and to contextualize the setting; structural questions provided him with the units of cultural knowledge necessary to make sense of the setting; and finally, contrasting questions helped to illuminate the difference between cultural units or terms (Spradley, 1980). Although these categories of questions are useful in explaining the types of questions he could ask, they were not delivered in an organized fashion. Instead, he would merely engage the bar staff and/or patrons in casual conversations on a topic. Then he would deliver the questions asking Jack, for example, to tell him about two-stepping at Saddlebags bar (descriptive); the roles of each two-stepper in the dance (structural); and the differences between two-stepping and line-dancing (comparison) (Johnson, 2005).

The unstructured interview offered an opportunity to gather important perspectives about the culture from the point of view of the participants in the site (compare with Madison, 2012). Ethnographic interviews are easier to conduct than formal interviews because they are not directed by specific questions and are much more conversational, but still need to be thoughtfully planned and executed as part of the conversation; too much questioning or inflexibility could create awkward or unsuccessful interviews. As a result, the researcher will quickly became aware of how to interview more subtly, always paying close attention to the participant's timing, tone, and body language. Although unstructured interviews are not usually recorded, these conversations become part of one's fieldnotes as the product of those conducting participant observation.

Participant Observation

Participant observation is one of the primary methods used in ethnography and case study research, but is also used as a data collection method in other designs. According to Spradley (1980), the participant observer comes to a social situation both to participate in activities appropriate to the culture and to observe the people, activities, and context of the social situation. Immersion in the *field* is necessary to see, hear, and experience "reality" similar to that of the study participants. As a result, there is a need to balance being both an insider and outsider in the cultural context. On the one hand, a researcher will participate in everyday experiences to see what goes on in the context and to become immersed in the culture. On the other hand, the researcher will document and describe the culture as a detached observer, attempting to understand, question, and critique the culture. Thus, researchers need to be able to alternate between the insider/outsider subjective positions, and be an insider and outsider simultaneously (Spradley, 1980), which is a difficult balance to maintain.

Since participant observation requires an immersion in the culture of study, the duration and frequency of visits is important. Some researchers go into the field for intense but short periods of time;

some go sporadically for years. The length and intensity of immersion in the research context will vary and should be considered in relation to the scope of the study, the practicality of the researcher's life, and access to the field. For example, in Corey's study of the country-western gay bar, he planned his visits over the course of fourteen months so that he could spend both brief and long periods of time in the bar. He spent brief periods of time (one to two hours) in the bar every two or three weeks, becoming comfortable with his role as a participant and a researcher. Then he slowly increased his time in the field, spending between eight and fifteen hours per week conducting participant observations. He used a spreadsheet software program to chart his observations according to the date, time he arrived, time he departed, amount of time spent in the site, who if anyone accompanied him to the site, the focus of his observations/purpose of his visit, and what type of writing he did upon leaving the site. He also used the information in this spreadsheet to identify gaps or disparities in his observation times and dates to ensure good observation sampling according to the time of day, day of the week, and time of the year. As the frequency of his participant observations increased, he began to funnel his observations, moving from a macro focus on the bar as a cultural site for examination toward a micro focus on the cultural activities (i.e., dancing) and individual behaviors (i.e., how men dressed) that were more relevant to his research questions.

Though systematically structuring time in the field is important, the actual documentation of it in a rigorous and systematic way is critical. The goal should be to create a record of observations, experiences, feelings, reactions, and reflections to serve as a data source. Moreover, while there is no one way to create or maintain this written record, we affirm the advice of experienced fieldworkers (compare Emerson, Fretz, & Shaw, 2012; Spradley, 1980) who suggest taking jottings in the field, expanding fieldnotes, and maintaining a research journal.

These days most researchers use voice recorders to capture "jottings" or key words, phrases, and ideas to remind them of important events or to stimulate their memory of scenes and interactions, thick characterizations (not generalizations) of participants, concrete details about actions and talk, sensory details about the scene, and impressions or feelings about the significance of events. Once removed from the field, researchers transform their jottings into expanded fieldnotes. For example, during one night in the field, Corey spoke the words "blue hanky performance awareness" into his digital voice recorder; later, that transformed into:

The man with the blue bandanna in his pocket had just arrived. He ran straight to the dance floor and asked Dirk to dance. As they began to dance, he constantly looked around the room. He seemed acutely aware of everyone watching him as he fumbled through the awkward movements of the two-step. Dirk, however, seemed to have little recognition of the crowd around him as he belted out the words to the song and led the man forward around the dance floor, in a cadence of quick-quick, slow-slow.

Fieldnotes are perhaps the defining feature of participant observation. Learning to take fieldnotes does not come easily to everyone, so researchers should expect to spend some time figuring out a system that is effective and comfortable. The following questions can guide initial participant observations:

- What is happening in that site?
- What are the behaviors, norms, and values performed in the site?
- Who are the people (actors) in the site and how do they interact with each other and with others who enter the site?
- How are emotions communicated?
- How do people use tools and artifacts in the site?
- How is power displayed in the site?
- What preliminary cultural themes, patterns, or connections are emerging in the data? What else seems interesting or important?
- As observations continue in this setting, what questions/topics should be considered in planning the next observation?

Researchers need to plan for time to write up fieldnotes in the field or immediately upon leaving. If there is one rule of thumb for good fieldnotes, it is not to postpone writing them. Any delay causes a significant loss of detail, mistakes in reporting, and distortions of the experience. Fieldnotes will include notes from observation and from informal conversations with informants. They will include any samples of print media, photos, and other artifacts from the study site. They might also include the ongoing process of analysis and interpretation, including a record of what was done and when; thoughts on those actions; decisions made about ongoing data collection and plans for what to do next; hunches, questions, and commentary about what is happening; a record of what is known about the site and what is not yet known or is necessary to understand; and personal notes about who to talk with and what to talk with them about.

Researchers who use participant observation as a method usually also keep some sort of separate researcher journal that documents the more personal experiences, ideas, mistakes, dilemmas, epiphanies, reactions, and thinking about the site both in and out of the field. Of course, these journals not only contain personal entries about time in the field, but also interrogate the theoretical and methodological tensions encountered to exemplify and document any subsequent decisions made.

Document Acquisition

Documents (texts and other artifacts) are often overlooked as important data sources in the social sciences, but often serve as the primary data source in the humanities, communication studies, rhetorical criticism, and history. Documents can include those produced without any direct involvement from the researcher, usually for other purposes and priorities, or those that involve the researcher in the production of the document (McCulloch, 2004). Regardless, when considering documents as a source of data, scholars need to be sure to consider the document as multifaceted.

For example, if working in a school setting, there are many forms of documents that could be collected and interpreted, including mission statements, schedules, teachers' planning books, bulletin board content, student papers, etc. If engaged in historical research, archival data could include court records, letters, diaries, maps, photographs, and similar types of documents.

Sometimes, as is the case in rhetorical studies, the documents serve as the primary data source, and researchers generate questions around them specifically. For example, noting the "girls kick ass on television" phenomenon occurring in the late 1990s, Corey sought to examine the third season of his all-time favorite television series "Buffy the Vampire Slayer" for characterizations of masculinity and how that masculinity was used to either transform or reinforce dominant cultural values (Johnson, 2000).

More frequently in the social sciences, documents exist to supplement other data. For example, in Diana's study exploring women's experiences with infertility, she looked at brochures from different medical clinics on various infertility treatments such as in vitro fertilization (IVF), popular press articles on women's experiences with infertility, and advertisements that in her view reflected a pronatalist ideology, but also items that women brought to the interviews, including basal body temperature charts.

Regardless of what documents are chosen for analysis, and whether they are primary or secondary data source, the field, frame, or network of action always need to be considered for how the document is to be analyzed.

Forms of Data Analysis

Data analysis is the systematic effort toward describing, interpreting, and theorizing the data collected. Described as both and art and science, analysis is a recursive process that happens in conjunction with data collection. It often begins with "writing" data either in transcription of interviews, constructing fieldnotes, journaling, memoing, or even discussing ideas with friends and colleagues. Although this inductive analysis is important, we usually demarcate analysis as beginning with the organizing or redeployment of data to attend to the specific research questions (Schwandt, 2007).

Data analysis in qualitative inquiry is often the most uncomfortable and perplexing territory for novice researchers because so few have had formal training and have developed expertise in applying a variety of analytic techniques (Wertz, Charmaz, McMullen, Josselson, Anderson, & McSpadden, 2011). This is confounded by the fact that data analysis in qualitative research is much more varied than methods of data collection, including phenomenological analysis (Wertz, et al., 2011), constant comparison (Charmaz, 2006), discourse analysis (Fairclough, 2013), narrative analysis (Reissman, 2008), schizoanalysis (Biddle, 2010; Ringrose, 2011), thinking with theory (Jackson & Mazzei, 2012), and others; the list can go on and on. Of course, just like with data collection, theoretical orientation, research questions, and methodological choice might make some forms of data analysis more appropriate than others. For example, grounded theory almost always uses constant comparative analysis, whereas schizoanalysis might only be suitable if poststructural theory is used as a theoretical framework.

Regardless, what is most important when engaging data analysis is a detailed account of how these different procedures are carried out, what kinds of findings they make possible, and how they compare and relate to each other, including their potential compatibility and integration (Wertz et al., 2011).

Building Authenticity

So how do we judge the merits of qualitative research? Well, the truth is that it will vary according to tradition; discipline; epistemological, ontological, and theoretical orientations; methodological choices;

and cultural context. Following Lincoln and Guba, Schwandt (2007) believes we need to develop procedures that ensure

1) fairness: participants' different concerns, values, and perspectives are represented in a balanced way;

2) ontological authenticity: participants' understandings of their own lives are improved and/or more informed because of their participation in the study;

3) educative authenticity:participants have a more rich understanding or appreciation of the extent to how others see them as a result of their participation;

4) catalytic authenticity: action is a result of the inquiry; and finally

5) tactical authenticity: participants are empowered to act.

We feel these criteria are well suited to the endeavor of social justice. The procedures employed to achieve these criteria are subjective, but often include member-checking, triangulation of data, crystallization, triangulation of methods, advisory panels, policy suggestion, and advocacy efforts, to name a few. These various modes of quality control may demonstrate a tendency on the part of researcher to engender an accurate or "true" account of the knowledge constructed through inquiry. However, the next section of this chapter addresses the impossibility of creating a "true" account and the necessity of reflexivity for attending to the assumptions, intentions, and motivations of a researcher. In short, the crisis of representation thoroughly troubles how researchers working within a social justice paradigm position their work within a larger onto-epistemological framework.

Writing for Social Justice: Implications for Representation

> Representing other people's lives is a risky and difficult business, but it is also profoundly rewarding and worthwhile. (Ezzy, 2002, p. 156)

Research investigating lived experience seeks to understand from many perspectives how experiences emerge within material, social, economic, and/or cultural conditions (Olesen, 2005). As we have argued elsewhere (Parry & Johnson, 2007), social scientists traditionally assumed that adopting the proper research methods would enable them to accurately observe, understand, and represent the interactions, intentions, and meanings of research participants. However, the crisis of representation, something extremely sensitive to social justice scholars, challenged the assumption that a genuine, valid account of lived experience exists and that such an account can be understood, captured, and/or represented. In short, the crisis of representation centered on "the uncertainty within the human sciences about adequate means of describing social reality...aris[ing] from the (noncontroversial) claim that no interpretative account can ever directly or completely capture lived experiences" (Schwandt, 2007, p. 48). Researching lived experiences clearly is a complex undertaking.

Why is it so complex? First, research that engages participants' lived experience creates an "Other." Most social scientists want to know or understand an Other (e.g., people, histories, traditions, ancestors; Schwandt, 2007). According to Fine (1994), researchers create a social science that includes the Other by "self-consciously working the hyphen" between the Self (i.e., the researcher) and Other (i.e., the participant). She explains:

> The task at hand is to unravel, critically, the blurred boundaries in our relation, and in our texts; to understand the political work of our narratives; to decipher how the traditions of social science serve to inscribe; and to imagine how our practice can be transformed to resist, self-consciously, acts of othering. (p. 75)

Traditionally, the creation of the Other has suggested a distinction between the "researched" and the "researcher," which is typically manifest in the narrative voice of the text. As Dupuis (1999) notes, many scholars have traditionally used the third person to write up their research, which furthers the illusion of objectivity.

Second, the unquestioned authority of the text is complex. The separation of the researched from the researcher suggests the researcher stands above the participants as a godlike or all-knowing person. In turn, the researcher is privileged over the participants in the construction of knowledge, which may unwittingly encourage researchers toward reductionist and over-generalizing gestures in the production of their textual presentations of the research.

The separation of the researched and the researcher points to the third reason research that explores lived experience is complex: the alienation of the human side of a researcher (Dupuis, 1999). Richardson (1997) explains that "by objectifying ourselves out of existence, we void our own experience. We separate our humanity from our work. We create conditions of our own alienation" (p. 19).

In response to the complexity of alienation, scholars began problematizing issues connected to representing lived experience. For example, in the 1980s, many social inquirers started questioning gender, race, and class privilege as researchers and in the research process itself. They struggled with how to locate both themselves and their participants in reflexive texts (Denzin & Lincoln, 2005). Richardson (1997) asked, "How then do we write ourselves in to our texts with intellectual and spiritual integrity? How do we nurture our own voices, our own individualities, and at the same time lay claim to knowing something?" (p. 2). Finley (2005) continued to advance reflexive questioning by asking:

> How should research be reported? Are the traditional approaches to dissemination adequate for an expanding audience that includes a local community? What forms should research take? How can researchers make their work available and useful to participants rather than produce reports in the tradition of academics writing for other academics or policy makers? (p. 682–683)

These questions have created a crisis of representation for many scholars. The outcome of the crisis of representation was the realization that representing experience as it is actually lived is impossible (Denzin & Lincoln, 2005; Schwandt, 2007), and that any attempt to do so is partial, incomplete, and written by a particular scholar who comes from a particular standpoint and who wants to advance knowingly or unknowingly a particular cause or interest (Richardson, 2000). Lived experience is constructed in the text when the researcher writes it (Denzin & Lincoln, 2005). Thus, the "totalizing vision" or formulaic writing traditionally found in social science can be replaced by novel forms of expressing lived experiences (Richardson, 1997). In the end, "no research methodology can provide a perfect balance for telling and representing.... Each story and the accompanying data collection and analytic process is a balancing act" (Johnson-Bailey, 2004, p. 138).

Moving Forward

Now that we have established a purview of both the philosophical tenets and theoretical orientations typically associated with a social paradigm and a broad overview of the common elements of qualitative inquiry, we turn to some of the most common methodological strategies used in the social sciences. We assert that fairly traditional approaches and social justice is necessarily and beneficially changing them, and the chapters that follow document this evolution. In each instance, we have asked the contributors to this volume to discuss the methodologies' history and disciplinary roots, strategies for data collection, and analysis and implications for social justice, keeping their discussion close to their own empirical work. We hope these chapters are descriptive, relevant, and exemplary. In the next seven chapters, readers may find one or more methodologies that resonate, and a social justice issue to tackle.

REFERENCES

Barnett, J. T., & Johnson, C. W. (2013). We are all royalty: Narrative comparisons of a drag queen and king. *Journal of Leisure Research, 45*(5), 677–694.

Barone, T., & Eisner, E. (2006). Arts-based educational research. In J. L. Green, G. Camilli, & P. B. Elmore (Eds.), *Handbook of complementary methods in education research* (pp. 95–109). Mahwah, NJ: Erlbaum.

Bernard, H. R. (2006). *Research methods in anthropology: Qualitative and quantitative approaches.* Lanham, MD: Altamira Press.

Biddle, E. (2010). Schizoanalysis and collaborative critical research. *Aporia, 2*(3), 18–23.

Charmaz, K. (2006). *Constructing grounded theory: A practical guide through qualitative analysis.* Thousand Oaks, CA: Sage.

Costa, L., & Matzner, A. (2007). *Male bodies women's souls: Personal narratives of Thailand's transgendered youth.* New York, NY: Hawthorne Press.

Creswell, J. W. (2014). *Research design* (4th ed.). Thousand Oaks, CA: Sage

Dahlberg, K., Dahlberg, H., & Nyström, M. (2008). *Reflective lifeworld research* (2nd ed.). Lund, Sweden: Studentlitteratur.

deMarrais, K., & Tisdale, K. (2002). What happens when researchers inquire into difficult emotions? Reflections on studying women's anger through qualitative interviews. *Educational Psychologist, 37*(2), 115–123.

Denzin, N. K., & Lincoln, Y. S. (2005). Introduction: The discipline and practice of qualitative research. In N. K. Denzin & Y. S. Lincoln (Eds.). *Handbook of qualitative research* (pp. 1–33). Thousand Oaks, CA: Sage.

DeWalt, K. M., & DeWalt, B. R. (2011). *Participant observation: A guide for fieldworkers.* Lanham, MD: Altamira.

Dupuis, S. (1999). Naked truths: Towards a reflexive methodology in leisure research. *Leisure Sciences, 21,* 43–64.

Ellis, C. (1991). Sociological introspection and emotional experience. *Symbolic Interaction, 14*(1), 23–50.

Emerson, M., Fretz, R. I., & Shaw, L. L. (2012). *Writing ethnographic fieldnotes.* Chicago, IL: University of Chicago Press.

Ezzy, D. (2002). *Qualitative analysis: Practice and innovation.* London: Routledge.

Fairclough, N. (2013). *Critical discourse analysis.* New York: Routledge.

Fine, M. (1994). Working the hyphens: Reinventing self and others in qualitative research. In N. K. Denzin & Y. S. Lincoln (Eds.), *Handbook of qualitative research* (pp. 70–82). Thousand Oaks, CA: Sage.

Finley, S. (2005). Arts-based inquiry: Performing revolutionary pedagogy. In N. K. Denzin & Y. S. Lincoln (Eds.), *Handbook of qualitative research* (pp. 681–694). Thousand Oaks, CA: Sage.

Foucault, M. (1995). *Discipline and punish: The birth of the prison*. New York: Vintage Books.

Freire, P. (1970). *Pedagogy of the oppressed*. New York: Herder & Herder.

Goodall, H. L. (2000). *Writing the new ethnography*. Lanham, MD: Altamira Press.

Groenwald, T. (2004). A phenomenological research design illustrated. *International Journal of Qualitative Methods, 3*(1), 1–26.

Gutting, G. (2003). Michel Foucault. In E. N. Zalta (Ed.), *The Stanford encyclopedia of philosophy* (Fall 2012 edition). Retrieved from http://plato.stanford.edu/archives/fall2012/entries/foucault/

Heidegger, M. (2002). Hermeneutical phenomenology and fundamental ontology. In D. Moran & T. Mooney (Eds.), *The phenomenology reader* (pp. 243–308). New York: Routledge.

Jackson, A. Y., & Mazzei, L. A. (2012). Thinking with theory in qualitative research: Viewing data across multiple perspectives. London: Routledge.

Johnson, C. W. (2000). *Representations of masculinity in* Buffy the Vampire Slayer. Paper presented at the National Recreation and Park Association's Leisure Research Symposium, October 14–16, Phoenix, AZ.

Johnson, C. W. (2005). "The first step is the two-step": Hegemonic masculinity and dancing in a country-western gay bar. *International Journal of Qualitative Studies in Education, 18*(4), 445–464.

Johnson, C. W. (2008). "Don't call him a cowboy": Masculinity, cowboy drag, and a costume change. *Journal of Leisure Research, 40*(3), 385–403.

Johnson, C. W., Singh, A. A., & Gonzalez, M. (2014). "It's complicated": Collective memories of LGBTQQ youth. *Journal of Homosexuality, 61*(3), 419–434.

Johnson-Bailey, J. (2004). Enjoining positionality and power in narrative work: Balancing contentious and modulating forces. In K. deMarrais & S. D. Lapan (Eds.), *Foundations for research: Methods of inquiry in education and the social sciences* (pp. 123–138). Mahwah, NJ: Lawrence Erlbaum Associates.

Johnston, J. S. (2009). *Deweyan inquiry: From education theory to practice*. Albany, NY: State University of New York Press.

Kendall, G., & Wickham, G. (1999). *Using Foucault's methods*. London: Sage.

Kvale, S., & Brinkmann, S. (2009). *Interviews: Learning the craft of qualitative research interviewing*. Thousand Oaks, CA: Sage.

Madison, D. S. (2012). *Critical ethnography: Method, ethics and performance*. Los Angeles, CA: Sage.

Mattingly, C., & Lawlor, M. (2000). Learning from stories: Narrative interviewing in cross-cultural research. *Scandinavian Journal of Occupational Therapy, 7*, 4–14.

McCulloch, G. (2004). *Documentary research: In education, history and the social sciences*. New York: Routledge.

McIntyre, A. (2006). Constructing meaning about violence, school, and community: Participatory action research with urban youth. *Urban Review, 32*, 123–154.

Miller, D. (1999). *Principles of social justice.* Cambridge, MA: Harvard University Press.

Moran, D. (2002). Editor's introduction. In D. Moran & T. Mooney (Eds.), *The phenomenology reader* (pp. 1–26). New York: Routledge.

Olesen, V. L. (2005). Early millennial feminist qualitative research: Challenges and contours. In Denzin, N. K. & Lincoln, Y. S. (Eds.), *Handbook of qualitative research* (pp. 235–279). Thousand Oaks, CA: Sage.

Parry, D. C., & Johnson, C. W. (2007). Contextualizing leisure research to encompass complexity in lived leisure experience: The need for creative analytic practice. *Leisure Sciences, 29*(2), 119–130.

Peshkin, A. (1988). In search of subjectivity—One's own. *Educational Researcher, 17*(7), 17–21.

Richardson, L. (1997). *Fields of play: Constructing an academic life.* New Brunswick, NJ: Rutgers University Press.

Richardson, L. (2000). Evaluating ethnography. *Qualitative Inquiry, 6*(2), 253–255.

Riessman, C. K. (2008). *Narrative methods for the human sciences.* Los Angeles, CA: Sage.

Ringrose, J. (2011). Beyond discourse? Using Deleuze and Guattari's schizoanalysis to explore affective assemblages, heterosexually striated space, and lines of flight online and at school. *Educational Philosophy & Theory, 43*(6), 598–618.

Roulston, K. (2010). *Reflective interviewing: A guide to theory and practice.* Thousand Oaks, CA: Sage.

Schwandt, T. (2007). *The Sage dictionary of qualitative inquiry* (3rd Ed.). Thousand Oaks, CA: Sage.

Sokolowski, R. (2000). *Introduction to phenomenology.* New York: Cambridge University Press.

St. Pierre, E. A. (in press). *Post qualitative research.* Walnut Creek, CA: Left Coast Press.

Spradley, J. P. (1980). *Participant observation.* New York: Holt Rinehart and Winston.

Stake, R. E. (1998). Case studies. In N. K. Denzin & Y. S. Lincoln (Eds.), *Strategies of qualitative inquiry* (pp. 86–109). Thousand Oaks, CA: Sage.

Stuhlmiller, C. M. (2001). Narrative methods in qualitative research: Potential for therapeutic transformation. In K. Gilbert (Ed.), *The emotional nature of qualitative research* (pp. 63–80). Boca Raton, FL: CRC Press.

Tuck, E. (2009). Re-visioning action: Participatory action research and indigenous theories of change. *Urban Review, 41*(1), 47–65.

Vagle, M. D. (2010). *A post-intentional phenomenological research approach*. Paper presented at the annual meeting of the American Educational Research Association, Denver, CO, April 29th-May 1st, 2010

Vagle, M. D. (2014). *Crafting phenomenological research*. Walnut Creek, CA: Left Coast Press.

Wall, S. (2006). An autoethnography on learning about autoethnography. *International Journal of Qualitative Methods, 5*(2), 1–12.

Wang, H. (2001). Aesthetic experience, the unexpected, and curriculum. *Journal of Curriculum and Supervision, 17*(1), 90–94.

Wertz, F. J., Charmaz, K., McMullen, L. M., Josselson, R., Anderson, R., & McSpadden, E. (2011). *Five ways of doing qualitative analysis*. New York: Guilford Press.

Yin, R. K. (2009). *Case study research: Design and methods* (4th ed.). Thousand Oaks, CA: Sage.

Discovering Grounded Theories for Social Justice

Denise L. Levy

When "Mark" told his mother that he might be gay during his senior year in high school, she rushed to her car to retrieve the publications about sexuality that she had assembled from their church. She did not realize that Mark had already spent hours studying these same articles. She was not aware that he had desperately tried to change his sexuality, praying that God would make him straight, like the articles said. After this confession, Mark's relationship with his mom and his sister became strained; he became "an alien" in his own home. As he began to accept himself, his family slipped further away. And then Mark's deepest fear came true: when he boldly came out to them as a gay man, they chose their religion over him. In a process called "disfellowshipping," they shunned him and refused to talk to him in an effort to bring him back into the church. Now, at twenty-nine years old, Mark relives the moment when he was "invited to leave" his house by his mother when he graduated from high school. Talking through the tears, he says:

> It was really apparent that I had no place there. And so one day, when everybody was gone, I took the clothes that I had and I put them in my car.... I had to go to Wal-Mart to get one of those little hangers that spanned the back of the car. And I was terrified for months that my mom would report the car stolen and have me arrested. I literally took nothing but clothes.... I started over.

Eleven years later, he has only interacted with his mother and sister a few times. His mother says she pretends he is dead. Mark wants her to realize that he is happy and whole, and that he is a good person

Corey W. Johnson and Diana C. Parry, editors, "Discovering Grounded Theories for Social Justice" in *Fostering Social Justice Through Qualitative Research: A Methodological Guide*, pp. 71-99. © 2015 Left Coast Press, Inc. All rights reserved.

living a good life. He wants her to know that he resolved the conflict he once had between his sexual identity and religious beliefs, and that it is possible to be both gay and Christian.

Mark was the first person I spoke with as I started examining the process of resolving conflict between sexual identity and religious beliefs. Like Mark, other people I interviewed shared deep pain and anguish as well as hope, resilience, and resolution. There is much to be learned from them.

Years before I met Mark, as a clinical social worker, I counseled a young boy whose preacher told him that his same-sex attractions were "dirty and immoral." He was devastated and confessed to me that he often thought about running away from home. I turned to the literature to see what it said about the process by which people resolve conflicts between sexual identity and religious beliefs. I thought that if I could find out more about how others resolved conflicts, it would be helpful to my client. Although I learned about the religious and spiritual beliefs of gay and/or lesbian populations and the importance of gay-positive churches for some individuals (Levy, 2008), at that time, only a handful of studies addressed the *process* of resolving conflict between sexual identity and religious beliefs, and none specifically delineated this process. Further, studies focused mostly on the gay population, and none included both Christians and those who left Christianity (Levy, 2008). This gap in the literature eventually became my line of inquiry.

My research focuses on the process by which lesbian, gay, bisexual, transgender, and queer (LGBTQ) individuals with a Christian upbringing resolve conflict between sexual/gender identity and religious beliefs. Growing up in rural southern Georgia, I had several gay friends who were ostracized and condemned by their families, friends, and faith communities. As I bore witness to their experiences, I was compelled to do something. Being an ally who promotes social justice is important to my personal and professional identity, and my research is one avenue for "doing something."

An ally is a member of a privileged group who advocates for equality and social justice. Allies may, for example, interrupt discrimination or educate others about oppression. Sometimes, allies voluntarily give up their unearned privileges to call attention to them. For instance, as straight allies to the LGBTQ population, my partner and I have decided not to marry until same-sex marriage is legal in the state where we live. Our decision calls attention to unjust marriage laws and demonstrates solidarity with LGBTQ people.

I have used grounded theory to study sexual identity (Levy, 2011; Levy & Reeves, 2011) and gender identity (Levy & Lo, 2013). Both studies explored the process of resolving conflict between two aspects of identity. The resolution process is deeply personal; as such, it is important to hear participants tell their stories in their own words. With those values in mind, grounded theory was a natural methodological choice because it helps answer questions about processes (Charmaz, 2006).

First described in the 1960s by sociologists Barney Glaser and Anselm Strauss, grounded theory is one of the most widely used research methodologies today (Birks & Mills, 2011; Bryant & Charmaz, 2007). Rather than testing existing theories or hypotheses, grounded theory researchers generate new theories from their data (Birks & Mills, 2011). In other words, they develop theories that are "grounded" in data. These theories are either substantive or formal. Substantive theories, like those developed in my studies, are specific to a place or group and are written by researchers who have in-depth knowledge of a specific population or issue (Creswell, 2013). Formal theories, on the other hand, are developed from a wide range of cases or substantive theories and have broad applicability or generalizability (Bryant & Charmaz, 2007). In addition to the theories that emerge from grounded theory research, a core category is a key feature of this methodology.

> Core categories are central concepts that frame grounded theory studies; they bring together and relate to all of the other categories. Identified during the advanced coding stage of data analysis, a core category can be "a process, a typology, a continuum, a range, dimensions, conditions, consequences, and so forth" (Bryant & Charmaz, 2007, p. 279).

In addition to discussing essential elements of grounded theory research such as core categories, this chapter includes an overview of the historical and disciplinary roots of grounded theory research and details how grounded theory research can advance an agenda for social justice. Throughout this chapter, I incorporate examples and tips based on my own research and the research of other grounded theorists who study justice-related topics. In particular, I draw from Melendez's (2008) grounded theory study of African-American football players at a predominately white university to add a case of comparison.

Historical and Disciplinary Roots

During a time when qualitative research was considered unsystematic and subjective (Hall, Griffiths, & McKenna, 2013), grounded theory emerged from Glaser and Strauss's (1967) research on the awareness of death in terminally ill hospital patients. Interestingly, Glaser and Strauss's theoretical roots were quite divergent. Trained at Columbia University, Glaser's background was in the positivist tradition, including what has been called "dispassionate empiricism [and] rigorous codified methods" (Charmaz, 2006, p. 7). Strauss's roots were in pragmatism and symbolic interactionism, which focused more on subjectivity and socially constructed meanings (Charmaz, 2006).

> Pragmatism troubles the notion of an objective reality and instead explains that knowledge is created based on its usefulness or practicality (Hall, Griffiths, & McKenna, 2013). Grounded in this pragmatist philosophy, symbolic interactionism attends to the meaning people make in their social interactions based on their interpretations of symbols (language and objects) (Hall, Griffiths, & McKenna, 2013).

In their groundbreaking work *The Discovery of Grounded Theory*, Glaser and Strauss (1967) proposed using inductive analysis to develop theories based on, or grounded in, the data. These founders were some of the first scholars to legitimize inductive analysis and qualitative methodology. In fact, prior to this work, qualitative research was undervalued and taught orally, if at all (Hallberg, 2006). In addition to their focus on generating theory from data, Glaser and Strauss emphasized the importance of constant comparisons and simultaneous data collection and analysis (Bryant & Charmaz, 2007).

Since the 1960s, there have been several developments in grounded theory. The founders, once collaborators, notably disagreed on methodological procedures. Glaser maintained that a purely inductive analysis can be objective, and Strauss acknowledged the role of subjectivity, flexibility, and verification (evaluating for trustworthiness) in grounded theory (Hall, Griffiths, & McKenna, 2013). Later, Strauss collaborated with Juliet Corbin in proposing a more pragmatic and methodical type of grounded theory (Hallberg, 2006). Using a systematic coding process, Strauss and Corbin "rejected the positivist view that theory is 'out there,' waiting to be discovered, and instead assumed reality is a product of interpretation and construction by the enquirer" (Hall, Griffiths, & McKenna, 2013, p. 20). Criticizing their work, Glaser continued to adhere to his original or classic approach to grounded theory, maintaining that the researcher could be objective (Charmaz, 2006; Creswell, 2013; Hall, Griffiths, & McKenna, 2013; Hallberg, 2006).

A third type, and one of the newest developments in this methodology, is Charmaz's (2006) constructivist grounded theory. This approach recognizes that studies are affected by researchers and their relationships with participants (Birks & Mills, 2011). It acknowledges the importance of context in research, assuming "that any theoretical rendering offers an *interpretive* portrayal of the studied world, not an exact picture of it" (Charmaz, 2006, p. 10, original emphasis). In other words, the theories generated in grounded theory research are interpretive, emergent, co-constructed, and multidimensional (Charmaz, 2006).

In my research, I used Charmaz's constructivist grounded theory, acknowledging the context in which I conducted my research, including the general location for the research (the southeastern United States, rural Appalachia), the interview location (my office, participants' offices, participants' homes), my identity (white, cisgender, female, straight, raised Catholic with experience in various Christian denominations, currently spiritual/not religiously identified), and the participants' identities (various but including categories like white, Filipino American, biracial, LGBTQ, agnostic, atheist, Catholic, Christian, Church of Christ, Episcopal, spiritual, and Wiccan). In both studies, the grounded theories were fluid, multidimensional, and co-constructed. Using a constructivist epistemological perspective, I acknowledge that in another context, such as with a researcher who *had* experienced conflict between sexual/gender identity and religious upbringing, the emerging theory would have been different.

The term *cisgender* indicates congruence between one's gender identity and sex assigned at birth. For instance, as a cisgender woman, my birth certificate says that I am a female and I have always identified as a female.

Similar to my own approach, Melendez (2008) acknowledges the importance of context to his research on African-American football players at a predominately white institution by describing the setting of his study: a large, private, predominately white university located in a predominately white city in the northeastern United States. Given the topic of his research, context is critical. Edwards and Jones (2009) explain that using a constructivist perspective methodology allowed them to examine "processes, structure, and context, all of which are key tools in broadening rather than narrowing the inquiry and exploring identity as socially constructed phenomenon in the context of hierarchal social structures such as patriarchy" (p. 212).

Although there are various approaches to employing grounded theory methodology, researchers identify the following key concepts: simultaneous data collection and constant comparative analysis, theoretical sampling, semistructured and in-depth interviewing, hierarchical coding of data, inductive analysis in which categories are generated from data, identification of a core category, and ongoing memo writing (Birks & Mills, 2011; Charmaz, 2006; Hallberg, 2006). The key concepts of grounded theory are detailed below following the format of Figure 3.1.

FIGURE 3.1

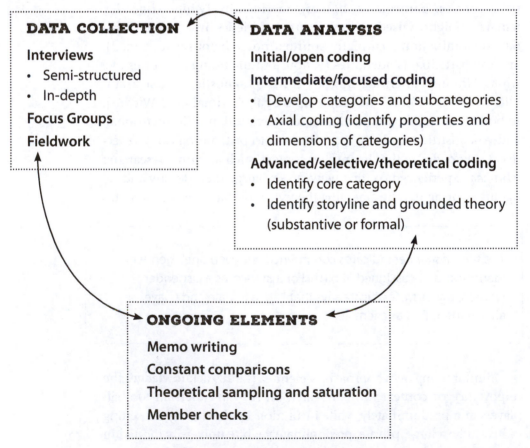

DATA COLLECTION

Interviews
- Semi-structured
- In-depth

Focus Groups

Fieldwork

DATA ANALYSIS

Initial/open coding
Intermediate/focused coding
- Develop categories and subcategories
- Axial coding (identify properties and dimensions of categories)

Advanced/selective/theoretical coding
- Identify core category
- Identify storyline and grounded theory (substantive or formal)

ONGOING ELEMENTS

Memo writing
Constant comparisons
Theoretical sampling and saturation
Member checks

Strategies of Data Collection

To Review or Not To Review?

Although many projects begin with a thorough review of the literature, there is debate as to whether or not this should occur in grounded theory research. Because the theories generated should be grounded in the data, it is important for researchers to view data from a fresh perspective that is not informed or "biased" by prior reading or study. Some view literature reviews as "potentially stifling the process of developing a grounded theory and thus something that could detract from the quality and originality of the research" (Dunne, 2011, p. 114).

Others believe that it is possible to complete a literature review at the beginning of a grounded theory study without negative impact, and that a focused review of the literature can be helpful (Birks & Mills, 2011). In my study on sexual identity, I completed a comprehensive literature review prior to undertaking the research. In my gender study, I did a more focused review, looking only at theories of gender identity development and methodological choices made by researchers studying similar topics. In both studies I employed strategies such as memo writing to assist with acknowledging assumptions. I found these literature reviews useful, and I suggest a more comprehensive review for those who are unfamiliar with theory and research on their topic.

Interviews

Most grounded theorists conduct interviews as the primary or sole method of collecting data because they seek to understand participants' perspectives (Birks & Mills, 2011). In qualitative research, interviewing has been described as having purposeful conversations (Bogdan & Biklen, 2007). In-depth or intensive interviews work well in grounded theory because they are "open-ended yet directed, shaped yet emergent, and paced yet unrestricted" (Charmaz, 2006, p. 28). Because the grounded theory emerges from researchers' interpretations of the data, short and unstructured interviews typically do not provide the rich data needed for theory development.

Qualitative interviews can range from highly structured to unstructured based on the number of preset questions and flexibility in the interview guide. In my research, I used a semistructured interview format and developed a flexible interview guide. Charmaz (2006) encourages researchers to "devise a few broad, open-ended questions. Then you can focus your interview questions to invite detailed discussion.... By creating open-ended, non-judgmental questions, you encourage unanticipated statements and stories to emerge" (p. 26). My interviews were structured enough that I was able to obtain common information to compare across participants. However, I was flexible enough with my questions to capture the unique experiences of each participant. I began with more impersonal topics by asking interviewees about their childhood church(es). My interview guide also included overarching questions such as "How did the conflict between religious beliefs and sexual identity impact your life?" and "How did you move from experiencing conflict to resolving conflict?"

Tips for Developing a Semistructured Interview Guide in Grounded Theory

- Start with a few background questions.

- If the study includes research questions or particular areas of theoretical inquiry, organize the remaining interview questions by these areas. For instance, Melendez (2008) organized his interview questions into three topical areas to learn about experiences that football players had within the team, university, and city.

- Use open-ended rather than closed (yes/no) questions.

- Ask one question at a time.

- Make sure the questions do not assume a certain type of answer.

- Avoid jargon unless using terms already spoken by the participants.

- Add questions that will assist in developing emerging categories and theories.

- Remember, it is just a guide; listen and respond to participants in the moment.

Birks and Mills (2011) explain that researchers may need to modify the interview guide as the study progresses. I viewed my guide as a flexible reference to change and development based on what I learned. For instance, I found it helpful to ask about certain areas of the theory that were emerging, such as the personal factors that were helpful to participants as they resolved conflicts.

Other Methods of Data Collection

In addition to interviewing, data may be collected through focus groups and fieldwork (Birks & Mills, 2011). For instance, Eyles' study on homeopathic consultation used data from observations (field-notes) and documents (practitioner diaries) in addition to interviews (Eyles, Leydon, Lewith, & Brien; 2011; Eyles, Walker, & Brien, 2009). Melendez (2008) used field notes in his study on African-American football players. In addition to notes and memos on team meetings, practices, and study halls, Melendez collected data through individual and group interviews. In both Eyles's and Melendez's studies, field notes and memos seemed to supplement interview data rather than stand alone.

Although most grounded theorists primarily use interviewing, they will "undertake work in the field, even if it is only to interview participants in their own environment" (Birks & Mills, 2011, p. 77). As expected, I completed some fieldwork in both of my studies. In addition to interviewing some participants in their homes, I attended several services or ceremonies at welcoming churches where I was able to witness the supportive environments described by participants. Further, I reviewed and analyzed almost 20 denominations' sexuality-related policies for a recent book chapter (Levy, 2014). Obtained from religious texts, official websites or materials, conference meeting minutes, and news sources, denominations' policies focused on sexuality, gay or lesbian clergy, same-sex ceremonies, inclusion of sexual orientation in hate crime laws, and other topics. During this review, I was surprised at how far-reaching some policies were. For instance, the Southern Baptist Convention (1997) encourages its members to avoid purchasing or associating with the Disney Company based on the company's perceived promotion of "homosexuality." The review also assisted me in understanding the complexity of denominations' policies, the changes in policies over time, and the ways that policies may or may not affect individuals who are part of that denomination. After all, how many Southern Baptists are aware of the Disney policy?

Data Analysis

As grounded theorists collect data, they simultaneously analyze transcripts and fieldnotes. Given the recursive process between data collection and analysis, I suggest scheduling interviews so that transcription and analysis can take place between each one.

Initial Coding

Although Glaser and Strauss did not thoroughly detail coding in *The Discovery of Grounded Theory*, other grounded theorists have since described it (Birks & Mills, 2011). The process begins with *initial* or *open coding*, in which researchers identify key words by reviewing transcripts word by word and line by line. *In vivo codes* use participants' own words (Birks & Mills, 2011), and are particularly important in justice-related research to give voice to marginalized populations. Researchers who are not part of the population of study may depend heavily on in vivo codes to avoid misrepresentation or misinterpretation.

Research should rely on the data during open coding rather than bringing in preconceived notions or ideas. To keep codes grounded in the data, Charmaz (2006) advises to "remain open, stay close to the data, keep your codes simple and precise, construct short codes, preserve actions, compare data with data, [and] move quickly through the data" (p. 49).

Example of Open or Initial Coding (Study 2)

Participant discussing his childhood experience in a faith-based daycare program:

I remember being there in the morning one time and playing with some stuff and for some reason I had this urge to go over and play with some of the girls' dolls with the girls. I'm not going to say that I was one of those kids that wanted to play with the Barbies, but to some extent it looked fun. All they had over here were some monster trucks and dump trucks and stuff, and I was kind of bored with that. So I went over and tried to play with them and play with the girls, at the same time as playing with whatever they were playing with. Like I said, it wasn't even a super-feminine thing (like I'm going to dress up all the Barbies or anything like that). I was just playing with the girls with what they were playing with—their toys. Someone came over and stopped me. "No, you have to—you should go over here and play with that stuff." And I was like, "Why?" I remember asking why, what's the big deal? It was like, "You just have to. This is what you're supposed to do." I wasn't going to fight it or anything. I was never really one of those kids to try and fight the system, but little things like that kept happening.	*playing* *wanted other toys* *girls' toys—dolls* *not one of those kids** *girls' toys looked fun* *boys' toys-trucks* *bored with boys' toys* *played with girls' toys* *was not super-feminine** *did not dress up Barbies* *playing with the girls** *teacher intervened* *redirected to boys' toys* *asked why* *didn't understand* *supposed to do** *didn't fight the system** *it kept happening**

*In vivo codes.

Melendez (2008) used open coding in his study, reviewing each individual transcript line by line several times to identify key themes. However, he also coded transcripts for the "types of situation observed; perspectives and viewpoints of subjects; processes, activities, events, strategies, and methods observed; and social structure and relationships" (Melendez, 2008, p. 430). His initial coding highlights the multiple ways that codes can be used.

Intermediate Coding

Intermediate or *focused coding* includes identifying the more frequent and/or significant initial codes (Charmaz, 2006). In intermediate coding, researchers begin to develop categories and subcategories. Categories should be identified from the data rather than being forced upon the data (Bryant & Charmaz, 2007). I find it helpful to review a list of initial codes and sort them into categories and subcategories. Look back at the example of initial coding from my gender study. In this small excerpt from the transcript, what categories and subcategories can be found? Socialization? Gender norms? Choosing toys? Others?

It is not until the most advanced type of intermediate coding, called *axial* or *theoretical coding*, that researchers begin to examine categorical relationships (Birks & Mills, 2011; Charmaz, 2006). Defined by Strauss and Corbin (1998), axial coding identifies the dimensions and properties in categories. Theoretical coding, described by Glaser, relates codes to one another and integrates these codes into a theory (Charmaz, 2006). In both types, researchers examine the relationship between categories and subcategories rather than simply naming them.

In Melendez's (2008) study, axial coding reframed categories and highlighted relationships between them. In particular, axial coding focused on the context of participants' experiences and the similarities and differences in their experiences with the team, university, and city. Similarly, as my study progressed, axial coding assisted in identifying categories and subcategories and the relationships between them. For instance, three subcategories emerged under the category of defying gender norms: choosing clothes, choosing toys, and performing. For the subcategory of choosing toys highlighted in the transcript excerpt, axial coding revealed that participants started playing with toys typically associated with the "other gender" in childhood. One participant explained, "I was doomed from the start.... I didn't fit their mold.... I was always more interested in scones than scores." Like the other subcategories, choosing toys was a way that participants defied gender norms learned during socialization.

FIGURE 3.2. Process of resolving conflict between gender identity and religious beliefs. First published in Levy and Lo (2013) and reprinted by permission of Taylor & Francis, Ltd.

Experiencing Gender Socialization
- ○ **Family**
  - — Acceptable clothing and behaviors
  - — Limited connection or understanding
- • **Community**
  - — Strict gender roles
- • **Church**
  - — Messages about sexuality and gender
  - — Observable gender roles

Having Conflict Between View of Self and Socialized Gender
- • **Dreaming about being the "other gender"**
- • **Trying to fit in**
- • **Experiencing isolation and depression**

Defying Gender Norms
- • **Choosing clothes**
- • **Choosing toys**
- • **Performing**

Exploring Gender and Religious Identities
- • **Doing research**
- • **Talking to others**
  - — Family
  - — Community
  - — Church
- • **Forming new identities**

Continually Resolving
- • **Gender Identity**
  - — Still forming
  - — Becoming comfortable with self
- • **Religious identity**
  - — Maintaining core beliefs
  - — Personalizing faith
  - — Not regularly attending church

Advanced Coding

Advanced coding, the final type of coding, is sometimes called *theoretical* or *selective coding*. Regardless of the terminology, advanced coding takes the categories and subcategories developed in intermediate coding and weaves them into a storyline or theory (Birks & Mills, 2011; Charmaz, 2006). For instance, in my gender study (Levy & Lo, 2013), five fluid "stages" of the conflict resolution process emerged (Figure 3.2). Likewise, by incorporating all of the data in his study, Melendez (2008) developed an illustrative model of the experiences of African-American football players in college. His model highlights categories of "judgment, double standards, values, integration, stigma of the Black athlete, living in an inhospitable city, and unwritten rules" (Melendez, 2008, p. 433), with an overarching core category of mistrust.

During this advanced stage, researchers identify a core category through an iterative process of coding, memoing, and sampling. In my study on sexual identity (Levy, 2011), I questioned whether or not there could be more than one core category when advanced coding revealed two core categories: personal and contextual factors (Figure 3.3). These two core categories were related to each other, yet distinct. Although both factors influenced the resolution process, many participants resolved conflict by changing one or more of the contextual factors. For instance, they moved to a new area or left their childhood churches. Personal factors, on the other hand, were more consistent.

FIGURE 3.3. Process of resolving conflict between sexual identity and religious beliefs. First published in Levy and Reeves (2011) and reprinted by permission of Taylor & Francis, Ltd.

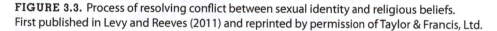

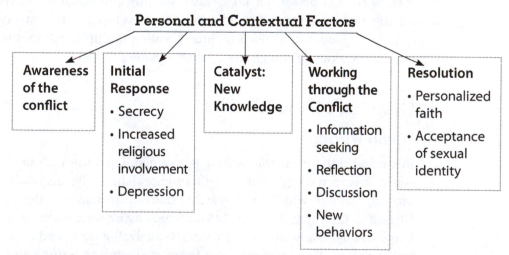

Personal and Contextual Factors

Awareness of the conflict	Initial Response	Catalyst: New Knowledge	Working through the Conflict	Resolution
	• Secrecy		• Information seeking	• Personalized faith
	• Increased religious involvement		• Reflection	• Acceptance of sexual identity
	• Depression		• Discussion	
			• New behaviors	

Personal factors: reflective abilities, strength and resiliency, anger, creativity, and humor
Contextual factors: family, community, and church.

> Personally, I find advanced coding to be the most difficult, likely because it seems so final. I want to get it "right," and I often need to cycle between complete immersion in the data and stepping away from the data. While "away," I spend time theorizing and writing memos until a core category and theory emerge.

It is also during this advanced coding stage that a theory, grounded in the data, is constructed. Because data collection and analysis occur simultaneously, grounded theorists may find that theories develop and change as the research progresses. In my sexual identity study, analysis led to a theory about the process by which gay, lesbian, and queer individuals with a Christian upbringing resolve conflict between sexual identity and religious beliefs. My grounded theory asserts that the resolution process includes five fluid "stages" that are influenced by personal and contextual factors (see Figure 3.3). According to the theory, sexual identity development and faith development are intertwined for these individuals, and resolving conflict is easier for those who are in more welcoming environments or contexts (Levy, 2008).

As noted in the chapter introduction, grounded theorists discuss theory as either substantive or formal. In grounded theory, we typically see substantive theories (Bryman, 2012). This is because the theories are specific to a certain situation. Formal theories, developed based on a wide range of situations or substantive cases, are more abstract and generalizable (Bryman, 2012). Although my theories of resolving conflict between gender/sexual identity and religious beliefs are substantive theories, I could potentially develop a formal theory of resolving identity conflicts by incorporating multiple, substantive theories generated from grounded theory studies.

Ongoing Methods

Memo Writing

In grounded theory, memo writing is essential. Used throughout the study, memo writing is the "methodological link, the distillation process, through which the researcher transforms data into theory" (Bryant & Charmaz, 2007, p. 245). Memos assist researchers in acknowledging assumptions and contexts, analyzing data, and developing theory. They may take the form of structured writing from prompts, free writing, charts, drawings, lists, questions and answers, or a combination of these.

During data collection, I used memo writing to consider the contextual forces affecting the study and to examine my positionality as a researcher (Bryant & Charmaz, 2007). For instance, I examined issues of power and privilege in the research relationship and wondered if the data and resulting analysis would be different if I were LGBTQ rather than an ally who is straight and cisgender (Levy, 2013). I often used one of the following prompts in writing memos after each interview: What did the participant say that I agreed or disagreed with during the interview? How are the participant's experiences similar or different from my own? What issues of power or privilege were highlighted in this interview? In one memo, I began exploring these issues:

> Even though I'm an ally, I'm still a privileged researcher studying a population that has been marginalized and oppressed. As such, I think it will be important to continue to journal about how issues of power and privilege are at work in this study and to do what I can to equalize the researcher–participant relationship. In addition to sending a summary of the findings to participants for review, should I also send the entire document?

During data analysis, memo writing allowed me to write freely about the emerging categories without the pressure of formally presenting a grounded theory. I used memos to test my ideas and assumptions, and to conceptualize the substantive theory and core categories. Melendez (2008) also used memos in his study of African-American football players, and he categorized his memos into two types: *content memos* and *process memos*. Content memos highlight themes and patterns from interviews and lead to development of initial categories, and process memos focus on the feelings and thoughts of the researcher to monitor subjectivity and potential misinterpretation of data (Melendez, 2008).

Constant Comparison

Throughout the process of collecting and analyzing data, grounded theory researchers constantly compare data. Glaser and Strauss (1967) used constant comparisons to identify similarities and differences in data. Researchers can compare codes within one transcript as well as across transcripts. Bryant and Charmaz (2007) explain that the process of constant comparison assists in establishing and elaborating concepts until a theory emerges.

Each time I complete open coding on a transcript, I compare the initial codes throughout the transcript and then compare these codes to other transcripts. Sometimes, I find similar codes that are worded slightly differently, and I then compare transcripts to see if one code better illustrates the data. In the sexual identity study, for example, I had several codes that I eventually labeled as "creativity." These included: theatre, visual art, creative writing, creative outlets, personal creativity, artistic outlets, and artistic performances. I have also used this method to compare the overall results and grounded theories from each of my two studies discussed in this chapter (Levy & Edmiston, 2014).

Theoretical Sampling and Saturation

Theoretical sampling is a key concept in grounded theory. In this type of sampling, researchers recruit and select participants who can contribute to the development of analytic categories and of the overall grounded theory (Bryant & Charmaz, 2007). Because data collection and analysis occur simultaneously, it is possible to modify criteria for participation as the study progresses to gain specific knowledge. In fact, the iterative process in grounded theory includes "movement backwards and forwards between sampling and theoretical reflection" (Bryman, 2012, p. 420). Participants selected by theoretical sampling might answer specific questions to assist researchers in refining their emerging theories. In my study on sexual identity, for instance, the majority of the participants identified as white. As the study progressed, I sought out more diverse participants and specifically asked them about the impact of culture on their experiences. For racially and ethnically diverse participants, culture was part of the family and community contexts affecting their experiences. For instance, "Chad" shared that his mom, who is Korean, took "some of the heat off of herself" by saying "we don't have gay people" in Korea.

Qualitative researchers often continue sampling until they research a point of saturation, which means that continued data collection will not provide any new information or insight. In grounded theory, theoretical saturation of categories occurs when no new properties or dimensions evolve in the analytic process (Bryant & Charmaz, 2007). Constructivists recognize that the larger sample sizes required by positivist researchers may not provide additional insight, and saturation supersedes the size of the sample (Charmaz, 2006). In my study on sexual identity, I was required to initially estimate the number of participants for my application to the institutional review board (IRB). Based on numbers of participants from other grounded theory studies I reviewed at that time, I planned to interview approximately fifteen to eighteen individuals. However, once I interviewed thirteen participants, I found that I no longer gained new information or insights for my categories. Just to be sure, I interviewed two additional participants.

In my gender study, I initially planned to interview approximately the same number of people as I did in my first study. This study, unlike the other, took place in rural Appalachia. Ideally, I hoped to recruit about fifteen transgender, transsexual, gender queer, or similarly identified individuals with a Christian upbringing from the surrounding rural areas. Despite my best efforts in contacting stakeholders, meeting with individuals and groups, sending information to listservs, and connecting with people who were interested in the project, I was not able to recruit nearly the number of participants that I initially estimated. In fact, out of the total number of participants in the study (five), two were located outside of the general area I originally had in mind. Although I did not mind traveling, interest in the study seemed to suddenly halt. Recruitment of participants from marginalized and oppressed populations proved difficult (Levy & Johnson, 2012).

I continued to try to recruit for several months while simultaneously moving forward with more advanced analysis of the interviews that I had already conducted. As categories and a theory emerged, I found that the existing data were quite rich and that I was able to draw several conclusions from the five in-depth interviews. Although the sample size was not ideal and is certainly on the lower end of what is expected for a grounded theory study, I drew the study to a close. I cannot be certain, but I do not believe theoretical saturation was perfectly achieved for every single category in this study. I suspect that I will continue to refine and develop the resulting grounded theory as I complete additional studies in the future.

I learned several important lessons from this experience. First, things will not always go as planned. In fact, in grounded theory research, we want to remain open to whatever might come up in the research process. Second, we cannot always answer all of our research questions in one study. In grounded theory, our research questions will change as the study progresses. Third, we will make mistakes as researchers. If these mistakes are recognized while the study is ongoing, we can sometimes work to rectify them. In this case, I realized after the fact that I could have reached out to participants from other areas of Appalachia that I had not considered. I later met someone at a conference who said that she would have participated via Skype if I had not been able to travel to her remote location. Although I much prefer face-to-face interviews, I have started to consider other platforms. These could broaden my work into other areas of the country and even internationally. Finally, having only lived in the area for a couple of years, I did not take into account the cultural factors present in Appalachia and the importance of laying the groundwork for this type of research. In Appalachian culture, there is a spirit of independence and loyalty to family (Messer, 2007) that may result in individuals avoiding discussion of personal or family problems with "outsiders." It may take months or even years to build relationships with stakeholders and to make connections with individuals who want to share their stories.

Member Checks

Member checking involves sending tentative findings to participants for feedback. This may occur at any point during data collection and analysis, and sometimes at multiple points. Although it can be used to validate findings (Birks & Mills, 2011), member checking may also provide useful information to researchers. Although he did not use the specific term, Melendez (2008) obtained "participant feedback from key informants regarding perspectives and themes emergent in the data" (p. 430). Melendez explained that this feedback was incorporated to minimize his own influence and to facilitate a focus on the participants.

In my first study on sexual identity, I sent participants their page-long participant descriptions, a summary of the grounded theory, and a draft of the entire report. As a result, I was alerted to two minor errors in the participant descriptions, and several participants shared that they experienced aspects of the conflict resolution process that they did not originally mention during their interviews. For instance, although they did not indicate humor as a personal factor during the initial interview, several identified it after reading the full report. Member checking is an important way to clarify details, gain further insight, and—in some cases—collect new data.

Grounded Theory Research and Social Justice

Advocating for social justice is an integral part of the social work profession and my life. As a social worker and researcher, my conceptualizations of social justice are primarily shaped by two texts. First, the National Association of Social Workers' (2008) *Code of Ethics* instructs social workers to challenge social injustice and explains that "social workers pursue social change, particularly with and on behalf of vulnerable and oppressed individuals and groups of people" (Ethical Principles section, para. 3). Second, in John Rawls' (1999) seminal text *A Theory of Justice*, he defines social justice as "the basic structure of society, or more exactly, the way in which the major social institutions distribute fundamental rights and duties and determine the division of advantages from social cooperation" (p. 6). Among other things, Rawls outlines a thought experiment that can assist with determining what is just. He encourages people to consider what might be just in a hypothetical society in which they do not know their eventual position; in other words, what societal rules would we endorse if we did not know our race, ethnicity, socioeconomic status, sexual identity, gender identity, and so forth? (Rawls, 1999).

As a social work researcher, I hope my research will make a difference in the lives of participants, their communities, and greater society. As a grounded theorist, I hope to critically examine social inequality and discover ways to promote social justice. Toward this end, I have presented information on culturally competent practice with LGBTQ clients to social work students and practitioners, some of whom were never exposed to this information in their previous education and training. I have also led discussions with faith-based practitioners who were struggling with their personal and professional values related to this topic. My goal in all my publications and presentations is to promote respect, understanding, and equality for LGBTQ individuals.

Denzin and Giardina (2009), in their book on social justice and qualitative research, explain that they "seek forms of qualitative inquiry that make a difference in everyday lives by promoting human dignity and social justice" (p. 13). Focused specifically on grounded theory, Charmaz (2013) describes research that promotes equality, access, human rights, and justice. Charmaz explains that social justice inquiry should not only study instances of social injustice, but should also critically examine the social structures that create that injustice. In grounded theory research, theories emerge that are grounded in the data. Thus, it is a natural fit for researchers who are attempting to critically analyze social inequality and discover new ideas (Charmaz, 2013).

It is important to note that grounded theory methodology is often influenced and changed when used in research focused on social justice. For instance, justice-related grounded theories often assume that a group of people have been marginalized and disenfranchised, or that there is some type of injustice present. In these situations, grounded theorists should take special care to attend to reflexivity and power during the study, involve participants and stakeholders in every step of the research, and disseminate results with advocacy and positionality in mind. The goal of the research is not only to generate a justice-related grounded theory, but also to promote social justice throughout the study.

Naturally, my own grounded theory methodology has been informed and affected by my social justice work. From identifying research questions at the very beginning to generating grounded theories near the end, the study is intended to further social justice. For instance, my grounded theory studies have been affected by my ally status and by my belief that faith groups often marginalize LGBTQ individuals. My justice orientation and framework lead me to ask research questions about how LGBTQ individuals resolve faith conflicts, to frequently highlight participants' own words by using in vivo coding, to generate theories that promote equality, and to advocate for understanding and change.

Similarly, Melendez's (2008) study of African-American football players' experiences was affected by the focus on social justice. In fact, this research was part of a larger study that sought to understand the experiences of several different underrepresented groups at the predominately white university (Melendez, 2008). Incorporating a social justice approach, Melendez's suggested implications expand the study's results to highlight the importance of, and need for, educational and emotional support for underrepresented groups in a university setting. This is one of many examples of how social justice affects grounded theory studies. Using additional illustrations from my research and the grounded theory literature, I now provide additional information about how social justice influences grounded theory methodology.

Reflexivity as the Researcher

Glaser and other first-generation grounded theorists tended to disregard reflexivity and believed that participant data could be collected objectively (Birks & Mills, 2011). Contemporary and constructivist grounded theorists, especially those who are studying justice-related topics, acknowledge the impact of the researcher–participant relationship and attend to reflexivity and power (Birks & Mills, 2011). Memo writing is especially useful in this endeavor, and Le Gallais (2008) suggests writing a short autobiography. In both of my studies, I wrote a subjectivity statement in the beginning phases of the study, and then revisited this topic in memos. In my initial statement, I examined my own identity, and I wrote about my experiences of privilege and of discrimination. Reviewing this information throughout the study was important because I found that my beliefs and ideas were shaped by the stories I heard in the interviews. When I found myself making assumptions about certain Christian denominations that I perceived as fundamentalist and exclusionary, I wrote memos to examine and challenge my biases.

Excerpts from a Sample Subjectivity Statement*

Growing up in the southeastern United States, I was surrounded by individuals who believed that being a gay was a choice and a sin. These beliefs were often tied to religious convictions and church affiliations. At the same time, I had multiple friends who were Christian, gay, and afraid to disclose their sexual orientation. When these friends did come out, there were devastating consequences. They experienced rejection from many people, including family members, friends, and people at their churches. My concern for these friends and my horror at discrimination in the name of religion grew into a desire to understand their unique situations.

As a child, I was raised in the Catholic Church with a Catholic mother and an Episcopal father. Although I was born and lived in the primarily Catholic state of Louisiana, we moved to Georgia when I was 10 years old. During adolescence, my religious beliefs transformed to become more like the Southern Baptist and Pentecostal beliefs of my friends in Georgia. I was very involved in church, and religion was woven into every aspect of my life.

I continued to be involved in a religious organization in college, and spent a year volunteering for a Christian group after I graduated. That year was a time of personal growth in which I reflected upon and sincerely questioned my religious beliefs, something I had never done before. This questioning was due, in part, to my discontentment with the social and political beliefs promoted by Christianity, including my church's stance on homosexuality. During this time I not only examined my church's stance on social issues, but I also began to question my belief in a higher power. I sought answers through personal reflection, talking to friends and spiritual leaders, reading books, and learning about other worldviews.

Ultimately, I emerged from this experience believing in an interconnectedness of all beings without aligning myself with any one religion. I identify with concepts that are common to many religions, including peace, social justice, goodwill, and human rights. Today I continue to ponder my spiritual journey, making time to learn about new ideas and ways of knowing.

*Taken and modified from Levy (2008, pp. 100–102).

Participants and Stakeholders

Qualitative researchers can promote social justice and human rights simply by treating participants respectfully and informing them about the purpose of the study (Erickson, 2010). In grounded theory, many researchers involve participants in all aspects of the study; this is especially important when working with populations who have been marginalized and overstudied. Rather than viewing participants as different, objects, or others, researchers can partner with participants to co-construct the study (Krumer-Nevo, 2012). In constructivist grounded theory, researchers do just that. They not only involve participants, but they also invite participants to contribute as co-researchers (Charmaz, 2013).

When talking with stakeholders or participants, it is vital to disclose the study's purpose and your position as the researcher. Because many LGBTQ people have been deeply hurt by religious individuals, it is important for me to explain that I am an ally and an advocate. This is especially true when groups such as NARTH (The National Association of Research & Therapy of Homosexuality) continue to use "research" to marginalize this population and support reorientation therapy. One participant in my sexuality study was taken by her parents to a convention founded on NARTH's ideas, and this experience was emotionally devastating. For her and for others, it was important to know that they were participating in a study conducted by an ally and advocate who affirms their LGBTQ identity.

Reorientation therapy, also called *reparative* or *conversion therapy*, is designed to "change" one's sexual orientation to heterosexual. It has been condemned as ineffective, unethical, and harmful by all major counseling organizations (Blackwell, 2008; Jenkins & Johnston, 2004). This type of individual or group therapy has used aversion conditioning (using shock treatment and medications), promotion of celibacy, analysis and blame for what "caused" same-sex attractions, and attempts to stimulate arousal from heterosexual images or videos (Blackwell, 2008).

Participants and stakeholders should be involved in all aspects of the study. For instance, as I started preparing for my studies, I met with stakeholders and those who were part of the population being investigated to discuss my ideas and obtain feedback. These meetings were integral to many of the research decisions I made. Initially, I was focused too broadly on the LGBTQ population as a whole, not considering the specific experiences of subgroups. After consultation, I realized that the transgender population, for instance, was unique in that most churches did not address this population in their policies and there was less information and knowledge on gender identity among people of faith. This information proved helpful in developing participant criteria for each study.

Data Collection and Analysis

There is a power differential assumed in the researcher–participant relationship. Researchers often decide what questions to ask, how to ask them, when to ask them, and who to ask. Because of this differential, grounded theorists make efforts to equalize relationships. During interviews or focus groups, researchers may need to attend to the "dynamics of power and professional status, gender, race, and age" (Charmaz, 2006, p. 27). In promoting equal exchange and establishing reciprocity (Birks & Mills, 2011), seek assistance from participants in forming interview protocols, research questions, and the grounded theories themselves. Not only does the equal exchange of information promote comprehensive data collection and analysis, but it can also give voice to marginalized and overstudied populations who have not historically played a part in the research process (Levy, 2013). I found it helpful to set a reciprocal tone early in my interaction with participants, explaining how important their voices were. I closed interviews by asking for feedback about the study and the interview process. Although most participants did not have any feedback, one individual from the gender study suggested recruiting additional participants by contacting a support group that was helpful to her.

In addition to providing information about the purpose of the study, researchers should take time to discuss the study with participants, answering any questions individuals have about their participation or about the study in general. It is also important to explain how confidentiality will be protected. For participants to be comfortable, I defer to their preferences for the interview location as long as it is a private or quiet space. Although some opt to come to my office, many prefer the privacy, safety, and comfort of their homes or offices.

During the interview, participants may become emotional when sharing their experiences. When this happens, I invite participants to take a break or end the interview if needed. I always have a list of trusted counselors in the area in case additional processing is needed after the interview concludes. In fact, many IRBs will encourage or require researchers to provide a resource list to participants as part of the process of obtaining approval for the study. Regardless, researchers studying injustice and discrimination should be aware of the impact it may have on participants to discuss their experiences, and participants' health should be the foremost concern.

Because analysis occurs simultaneously with data collection, it is often difficult to know when to begin consulting with participants regarding the emerging analysis. Researchers may elect to provide participants with copies of their interview transcripts for feedback (Bryant & Charmaz, 2007). As analysis progresses, I suggest providing some tentative results to participants once a theory begins to emerge, and allowing plenty of time for feedback before finalizing the results. Member checking, as described previously, can be used throughout analysis to involve participants in the process and in the development of the grounded theory.

Dissemination

According to Erickson (2010), qualitative research combats stereotypes, promotes human rights, and "affirms human dignity by seeking and telling the truth about what particular people do in their everyday lives and about what their actions mean to them" (p. 113). In other words, simply disseminating the results of our studies can be considered advocacy. We have the unique responsibility to honor participants through the retelling of their stories!

In dissemination, it is important to present the experiences of participants as fully and completely as possible, resisting the urge to oversimplify (Kruger-Nevo, 2012). Researchers might do this by writing in a more narrative style, including dialogue with participants and incorporating reflectivity into both the study and the write-up (Kruger-Nevo, 2012). For instance, Melendez (2008) included both the participants' own words as well as his perspective as the researcher in his final write-up, allowing for a balanced presentation of findings. In discussing the pressure to "sell out," Melendez explains that the players defined this as "giving up one's cultural values and beliefs and, in turn, accepting those of the majority culture" (p. 434). Melendez suggests that judgment and pressure to sell out along with the recent firing of the only African-American coach has led to an environment of mistrust.

Similar to disclosing researcher positionality when talking with participants and stakeholders, researchers should provide contextual information when disseminating findings. In constructivist grounded theory, the context of the study is an essential aspect of the results. This includes people and populations involved, time, place, space, culture, and other factors. For instance, I provide nonidentifying demographic information about participants as well as contextual information about the location in which the research took place. In my studies, the context (southeastern, Bible Belt region of the United States, and some in the Appalachian region) is particularly important in understanding how religion permeated all aspects of participants' lives.

Identifying power and positionality and promoting equality is vital in social justice–related research with marginalized populations. Melendez (2008) disclosed his identity as a male graduate student who had been a student-athlete; because his study focused on experiences of male student-athletes, his identification with this group is essential. Melendez notes several times throughout his article that he tried to eliminate any biases in the study by using process and content memos, obtaining feedback from participants, using more than one researcher to code transcripts, and collecting data from several different sources. Conversely, as a constructivist grounded theorist, I acknowledge that my subjectivity will be present in my research despite such efforts. As such, I begin presentations and publications of my research with information on my interest in the topic and my identity as a straight, cisgender ally. I have also troubled the notion of the insider/outsider researcher and suggested strategies, including some of those mentioned in this chapter, for those who consider themselves to be mostly outsiders to their population or topic of study (Levy, 2013).

Researchers have historically considered themselves to be either insiders or outsiders, based on their affiliations with the populations they study. Although insiders may be considered more trustworthy by participants, they are at risk for making assumptions about participants' experiences. In Levy (2013), I suggest that the insider/outsider dichotomy is overly simplistic and does not take into account the fluid and complex experiences of researchers and participants.

Because grounded theories may have wide implications, it is important for researchers to present their findings in a variety of settings. For instance, I have presented or published my research through several venues: national academic conferences (social work, sociology, and interdisciplinary), academic journals (social work, religion, and interdisciplinary), national and state conferences for practitioners (social workers and therapists), journals for practitioners (social workers and faith workers), regional PRIDE festivals, and local human service agencies. In these arenas, I try to connect participants' experiences with continued inequalities, and offer suggestions for advocacy.

As researchers, we are sometimes welcomed into spaces that might not be open to others. Several years ago, I presented my research at a conference for social work practitioners who are Christians, including people who held a wide range of beliefs about sexual orientation. I enjoyed leading what proved to be a very thoughtful discussion of social work practice with LGBTQ individuals. After the session ended, one attendee explained that he enjoyed the discussion and was struggling with the topic given his very conservative, Christian upbringing. He thanked me and said that he likely would not have been as open to hear the same information from someone who is LGBTQ.

Unfortunately, our research is not always welcomed. I once had an abstract accepted by a national Christian magazine only to be told that the full article, once completed, did not fit with the magazine's purpose. Even more disturbing, I recently attended a faith-based conference where the keynote speaker said how glad she was to be with a group of like-minded people, explaining that she had previously been reprimanded for saying that "God made Adam and Eve, not Adam and Steve" when speaking to a public school group. Most of the crowd started clapping and cheering; I walked out. Then, at the same conference, as I prepared my poster, someone moved my easel to the corner of the room and turned it around so that the title (based on my research) could not be read. These experiences remind me of the need for research that challenges social injustice.

Conclusions

Although Charmaz's constructivist grounded theory fits well with justice-oriented topics, researchers can also consider modifying Strauss and Corbin's pragmatic approach or Glaser's classical method. Across these traditions, there are several essential concepts to grounded theory, including simultaneous data collection and analysis, constant comparison, theoretical sampling, in-depth interviews, memo writing, hierarchical coding, identification of a core category, discovery of a theory that is grounded in the data, and member checks.

Grounded theory researchers have the opportunity to "play a vital role in producing new knowledge that provides a cultural context for social science theories with respect to diverse populations" (Bryant & Charmaz, 2007, p. 473). Those who study justice-related topics using grounded theory have the responsibility to involve participants and stakeholders in all aspects of the study and use their research to advocate for social justice. Through our research, we can make a difference in the lives of our participants, in our communities, and in society as a whole.

Like Mark, who opened our chapter, all of the participants in my studies deserve a safe space where they can freely share their experiences. In his final comment of an interview, Steve explained why a supportive community is so important to him:

> I really appreciate the fact that somebody is even bothering to try and do something like this [research this topic] because it does bother me that I don't feel like there is any place I can go to be comfortable. And I really wish that somebody would do something about that.... I want there to be some understanding where people can look at me and say "You're not some weird freak."

People like Mark, Steve, and the many others I have spoken with deserve to tell their stories and to be understood by counselors and social workers, by faith communities, and by those who judge them. They deserve respect, equality, and justice.

What other populations and groups have stories that need to be heard? What injustices need to be exposed? What societal structures need to be toppled? As you ponder these questions, consider using grounded theory as a way to explore justice-related topics and processes, in your own way and with the help of others, to change the world.

> It is from numberless diverse acts of courage and belief that human history is shaped. Each time a [person] stands up for an ideal, or acts to improve the lot of others, or strikes out against injustice, [that person] sends forth a tiny ripple of hope, and crossing each other from a million different centers of energy and daring, those ripples build a current which can sweep down the mightiest walls of oppression and resistance. —*Robert F. Kennedy*

REFERENCES

Birks, M., & Mills, J. (2011). *Grounded theory: A practical guide.* Thousand Oaks, CA: Sage.

Blackwell, C. W. (2008). Nursing implications in the application of conversion therapies on gay, lesbian, bisexual, and transgender clients. *Issues in Mental Health Nursing, 29,* 651–665.

Bogdan, R. C., & Biklen, S. K. (2007). *Qualitative research for education: An introduction to theories and methods* (5th ed.). New York: Allyn and Bacon.

Bryant, A., & Charmaz, K. (Eds.). (2007). *The Sage handbook of grounded theory.* Thousand Oaks, CA: Sage.

Bryman, A. (2012). *Social research methods* (4th ed.). New York, NY: Oxford University Press.

Charmaz, K. (2006). *Constructing grounded theory: A practical guide through qualitative analysis.* Thousand Oaks, CA: Sage.

Charmaz, K. (2013). Grounded theory methods in social justice research. In N. K. Denzin & Y. S. Lincoln (Eds.), *Strategies of qualitative inquiry* (4th ed.) (pp. 291–336). Thousand Oaks, CA: Sage.

Creswell, J. W. (2013). *Qualitative inquiry and research design: Choosing among five approaches* (3rd ed.). Thousand Oaks, CA: Sage.

Denzin, N. K., & Giardina, M. D. (Eds.). (2009). *Qualitative inquiry and social justice.* Walnut Creek, CA: Left Coast Press.

Dunne, C. (2011). The place of the literature review in grounded theory research. *International Journal of Social Research Methodology, 14*(2), 111–124.

Edwards, K. E., & Jones, S. R. (2009). "Putting my man face on": A grounded theory of college men's gender identity development. *Journal of College Student Development, 50*(2), 210–228.

Erickson, F. (2010). Affirming human dignity in qualitative inquiry: Walking the walk. In M. D. Giardina & N. K. Denzin (Eds.), *Qualitative inquiry and human rights* (pp. 112–122). Walnut Creek, CA: Left Coast Press.

Eyles, C., Leydon, G. M., Lewith, G. T., & Brien, S. (2011). A grounded theory study of homeopathic practitioners' perceptions and experiences of the homeopathic consultation. *Evidence-Based Complementary and Alternative Medicine, 2011,* 1–12.

Eyles, C., Walker, J., & Brien, S. (2009). Homeopathic practitioner's experiences of the homeopathic consultation: A protocol of a grounded theory study. *The Journal of Alternative and Complementary Medicine, 15*(4), 347–352.

Glaser, B. G., & Strauss, A. L. (1967). *The discovery of grounded theory: Strategies for qualitative research.* Chicago, IL: Aldine Publishing Company.

Hall, H., Griffiths, D., & McKenna, L. (2013). From Darwin to constructivism: The evolution of grounded theory. *Nurse Researcher, 20*(3), 17–21.

Hallberg, L. R.-M. (2006). The "core category" of grounded theory: Making constant comparisons. *International Journal of Qualitative Studies on Health and Wellbeing, 1*(3), 141–148.

Jenkins, D., & Johnston, L. B. (2004). Unethical treatment of gay and lesbian people with conversion therapy. *Families in Society: The Journal of Contemporary Social Services, 85*(4), 557–561.

Krumer-Nevo, M. (2012). Research against othering. In N. K. Denzin & M. D. Giardina (Eds.), *Qualitative inquiry and the politics of advocacy* (pp. 185–264). Walnut Creek, CA: Left Coast Press.

Le Gallais, T. (2008). Wherever I go there I am: Reflections on reflexivity and the research stance. *Reflective Practice, 9*(2), 145–155.

Levy, D. L. (2008). Gay, lesbian, and queer individuals with a Christian upbringing: Exploring the process of resolving conflict between sexual identity and religious beliefs. Doctoral dissertation, The University of Georgia, Athens, Georgia. *Dissertation Abstracts International, 69*(08), 282A. (UMI No. AAT 3326661)

Levy, D. L. (2011). The importance of personal and contextual factors in resolving conflict between sexual identity and Christian upbringing. *The Journal of Social Service Research, 38*(1), 56–73.

Levy, D. L. (2013). On the outside looking in? The experience of being a straight, cisgender, qualitative researcher. *Journal of Gay & Lesbian Social Services, 25*(2), 197–209.

Levy, D. L. (2014). Christian doctrine related to sexual orientation: Current climate and future implications. In A. B. Dessel & R. M. Bolen (Eds.), *Conservative Christian beliefs and sexual orientation in social work: Privilege, oppression, and the pursuit of human rights* (pp. 11–42). Alexandria, VA: Council on Social Work Education Press.

Levy, D. L., & Edmiston, A. (2014). Sexual identity, gender identity, and a Christian upbringing: Comparing two studies. *Affilia: Journal of Women and Social Work, 29*(1), 66–77.

Levy, D. L., & Johnson, C. W. (2012). What does the Q mean? Including queer voices in qualitative research. *Qualitative Social Work, 11*(2), 130–140.

Levy, D. L., & Lo, J. R. (2013). Transgender, transsexual, and gender queer individuals with a Christian upbringing: The process of resolving conflict between gender identity and faith. *Journal of Religion & Spirituality in Social Work: Social Thought, 32*(1), 60–83.

Levy, D. L., & Reeves, P. (2011). Resolving identity conflicts: Gay, lesbian, and queer individuals with a Christian upbringing. *Journal of Gay and Lesbian Social Services, 23*(1), 53–68.

Melendez, M. C. (2008). Black football players on a predominantly White college campus: Psychosocial and emotional realities of the Black college athlete experience. *Journal of Black Psychology, 34*, 423–451.

Messer, D. R. (2007). *Ablaze in Appalachia: A social approach to a forgotten culture.* Charleston, SC: BookSurge Publishing.

National Association of Social Workers. (2008). *Code of ethics.* Retrieved from http://www.socialworkers.org/pubs/code/code.asp

Rawls, J. (1999). *A theory of justice* (rev. ed.). Cambridge, MA: Harvard University Press.

Southern Baptist Convention. (1997). *Resolution on moral stewardship and the Disney company.* Retrieved from http://www.sbc.net/resolutions/amResolution.asp?ID=436

Strauss, A., & Corbin, J. (1998). *Basics of qualitative research: Techniques and procedures for developing grounded theory* (2nd ed.). Thousand Oaks, CA: Sage.

Leaning into the Ambiguity of Liberation: Phenomenology for Social Justice

Anneliese A. Singh

Between 8 and 11 years old, my uncle and brother sexually abused me. At the time, I believed that I somehow deserved the abuse. Growing up as a girl-child in India, I was not taught to value my body as my own. In my family, I learned that being female meant I was undervalued. This was reinforced by the patriarchal values of my South Asian family. The status of my uncle and brother was elevated in the family compared to mine. This made it difficult for me to disclose my abuse to my mother.

When I did disclose the abuse to my mother, I was told, "It (childhood sexual abuse [CSA]) happened, so now you have to try to move on and not talk about it, and not think about it." All that mattered was our family privacy. No one could know about the abuse. I had always grown up with a strong South Asian ethnic identity, but I began to question my ethnicity after I was encouraged to be silent about my abuse. My family immigrated to the United States when I was 12 years old. I began learning new values of independence and assertiveness—values that conflicted with the South Asian norms of interdependence and privacy in my family. In the United States, I was shocked to hear people talk openly about family violence. A friend of mine from school shared with me that her father had abused her. Not long after, I saw an after-school television show about CSA. The next day, I went to speak to my high school counselor. I talked about my sexual abuse outside of my family for the first time. I also shared what it felt like to be an immigrant in a strange new land.

—*Satyam*

Satyam's story was not unfamiliar to me. I had been volunteering in a local nonprofit organization that served South Asian immigrant and refugee women who had survived intimate partner violence. I facilitated a weekly support group for these women. My co-leader and I noticed rather quickly that the women did not just talk about intimate partner violence, but also talked extensively about experiencing childhood sexual abuse (CSA) and other types of family violence. The group members also talked about what it was like to be immigrants: to be in a new country, eat different food, and experience U.S.-style racism for the first time in a mostly black-white culture. As a South Asian woman myself, I understood how patriarchal values could stifle our voices. I had witnessed family violence in my community. Growing up in the deep South (southeastern United States), I had also experienced racism that breaks your heart and your spirit. I did not, however, know how to talk about CSA. I looked to the literature, and found nothing that assisted me in helping these women.

Striving to understand the essence of CSA for South Asian women and the resilience strategies that help them cope and/or heal, I also served as an activist for this group. I joined fellow community organizers to challenge the injustice of silence about CSA in our communities. Collectively, we visited religious institutions (e.g., mosques, temples, *gurdwaras*, churches) and community organizations (e.g., domestic violence, child abuse), and we sought to break the silence about CSA in our South Asian community. As a scholar/activist/counselor, I knew that one of the major components of social justice for South Asian women who are survivors of CSA was having the access to the empowerment and support services they needed to heal. Social justice also meant that these survivors experienced the validation and witnessing of their stories, knowing that the CSA they experienced was not their fault.

Phenomenology helps me works towards social justice in my research; it demands that I continually strive to identify the essence and meaning of phenomena under study (Moustakas, 1994). Phenomenological studies examine the depth of a phenomenon, as opposed to its breadth. In seeking a deeper level of understanding of South Asian women's experiences of CSA and resilience, social justice and empowerment become real possibilities because their voices can then guide healing interventions and CSA prevention strategies. As a researcher, once I have sought the phenomenological depth of a social justice issue, I am forever changed. For participants from historically marginalized groups, the time and attention that phenomenology requires often provide the first space to tell their story in depth. It may also be the first time they have been valued for telling it.

The search for the core meaning and understanding of a phenomenon is what makes phenomenological research distinct. Phenomenological researchers tend not to be concerned with goals that are important to other research methods, such as saturation of data or theory building (Hays & Singh, 2012). Rather, phenomenologists delve into the essence of what a phenomenon is to describe it to others. I commonly use prolonged engagement with individuals and communities to seek such depth in understanding. For instance, with South Asian women who are survivors of CSA, I spent a good deal of time in South Asian community centers and religious institutions, and other places women gathered to understand the context of their lives. Moreover, I endeavored to interview participants multiple times so that I gained the depth and meaning that the phenomena of CSA and resilience had in South Asian women's lives rather than a surface-level understanding.

In this chapter, I share examples from my phenomenological research with South Asian women survivors about their experiences of CSA and resilience. Along the way, I review the historical and disciplinary roots of phenomenology, discuss the social justice implications of phenomenology, and describe phenomenological approaches to data collection and data analysis I have used in my work. I also review considerations involved in phenomenology when working with historically marginalized people/communities in situations where the researchers hold social justice as both a process and an end goal. Throughout the chapter, I seek to illustrate how phenomenology helps researchers and participants lean into the ambiguity of liberation and social justice.

Historical and Disciplinary Roots

Phenomenology as a word has its origins in the Greek root of *phainomenon*, which translates as "appearance" (*Stanford Encyclopedia of Philosophy*, 2008). The word "phenomenology" also refers to the constructs or structures of consciousness (Moustakas, 1994; Patton, 2002). The roots of phenomenology are grounded in philosophy (Moustakas, 1994). The German philosopher Immanuel Kant proposed ideas that became the early foundations of phenomenology (Rockmore, 2011), articulating a division between phenomena or objects that humans could seek to understand through direct experience and objects that humans could not experience directly.

However, it was Husserl ([1913] 1931), a German philosopher, who furthered the tenets of phenomenology. Husserl asserted that phenomenology was a philosophy of living and consciousness. From

Husserl's perspective, phenomenology refers to what we may discover through our own reflection. Husserl used the word *lebenswelt*—life-world—to describe phenomenology's core recognition that as humans we perceive objects in the world simultaneously with our own experiences (e.g., of the body, of our relationships).

To understand the importance of these assertions, one should understand the political context in which Husserl's phenomenology emerged. After the massive turmoil and destruction of World War I, science as a discipline in Western Europe was reduced either to simple positivism or a subjectivism without an articulated foundation (Eagleton, 1983). As a result, Husserl was reacting against the positivist notion that objects existed independently from one another in the external world and that information about these objects was reliable (Groenewald, 2004). Instead, he argued that the certainty of understanding an object or phenomenon comes to a person only through one's own consciousness; therefore, to understand or know this object, one must exclude experiences outside of this personal consciousness (Groenewald, 2004).

From Husserl's ([1913] 1931) perspective, intentionality was a large component of phenomenology, in which structures of experiences such as imagination, memory, thought, and bodily awareness are interrogated. The emphasis is on the structure of the experience in first person. The "noema," Husserl's term for the core of an experience's meaning, is also included (*Stanford Encyclopedia of Philosophy*, 2008). Heidegger ([1927] 1962) expanded Husserl's ([1913] 1931) conceptualization of phenomenology, designating an "unfolding, breaking apart, and, ideally, revealing what is concealed about this, or any other, phenomenon" (Ziemba, 2007). Heidegger used the word *dasein*—meaning existence—to denote the temporality of phenomenology ([1927] 1962).

Thus, in the practice of phenomenological research, there are two major approaches resulting from Husserl's and Heidegger's philosophies (Vagle, 2013). The first is *descriptive phenomenology*, which draws from Husserl's philosophy. In this approach, the researcher explores the meaning of a phenomenon and describes this meaning to others (Vagle, 2013). Moustakas (1994) is an often-cited descriptive phenomenologist who developed transcendental phenomenology, which recognizes that our perception is a leading knowledge source through which the experience of a phenomenon is described. The second approach is *interpretive phenomenology*, which draws heavily from Heidegger. Whereas Husserl conceived of phenomenology as a whole philosophy unto itself, Heidegger described phenomenology as an ontology. From this perspective, researchers seek to interpret the meaning of a phenomenon, and they acknowledge that this process ultimately provides meaning to the phenomenon as well (Vagle, 2013). van Manen's (1997) work is a prime example of interpretive phenomenology. This is evidenced by his assertions that phenomenologist researchers must name their assumptions about a phenomenon to reduce their impact on the study's findings.

Other scholars have taken up phenomenology slightly differently, but always within an interpretive theoretical framework, or a way of not only describing a phenomenon, but also moving into a description of the meaning of a phenomenon (Denzin & Lincoln, 2011). There are several other scholars who have contributed to phenomenology, both as a philosophy (e.g., Merleau-Ponty, Sartre) and as a research tradition (e.g., Polkinghorne, 1989; Rossman & Rallis, 1998; Vagle, 2013)

Vagle (2010a) asserts the importance of identifying a phenomenon in its complexity of contexts. One can understand a phenomenon, he asserts, only if one considers the multiple, partial, and varied ways of understanding this same phenomenon. Embedded in this understanding is a recognition that one might not know exactly the phenomenon of investigation at the beginning of the research process; therefore, the researcher should remain open to the multiple, partial, and varied contexts influencing participants' experience of the phenomenon. In my phenomenological studies, for instance, the context of a phenomenon (e.g., South Asian, North American) is as important as an individual's description of CSA and resilience. From a social justice perspective, phenomenology provides a nice match as advocates endeavor to maintain awareness of our socialization and related stereotypes about various individuals and communities.

Strategies of Data Collection and Data Analysis

Because phenomenology invites researchers to dive into the deepest waters in understanding a phenomenon, we are able to unearth information that can be used to advocate for social justice. When I first began studying CSA among women in South Asian communities, the consensus of my colleagues was that I would not find participants willing to speak about their experiences. My colleagues' assumptions were indeed on target: women were hesitant to speak about their experiences for fear of further abuse or giving their families "a bad name." However, once I identified participants and earned their trust,

I found that CSA survivors were willing to share far more about their experiences than I anticipated. These women CSA survivors experienced a sense of justice and empowerment sharing their stories, and as a researcher, I was their witness. Listening carefully and respecting their voices, their interview data have given me a sense of what their resilience and healing "looks like" in the South Asian context. Understanding the essence and meaning of these phenomena prepared me to advocate for culturally responsive mental health resources for survivors of CSA. As a social justice-oriented phenomenological researcher, I recognize that I have power. Because I am committed to interrogating this power, I endeavor to have a process of accountability in terms of what I do and say about participant data. I also believe socially just research must acknowledge the cultural context to richly capture the essence and meaning phenomenology demands.

Bridling and Bracketing Researcher Assumptions

Regardless of context, every phenomenological study has a starting point, which is typically documenting one's subjectivity by bracketing and/or bridling (Singh, Garnett, & Williams, 2013). I have found bracketing/bridling helps me name my own socialization and stereotyping to learn more about other people and the complexity of my world. Without it, I might not question the very nature of my own assumptions and thus would struggle to understand the experience of others. In phenomenological research, bracketing/bridling is a strategy placed at the forefront of the research process and attended to in an ongoing basis. *Bracketing* (as Husserl [(1913)1931] named this epoché) involves researchers noting their assumptions and biases about a phenomenon before commencing research activities (Polkinghorne, 1996). The process of bracketing provides researchers with multiple opportunities to name and "keep an eye on" their assumptions, biases, and relationships with a phenomenon. Bracketing is— depending on the discipline—often viewed as a marker or indication of rigor in phenomenological studies. Chan, Fung, and Chien (2013) assert that phenomenologists should document their bracketing process using a reflexive journal, wherein the researcher regularly writes about research activities and her or his related thoughts and feelings to both challenge and interrogate them. As a result, the bracketing/ reflexive journal becomes a key component of data collection and is useful later in analysis and interpretation.

Bracketing researcher assumptions in these ways can be complicated. Questions such as whether one has bracketed "enough" inevitably arise, as well as how to handle the bracketing process as a data source. I believe there are two core components of bracketing that should be included in phenomenological research: describing the researcher assumptions at the beginning of a research study and noting how interview questions or other data processes are recursively shifted based on ongoing documentation of these biases. The following excerpt is from the reflexive journal I kept at the beginning of a phenomenological study exploring the resilience of South Asian immigrant survivors of CSA. This reflexive journal helped me continuously document and interrogate my values, biases, and assumptions about South Asian women, as well as those ideas I had about resilience and child sexual abuse:

> I visited a mosque today with some dear friends. We attended service and then were part of a health education fair where we handed out information on CSA. As I spoke with mothers, fathers, grandparents, and the Imam [Muslim religious leader], it was obvious to me that the community is still hurting from post-9/11 Islamophobia. I know how much the racism post-9/11 hurt my Sikh community, and it is SO intense to see the pain that is still in this community two years after 9/11. I realized today that even though I am keeping this journal and exploring my positionality as a researcher, there are so many things I will not be able to anticipate in this study of CSA. Today, I am reminded that one of these unanticipated factors is intergenerational trauma—and not just in families. Intergenerational trauma that derives from a larger, systemic, political context is what I am talking about. Today, I couldn't talk about CSA with Muslim community members without talking about 9/11. I was surprised by this—and then stumbled over my words at times. I learned that I will need to be open (and want to be open) in the research process to explore how a larger political context and historical events of oppression (maybe even colonization?) influenced families. This brings me back to how the British colonization and partition of India affected my own family—and how my Indian family members don't want to talk about family violence, and sometimes don't want to even talk about their experiences of partition growing up. If political and individual trauma is connected—and if it is intergenerational—then I myself will need to be mindful of the places I listen to carefully or tune out as I hear stories of trauma so I create as much space as possible for women survivors of CSA to tell their own stories in the way they need to tell them—not in the way I may want them to tell them. There won't be a lot of stories with fairytale endings for sure. Resilience and healing for these women may be like the colonization/ partition of India and post-9/11 racism. Messy, brutal, full of contradictions, and ultimately with pockets of hope. Maybe.

To further clarify how bracketing can be used in the phenomeno-logical research process, Vagle (2009) and Dahlberg (2006) explore the concept of *bridling*. Bridling is a form of bracketing that not only details researcher assumptions, values, and biases about a topic, but also develops an attitude of availability (Dahlberg, Drew, & Nystrom, 2008). This attitude of availability refers to the intentional openness of the researcher in seeking to describe a phenomenon. In the South Asian study, we bracketed our research team's assumptions about South Asian women, CSA, resilience, and healing to keep an eye on how these assumptions influenced our data analysis and interpreta-tion. Bridling was the next step we took as a team to nurture an atti-tude of availability. In this manner, we remained open to participants describing the phenomena of CSA and resilience as different, similar, or neither when examined in relation to our own researcher assump-tions. We maintained this form of bracketing/bridling throughout re-search activities so we could more closely interrogate our researcher assumptions as we sought to describe the meaning and essence of CSA and resilience for South Asian women survivors.

Vagle (2009) describes four stages of the phenomenological re-search process where bridling could be used. In the first step, he sug-gests the use of a research team. Vagle asserts that each additional team member offers "more to bridle [but] also means bringing more opportunities for us [as researchers] to bridle for and with one an-other" (2009, p. 355). In my South Asian study, our research team discussed our diverse perspectives and assumptions about the study topic. We made space to ensure we valued all of the perspectives and experiences of social justice and injustice that we brought to the re-search process. For instance, both South Asian and white women served on the research team who were able to explore how racism was experienced, witnessed, and/or enforced in the researchers' lives. These explorations allowed us to identify collectively how patriarchy influenced our lives across contexts and seek to understand how patriarchy did and did not influence the lives of participants ground-ed in the data. The second component of bridling is endeavoring to remain to true to the nature of phenomenological research, which is the description of a phenomenon and the relationship of the re-searcher to the phenomenon. In this component, tact is referred to as the patience involved in waiting and maintaining mindfulness of how researcher assumptions are affecting the description of a phe-nomenon (van Manen, 1991). In the South Asian study, this step en-tailed a deliberate discussion about the phenomenon of resilience and being mindful of the specific ways our assumptions were shaping both data collection and analysis.

The third step of bridling involves ongoing learning about phenomenology. Although this seems like a simple step, Vagle (2009) emphasizes that people come to phenomenology with different understandings, and therefore part of the rigor in the process is about expanding the boundaries of one's knowings about phenomenology as these influence the data-collection process. In our research team, the second author and I had significant understandings and experience of using phenomenology, whereas the rest of the team members did not. Therefore, we continually checked in with one another about whether we were staying true to the nature and goals of phenomenology, as well as expanding our previously held notions of what phenomenology "looks like" in practice. Finally, Vagle discusses holding the question of "Am [I] doing this right?" (2009, p. 361) to ensure bridling is an ongoing and critical part of the research process.

A brief snapshot of our process for this step is included below. This excerpt shows how phenomenology can create conversations related to social justice into the bracketing and bridling process:

Anneliese: Ok: we have 10 questions on our interview protocol. What is missing and how might we be leading with our assumptions about what resilience "looks like" for South Asian women survivors of CSA?

Sonali: We definitely have a bias in this one question that families don't support survivors. We need to rewrite that one.

Anneliese: I agree, and I have another question: Are we remaining true to phenomenology, or are we veering into other territory with our protocol? Are we seeking to describe the meaning these resilience strategies have for the women, or the ones that we feel most comfortable with? We may hear stories that don't fit with what our ideas of resilience are.

Sonali: Interesting point. I think we are mostly on track. The main challenge is going to come when we code the women's data. How are we going to ensure we are bridling our assumptions throughout the entire research process?

Anneliese: Good question! We should maintain our reflexive journals regularly. Let's journal before and after each interview we conduct, and then after our research meetings. We can include our reflexive journals as data sources themselves. That way we can talk about these journals and our assumptions along the way.

Ultimately, we heard stories of resilience that we would not have characterized as such! For example, participants talked about how they used their silence about CSA as a resilience strategy. One participant said:

> I think silence about my abuse has been a good thing because that's what helped me get through a lot of the hardship. I could make my world silent, and I could retreat…things made more sense or were bearable. This next half of my life is about breaking out of that silence, but choosing to do so, not having people telling me to do that. It has to come from myself.

If we had not kept a close eye on our assumptions, we would have missed a rich description of this resilience strategy.

For many scholars, the goals of phenomenological research from a social justice perspective might seem admirable; however, many critiques indicate it is unrealistic or undesirable to suspend judgment as the research process commences. Vagle (2009, 2010b) endorses some of these impossibilities and draws closer into the phenomenological research process with some guiding tenets of questioning, challenging, and interrogating researcher assumptions throughout the research process. As with any qualitative design, critics might note the subjectivity of phenomenological research and question the extent to which participants are able to describe the meaning making or multiple essences of a phenomenon. For the numerous tensions encountered in phenomenological research, I believe social justice as a framework gifts the researcher with the necessary critical questions to maintain the rigor of it being more than enough. Here, I note a few of the social justice-related questions we used in our study to guide us through the tensions of bracketing/bridling:

- Who benefits from the research?
- What are the findings that I might not be delving into because they represent challenges to society?
- How are my assumptions clouding what I can see about the meaning making of participants?
- Do I have enough data to draw social justice considerations and implications, such as information for experiences of societal oppression, recommendations for policy change, and challenging the invisibility of historically marginalized people and communities?

Most important, when we asked these types of questions, we embraced and leaned into our subjectivities and those of the participants. We sought to be mindful that bracketing and bridling are not one-time events, but should be continuously examined and uprooted in data analysis interpretation. How others document this bracketing and bridling reflects the trustworthiness of the study (Hays & Singh, 2012). Now that I have stressed the importance of bracketing and bridling, I'll discuss the methods of phenomenological data collection.

Entering the Phenomenological Field

When entering the phenomenological field, Vagle (2010b) suggests devising an overall process to collect data to illuminate a phenomenon. Vagle again draws on Dahlberg's (2006) ideas of phenomenologists relying minimally on the methods of phenomenological designs, but focusing on remaining open about the decisions that are required by a phenomenological approach. *Postintentionality* entails using the data sources called for to describe the multiplicities of a phenomenon (e.g., numbers, fiction writing) as opposed to solely relying on more traditional data collection methods such as interviews.

Staying close to the goal of phenomenology while remaining open to the essence and meaning of the phenomena of CSA and resilience for South Asian women, we used purposeful sampling to ensure the sample was both diverse and information rich (Hays & Singh, 2012). We believed that sampling decisions are related to issues of social justice and that phenomenology helps target decisions to locate information-rich cases. For this reason, we knew we wanted to interview adult South Asian women who were survivors of CSA and understand not only the phenomenon of their experience of CSA, but also the phenomenon of their resilience and how they healed. We also knew from a review of the trauma literature that memories of CSA can be unstable before the age of five years old, as the memories are often bodily memories difficult to describe verbally. Setting our purposeful sampling criteria helped make sure our participants would have thick descriptions of the phenomenon. I also used a maximum-variation purposeful sampling approach because I was interested in understanding the essence of resilience for South Asian women CSA survivors from a wide variety of backgrounds (e.g., religion, country of origin).

I was not dedicated to setting a predetermined number of participants in this study, but I do believe it is important to be prepared to thoughtfully explain your sampling strategy. Especially with hidden or historically marginalized groups, researchers may struggle with identifying participants willing to participate. No matter what the sample size, phenomenological researchers should not rely on the saturation of data as a standard of when to complete data collection. Instead, phenomenologists should ask themselves how they will know that they have interviewed "enough" participants to gain a rich, in-depth understanding of the essence and meaning of a phenomenon.

Researchers should also continually self-reflect on whether participants have been given the opportunity to share fully about the phenomenon studied. For instance, in the study with South Asian CSA survivors, there were no previous empirical studies of CSA or resilience for this group. Therefore, the invisibility of South Asian women survivors of sexual trauma in the field was an important social justice consideration that drove our decision to sample five participants with an in-depth interviewing protocol. We thought sampling fewer participants and conducting more in-depth interviews (or sometimes repeated interviews) would yield the type of information-rich description of the resilience strategies previously unknown. In this case, we decided to follow the individual interviews with a single focus group. Participants in the focus group told us that sharing their CSA experiences as South Asian women empowered them and facilitated further healing.

When we began this study, we did not know initially that we would sample fewer participants with more depth; rather, we let the participant data guide us to this final decision. Once we had sampled our first participant, it became evident that her story of resilience and healing from CSA could not be told in one or two interviews. We believed our sampling strategy remained true to phenomenology's goal of seeking the meaning of a phenomenon. Therefore, let the phenomenological sampling strategy in terms of "deciding the number" of participants be guided by the data itself. Institutional research boards (IRBs) and dissertations chairs may be nervous about this approach, but in my experience, it is the way to be most true to the goals of phenomenology and social justice.

Data Sources in Phenomenology

Individual interviews and focus groups are the typical methods of data collection in phenomenological research (Bradbury-Jones, Sambrook, & Irvine, 2009; Hays & Singh, 2012). Semistructured interview protocols are a good fit for phenomenological designs to ensure participants' voices are privileged in the data collection process (Hays & Singh, 2012). Ultimately, using a social justice lens, one must acknowledge that the roots of phenomenology are in Western philosophy; therefore, depending on the context and focus of the study and its related social justice implications, phenomenology might need to be adapted to address Eastern philosophical underpinnings. Gathering phenomenological data in India, I found the cultural context demands more of my voice in the data. Participants often interview me about topics of their interest as I am interviewing them. For instance, when I meet with participants, they want to have me in their homes to share afternoon chai. Our interviews began with their questions about me as a researcher, why I came to the research at hand, and also an expectation that I would share my reactions to their description of a phenomenon. Holstein and Gubrium (1995) call these types of interviews *active interviews*, as both the researcher and the participant are co-constructing the meaning of a phenomenon. When engaging in active interviews, the processes of bracketing and bridling are embedded in the development of questions before, during, and after the interview. For instance, when I have used active interviewing, I collaborate with participants prior to an interview and ask what types of questions they believe would allow them to best explore their experiences. During the interview, there is a continual question raised of whether there are other or better questions to seek the meaning of a phenomenon. Then, after the interview, the participants and I have an opportunity collaboratively to identify questions that were not asked—or questions that should have been asked—to illuminate the essence and meaning of a phenomenon.

Because the majority of my phenomenological research is with historically marginalized individuals and communities (Singh, 2012; Singh, Hays, Chung & Watson, 2010; Singh, Hays, & Watson, 2011; Singh, Meng, & Hansen, 2013, 2014), I have often used Seidman's (2006) phenomenological interviewing approach. Seidman's approach to interviewing involves multiple interviews aimed at developing the space participants need to make meaning of their experiences of a phenomenon. Again, it is the in-depth interview protocol that creates a structure necessary for participants to share their experiences of a phenomenon. In my CSA study, I followed Seidman's (2006) suggestion that three interviews are scheduled at least a week apart to facilitate participants' meaning-making process about a phenomenon.

I outline Seidman's interview protocol below, with data examples from the South Asian survivors of CSA study. Each of the three interviews has a different aim, but the overarching goal is to nurture the meaning-making process for participants:

Interview 1: I collected a focused life history regarding a phenomenon for participants. For South Asian women, the aim in the first interview was to gather a life history of the phenomenon of CSA and their resilience. Interview questions centered on the general life events and critical turning points in their experiences of CSA and their resilience across their lives:

Anneliese: What were the major events going on in your family around the time CSA happened to you?

Meera: My family was Muslim and we did *salat* [prayers] regularly. My mom and dad decided to send us to a religious school. It was a school near us and a private school, so my parents thought it was best for my brothers and I to go there. What they didn't know was that my religious teacher would abuse me while I was learning. My brothers were sitting right across the table from me, but they didn't know what was going on. I just remember the blue walls and the paper of the book under my hands while my brothers read out loud and the religious teacher abused me. I hated him, and I hated going to school, but I was too scared to tell my parents. My parents didn't have the best relationship. There was a lot of fighting at home. I felt so isolated and so ashamed. I disconnected from Islam for many years. I disconnected from my body too. Later in life when I came to the U.S., I became more spiritual. Not religious. But in my heart, I am always Muslim, no matter what that religious teacher did to me.

Interview 2: In this interview, I encouraged Meera to reconstruct details of experiencing the phenomena of CSA and resilience. Understanding how and when the CSA occurred allowed the structures of meaning to be drawn out of their experience. The details helped highlight the resilience strategies the women drew upon to heal.

Anneliese: How did you take care of yourself after the abuse?

Meera: Hmmm. Well, at first, I used my imagination a lot. I imagined my brothers would stand up and tell my religious teacher to stop what he was doing. I also imagined telling my parents. I dreamed of what it would be like to go to another school. I ended up telling my parents, my mom first. She didn't believe me, but she could see I was scared. I didn't have to go back to that school again.... Later in life, taking care of myself has meant talking to my brothers, talking to my mom about the abuse. Over the last few years, I have brought more and more up with them. I feel validated by them now, and I didn't realize that I needed their support as much as I did. Turns out my brother was abused too. Talking with him about the abuse, about our mom and dad, about Islam... these things have been healing.

Interview 3: In this interview, I invited Meera to reflect on the meaning CSA and resilience had for her in her life. The focus of this interview was on looking back at the first two interviews to enhance opportunities to describe and understand the essence and meaning that the CSA and resilience had for Meera.

Anneliese: Looking back at the experiences of CSA and resilience that you have had in your life, what meaning do these experiences have for you now?

Meera: That is an easy question! I cherish my self. I cherish my mind. I cherish my body. My body is like a shrine. Taking care of my body...it is so important...my body was connected to my past abuse. I do yoga. I draw from these ancient South Asian practices to heal—meditation, ayurvedic eating—these are my cultural heritage and birthright, and I use them to heal. I have closer friendships. I am a better listener. Obviously I am not saying CSA should have happened. And I am a more spiritual and grounded person now. I have boundaries and accountability in my relationships. I am a survivor, yes. And I truly love myself. And I have a community who reminds me of this when I forget.

One thing to be aware of when using a multiple-interview protocol in phenomenology is that there is not only intensity of knowledge and understanding of phenomena generated (Penny & Kinslow, 2006), but also an ethic of care. In my bracketing journal after the second interview with Meera, I wrote:

> When I left the interview with Meera today, I began to cry. Crying for her experiences and for the South Asian context that I know so well that brings me so much joy, and also so much anguish. My own father saw so much abuse in his own family, but this was only spoken about in whispers in my home. I want to honor my own feelings of grief coming up about a world where CSA does happen, and as Meera said, "It doesn't only happen in white families." I feel deeply privileged to spend time with these women who are truly courageous and breaking multiple silences as they share their experiences of abuse and resilience.

Vagle (2010b) gives permission for researchers to draw techniques from other qualitative approaches (ethnography, evocative inquiry, etc.), as they are required to illuminate the phenomenon. For instance, visual ethnography (e.g., use of photography, diaries, graffiti art) can provide the exact data source necessary to elucidate the core meaning of a phenomenon. This step is particularly well suited for social justice–oriented research, as understanding a social justice–related phenomenon—such as liberation strategies within a community—can extend beyond the boundaries of interviews. A common result of oppression is silencing voices, or distorting words. With the South Asian women I interviewed, they provided in-depth, thick descriptions of the phenomenon of CSA and their resilience strategies for healing. However, we often started or ended our interviews using some sort of media to explore these phenomena nonverbally. Integrating participant-generated media in data collection in this manner can acknowledge the limits that words have and create an opportunity for creative expression. Researchers who blend research techniques will need to ensure these techniques facilitate a depth of understanding of the phenomenon and that phenomenology is still at the core of the research process.

Deepening the Analysis of Phenomenological Data

It is challenging to describe the steps of phenomenological analysis, especially as many early phenomenologists were less inclined to detail linear steps guiding data reduction (Groenewald, 2004). Moustakas (1994) advises analyzing data using horizontalization. We used this approach in the CSA study and started by reading participant statements line by line. Vagle (2010a) similarly urges a reading of and writing through collected data systematically. The beginning of this step requires an overall read-through for general comprehension of a data source, followed by a more detailed subsequent reading of each line (similar to horizontalization) where one writes initial impressions of the data. Remaining questions for follow-up inquiry with participants should also be noted. In Nima's transcript below, I use underlining to denote my horizontalization of the data:

> Reconnecting to the South Asian community [after CSA] really brought me almost to tears, because it made me realize how important it was. See, I was still a member of that community as an individual, and not only that—I still wanted to belong. I needed to reconnect. I could not survive outside of the community.

In this excerpt, you see the nonoverlapping statements about resilience after CSA included her desire to reconnect to South Asian community, the salience and meaning of that reconnection, the individual in context, and the need for connection to the South Asian community as part of survival.

Moustakas (1994) describes the resulting notes (that a researcher might keep in the margin of a transcript) as denoting units of meaning related to the phenomenon. Taking another look at Nima's transcript shows how the researcher can code, tag, or label the data into units of meaning:

Reconnecting to the South Asian community [after CSA]	Connection to South Asian community is important
really brought me almost to tears, because it made me realize	
how important it was. See, I was still a member of that	Survivor is still a member of community
community as an individual, and not only that - I still	
wanted to belong. I needed to reconnect. I could not	
survive outside of the community.	Connection to South Asian community is part of survival

The third step entails a clustering of these meaning units that shift the process of horizontalization into more discrete subsets of the phenomenon. For this study, Nima's units of meaning noted above were compared with other participant transcripts to denote similarities, contradictions, tensions, and explanations. Some of these clusters across the data included *sense of hope, social support, self-care,* and *self-advocacy.*

In the fourth step, we looked individually and across participants to identify a structural or textural description of a phenomenon. The structural description includes the components of the experiences of a phenomenon, whereas the textural description denotes the setting in which participants experienced a phenomenon. For instance, a structural and textural description of the resilience strategy survivors described in terms of having a "sense of hope" was exemplified by the following participant data:

> My mom and my dad raised me with the belief of the intrinsic power of good in people and the world, which is really what helped me cope and survive [CSA]. That spark of "goodness" kept me alive then…the power of something bigger than me, bigger than the abuse.

At the end of data collection and analysis, we used a summary narrative to capture the entirety of participant data related to the phenomenon of CSA and resilience for South Asian women survivors. Vagle (2010b) denotes this as providing "tentative glimpses" of a phenomenon. This is the opportunity for the researcher to once more lean into the ambiguities, tensions, contradictions, and similarities within the data and draw upon creative analytic practice (Parry & Johnson,

2007; Richardson, 1998) to showcase these elements. We might have used poetry, fiction stories, experimental media, performance, visual images, or other creative analytic practice to highlight these elements as well (Parry & Johnson, 2007). Ultimately, the form that the researcher selects should portray the intensity and richness of the data, staying true to participant voices and culture. The summary narrative of the findings we used in the South Asian women survivors study not only exemplified the core elements within participant data about CSA and resilience, but also more importantly brought the phenomenon alive. Take for example the "composite" case of Pritham:

> Pritham identified South Asian cultural factors as influencing the resilience strategies she ultimately used to heal from CSA. She described not only being silenced about CSA, but also using this very same silence about her abuse enforced by South Asian culture as a place to actively heal. Pritham said that she used her external silence to mask her internal use of imagination and play to heal. She also described using the silence "subversively" as a way to observe her environment and attempt to keep herself away from her perpetrators. Pritham's cultural values carried a belief in people's "innate goodness," and she said that she began healing from CSA when she actively looked at the "good and worth" in herself and other people.
>
> Although Pritham described initially disconnecting herself from her South Asian community to protect herself from further abuse and the cultural values she believed "allowed" her abuse, she joined a South Asian organization at college that helped her in healing. In this organization, Pritham identified reconnecting to a progressive South Asian community, where she could talk about issues that affected her community (e.g., violence, immigration) as a liberating space for her where she could also "claim the good parts about her culture, like relationships." Pritham also described that once she had begun healing from her abuse, she wanted to "give back" to others through social advocacy. She began volunteering with environmental causes in high school and ultimately chose a career in a helping profession.
>
> Pritham shared that intentional self-care was an important resilience strategy for her; once she "began to value her experience and value herself," she also began establishing boundaries in relationships and reading books on abuse. She described this regular self-care as being critical to "taking care of her mind, body, and spirit."

Managing the Depth of Phenomenological Data

One of the surprising results of our sampling was that many participants responded to our study. We wrestled with how many we could interview and still maintain our search to describe the essence and meaning of South Asian women's CSA and resilience experiences. Therefore, we used the following data analysis contact sheet (adapted from Hays & Singh, 2012) to track the information of our sample and specifically document social justice considerations and implications during the research process:

Interviewer: Anneliese, **Interviewee:** Seema

1. What were the main descriptions of the phenomenon in this contact?

Seema described CSA by an uncle. She did not tell anyone about the abuse, as she thought at the time that nobody would believe her. Seema also described an extended family context growing up: her paternal side of the family (two aunts, one uncle) lived in the same home with her family of origin. She described her healing from CSA as using resilience strategies such as developing deep friendships, turning inward and using her imagination, feeling hopeful about the future, and providing *seva* (service) to her community.

2. What tensions, impossibilities, and/or contradictions did you notice in the participant's response?

Seema said that there was no way her mother and father would have known she was sexually abused, but simultaneously described her paternal side of the family "being all in their business." Wonder if the collectivist values of extended family living and relationships have unspoken rules for what you can talk to other family members about and what is off limits. Will follow up with Seema about this after I transcribe the interview.

3. Anything else that stuck out as salient, interesting, or important in this contact?

Seeing the resilience strategy of survivors using silence about CSA—the feeling that they can't or shouldn't talk about what happened to them—as a place of resilience. Seema talked about her uncle threatening her if she told anyone he abused her. He told her that she would never get married and bring shame upon the family if anyone found out about the abuse. Seema deliberately removed herself from situations with these men whenever she could by spending time in her room. She talked about comforting herself with imagining she had a family whom she could talk to and who stood up to her abusers. She talked about other ways she transformed the silence she was made to feel into her own world where she was safe and could begin healing. Still struggling if this is resilience or not and need to talk to research team about this!

4. General comments about how this interviewee's responses compared with other interviewees:

This was the second interview of three with the second participant. Seeing some commonalities about resilience and South Asian context across participants in terms of family response to CSA and nurturing a sense of hope. Differences have been about religion, social class, and who knew about the CSA.

5. What are the specific issues of social justice related to the phenomenon that the participant shared?

Each of the participants so far has described experiencing racism upon coming to the U.S. Some of their reactions (e.g., silence, shame, internalized racism) seem to mirror their CSA and trauma experiences. Definitely want to talk about this in our research team.

Another data analysis tool I have found helpful in phenomenological research is participant displays to track the meaning making of a phenomenon by (and across) participants. In a phenomenological study of the resilience and healing processes of African-American women survivors of CSA, I used individual participant displays to manage data from the ten participants in the study. These individual displays were helpful to identify social justice considerations embedded in data. Specifically, for this sample the experiences and intersection of multiple identities as women of color surviving CSA were pertinent. The case displays also provided a "snapshot" of the data for research team meetings, recursively revising interview questions and/or structural or textural descriptions. Later, as I gathered more participant data, I used cross-displays that contained summaries of the entire data set so the research team could more effectively view our data in its entirety.

Trustworthiness in Phenomenological Research

Issues of trustworthiness have been previously discussed in this text and within this chapter (e.g., bracketing, bridling, reflexive journals, research teams, internal auditor); however, there are some methods of trustworthiness not discussed thus far that I have found most helpful when

Table 4.1 is the first individual participant display from a phenomenological study of the healing processes related to sexuality of African-American women who had survived CSA. We used bold fonts to denote areas of a phenomenon that a participant did not talk about, but other participants had made meaning of, as well as to note areas for potential follow-up questions with participants and to help identify gaps in our interview protocol related to the phenomenon. We could also track important social justice issues (e.g., racism, sexism) influencing the context of their abuse:

TABLE 4.1. Individual Participant Display

Type of CSA	Multiple Identities	Sexuality
(Abuser(s), age of abuse, others abused, setting, did anyone know, frequency, duration, impact on family constellation, other abuses)	(Associated with race/ethnicity, gender, CSA, etc.)	**Short-Term Impacts** · Not described
· Uncle · Mother did not seek retribution when she told her · Family did not discuss it · Abuse occurred in the family home · Cannot remember details just knew it was wrong · Happened until she was 6 · Still has a relationship with her uncle	**Descriptions** · Sex was taboo · Sex is power: being in control · Sex is sexuality · Wants more from me than just sex · Race/ethnicity affects how others view me and how I carry myself publicly · Having her daughter and marriage were protective factors · Silence in family about the abuse · Ethnicity is part of sexuality **Needed to Heal** · Sexuality is my relationship with God: reclaiming religion · Family support · Dealing with racist and sexist stereotypes	**Long-Term Impacts (Empowerment)** · Never discussed it or told anyone else besides mom · Becomes a little uneasy whenever she hears his name mentioned · Realized abuse runs in her family (intergenerational) · Closely monitors her daughters · Sexuality is more a part of her resilience now · Sought out information on trauma survivors and healing

engaging in social justice–related research. Engaging in an external audit of data is also a way I have addressed trustworthiness of phenomenological data collection and analysis (Hays & Singh, 2012). The external auditor reviews the data materials, findings, etc. as an entirety to help note surprises, contradictions, or other gaps in the research process that should be addressed before commencing with publication or presentation. I have sometimes selected an external auditor who is familiar with the content area to facilitate a deeper reading of the data. However, there have also been times when as a research team we are "so close" to the data that an external auditor with no previous knowledge of the content area can provide the most helpful reading of the data. External auditors typically bring additional questions about data processes, materials, and other content that can be addressed by the research team. These questions facilitate a description of participant meaning making of a phenomenon, and also can help identify issues of social justice not previously identified by researchers. In the South Asian CSA study, the external auditor was able to provide important questions on how some of our cultural assumptions (that were challenging for us to identify!) were influencing the study findings.

Member checking also is a strategy of trustworthiness. Using both transcripts and study findings, researchers and participants can develop increased accountability (a large social justice issue) between themselves. For example, we elected to also share the composite summary of participant data to provide participants with an opportunity to agree with, refute, or revise the data. Our research team noted the sense of empowerment that the women had in reading the summary narrative, a kind of archetype of their experiences. The women described feeling very listened to, validated, and valued as a result of the design of this composite case.

Phenomenological Considerations Related to Social Justice: Making Social Justice Happen

Phenomenologists began their inquiries because they were interested in issues of consciousness, meaning, essence, phenomena, and the relationship between humans and objects. Using a social justice lens to lean into these same investigations shifts the entire research process. The very basis of how one designs phenomenological research questions becomes tailored not toward general phenomena, but toward special social justice–related phenomenon. A common theme in phenomenological inquiry is the lived experiences of phenomena. For instance, a social justice lens shifts that same inquiry about the specific lived experiences of phenomena towards examining privilege, investigating historically marginalized groups, and researching how specific oppression experiences shape the context of an experience.

Similar to how social justice shapes phenomenological research questions, this lens is integrated into every step of the research process, from identifying researcher positionality to designing data collection and analysis. Merging social justice with phenomenology essentially shifts the entire foci of the work, particularly the researcher's self-examination of privilege and oppression experiences. Social justice–oriented phenomenologists are also persistent in naming the "personal is political" in their research: the connection between individual experiences of phenomena and structural systems of oppression (racism, sexism, heterosexism, classism, etc.). A social justice lens even shifts how phenomenological researchers handle findings after data analysis. For instance, it may be important for social justice–oriented researchers to publish their findings, but it becomes most important to connect these findings with action and advocacy. As we delve into the basics of phenomenological data collection and analysis from a social justice perspective, it is important for researchers to ask themselves with each step how positive social change is at the center of their phenomenological inquiries.

I have integrated examples of social justice–related research in phenomenology and what it may "look like" in practice. These examples have highlighted a number of overarching social justice considerations to note when using phenomenological approaches. Kline (2008) asserts the importance of the coherence of research methods (staying true to a research method throughout all research activities) and presentational rigor (using the language of a research tradition to present the entire research study) in the process of qualitative research, and I believe this is a social justice issue of researcher integrity to be consistently aware of in phenomenology. Although I am mindful of Vagle's (2009) urging to draw from other traditions when phenomenology fails during the research process to help the researcher describe phenomenon, this must be done with utmost integrity. Social justice–minded researchers, therefore, should not piecemeal traditions because the work of understanding a historically marginalized group becomes challenging. Rather, in these instances, it is a social justice issue to deepen one's thinking about the gaps in understanding a phenomenon, gather additional data, and/or add research team members to assist with the overall research process.

In addition, the discussion of bracketing/bridling researcher assumptions and beliefs about the phenomenon studied cannot be overemphasized to ensure a study aims toward justice. It is the central role of accountability related to the researcher and the data sources, and should be taken seriously and placed intentionally throughout the research process. For instance, unpacking one's privilege (white privilege, male privilege, heterosexual privilege, economic privilege, etc.) in addition to the privilege of being a researcher must be a continuous component of the entire research process. I have noticed that novice phenomenologists tend to turn away from the places of confusion, aiming to "know" the next step in a study as opposed to leaning into the ambiguity inherent in phenomenological research. With social justice–related research, the researcher's ability to lean into ambiguity becomes even more important. As we are often working with participants and phenomenon that are understudied, we are also exploring the vulnerabilities of our participants and ourselves. Therefore, as researchers engaging in social justice, we must embrace, reveal, celebrate, and honor our own vulnerabilities during the research process. An example (described in Hays & Singh, 2012) of this vulnerability is captured as my co-researcher and I named our own experiences of violence and how those experiences facilitated and/ or obstructed what we saw in participants' meaning-making processes. Researchers change and grow during phenomenological research, namely this process and the related vulnerabilities that accompany it. It will be hard, but necessary.

Finally, so much research sits on dusty shelves. Instead, ensure that the entire research plan entails connection, sharing, and feedback on findings with community members from the group, not only with the participants, but also with the larger demographic group related to the study and those who need to be changed as a result of the findings. In addition, researchers should invite critique where there might be missed important essences (which surely we always do). Then, connect findings with recommendations for policy change and other systemic-level interventions. For instance, in addition to sharing the findings of my resilience studies with South Asian communities, I have also ensured white health care providers and South Asian domestic violence advocates are target audiences to facilitate understanding of South Asian cultural contexts. I have collaboratively worked with local and national nonprofits to integrate a focus on resilience in community forums about abuse, but also as a framework for advocacy and support that nurtures resilience and healing for South Asian women CSA survivors. I have used the findings from these studies to examine and initiate policy changes that should happen with health care services and community organizations serving South

Asian women, families, and communities. Previous understandings of South Asian women's mental health has been deficit focused and did not acknowledge the importance of South Asian cultural values and context on the experience of violence. Therefore, these activities have been critical methods of justice-oriented social change. As I have leaned into the ambiguity of social justice–informed phenomenology, it has challenged some of my very core assumptions I have about the world, the phenomenon at hand, and ultimately allowed me to lean into my own liberation:

> *Anneliese:* I cannot thank you enough for sharing your story with me today. I am reminded of how important it is to make sure we as South Asian women can talk more openly about our abuse experiences and have safer families and communities so this abuse does not happen as frequently.

> *Neha:* Sure. I made some important connections about what happened to me and how I healed as we talked. I learned I am more resilient than I give myself credit for sometimes. Please let me know about the findings when they are ready. I am curious, is it hard listening to these stories?

> *Anneliese:* That's a tough question to answer. Sometimes it is difficult, and sometimes inspiring and hopeful like in our interview now. I do know for sure that listening to these stories changed me. I am not the same person I was when I began this research, and for that I am grateful. I know so much more about myself and my own family's experience of trauma, and that makes me feel a lot more resilient and free to be who I truly am.

REFERENCES

Bradbury-Jones, C., Sambrook, S., & Irvine, F. (2009). The phenomenological focus group: An oxymoron? *Journal of Advanced Nursing, 65*(3), 663–671.

Chan, Z. C. Y., Fung, Y. L., & Chien, W. T. (2013). Bracketing in phenomenology: Only undertaken in the data collection and analysis process? *The Qualitative Report, 18*(59), 1–9.

Dahlberg, K. (2006). The essence of essences—The search for meaning structures in phenomenological analysis of lifeworld phenomena. *International Journal of Qualitative Studies on Health and Well-being, 1*(1), 11–19.

Dahlberg, K., Dahlberg, H., & Nyström, M. (2008). *Reflective lifeworld research* (2nd ed.).

Lund, Sweden: Studentlitteratur.

Denzin, N. K., & Lincoln, Y. S. (2011). *The Sage handbook of qualitative research* (4th ed.). Thousand Oaks, CA: Sage.

Eagleton, T. (1983). *Literary theory: An introduction*. Oxford, UK: Basil Blackwell.

Groenewald, T. (2004). A phenomenological research design illustrated. *International Journal of Qualitative Methods, 3*(1), Article 4.

Hays, D. G., & Singh, A. A. (2012). *Qualitative inquiry in clinical and educational settings*. New York, NY: Guilford Press.

Heidegger, M. ([1927] 1962). *Being and time*. New York, NY: Harper and Row.

Holstein, J. A., & Gubrium, J. F. (1995). *The active interview*. Thousand Oaks, CA: Sage.

Husserl, E. ([1913] 1931) *Ideas: General introduction to pure phenomenology*. London, UK: George Allen and Unwin.

Kline, W. B. (2008). Developing and submitting credible qualitative manuscripts. *Counselor Education and Supervision, 47*(4), 210–217.

Moustakas, C. (1994). *Phenomenological research methods*. Thousand Oaks, CA: Sage.

Parry, D. C., & Johnson, C. W. (2007). Contextualizing leisure research to encompass complexity in lived leisure experience: The need for creative analytic practice. *Leisure Sciences: An Interdisciplinary Journal, 29*(2), 119–130.

Patton, M. Q. (2002). *Qualitative research and evaluation methods* (3rd ed.). Thousand Oaks, CA: Sage.

Penny, C., & Kinslow, J. (2006). Faculty perceptions of electronic portfolios in a teacher education program. *Contemporary Issues in Technology and Teacher Education, 6*(4), 418-435.

Polkinghorne, D. E. (1989). Phenomenological research methods. In R. S. Valle & S. Halling (Eds.) *Existential-phenomenological perspectives in psychology* (pp. 41–60). New York, NY: Plenum.

Polkinghorne, D. E. (1996). Transformative narratives: From victimic to agentic life plots. *The American Journal of Occupational Therapy, 50*(4), 299–305.

Richardson, M. (1998). Poetics in the field and on the page. *Qualitative Inquiry, 4*(4), 451–462.

Rockmore, T. (2011). *Kant and phenomenology*. Chicago, IL: The University of Chicago Press.

Rossman, R. B., & Rallis, S. F. (1998). *Learning in the field: An introduction to qualitative research*. Thousand Oaks, CA: Sage.

Seidman, I. E. (2006). *Interviewing as qualitative research: A guide for researchers in education and the social sciences*. New York, NY: Teachers College Press.

Singh, A. A. (2012). Transgender youth of color and resilience: Negotiating oppression, finding support. *Sex Roles: A Journal of Research, March,* 1–13.

Singh, A. A., Garnett, A., & Williams, D. (2013). Resilience strategies of African American women survivors of child sexual abuse: A qualitative inquiry. *The Counseling Psychologist, 41*(8), 1093–1124.

Singh, A. A., Hays, D. G., Chung, Y. B., & Watson, L. S. (2010). South Asian immigrant women who have survived child sexual abuse: Resilience and healing. *Violence Against Women, 16*(4), 444–458.

Singh, A. A., Hays, D. G., & Watson, L. (2011). Strategies in the face of adversity: Resilience strategies of transgender individuals. *Journal of Counseling and Development, 89*(1), 20–27.

Singh, A. A., Meng, S., & Hansen, A. (2013). "It's already hard enough being a student:" Developing affirming college environments for trans youth. *The Journal of LGBT Youth, 10*(3), 208–223.

Singh, A. A., Meng, S., & Hansen, A. (2014). "I am my own gender:" Resilience strategies of trans youth. *Journal of Counseling & Development, 92*(2), 208–218.

Phenomenology, in *Stanford Encyclopedia of Philosophy.* (2008). . Retrieved from http://plato.stanford.edu/entries/phenomenology/

Vagle, M. D. (2009). Validity as intended: "Bursting forth toward" bridling in phenomenological research. *International Journal of Qualitative Studies in Education, 22*(5), 585–605.

Vagle, M. D. (2010a). A post-intentional phenomenological research approach. Paper presented at the annual meeting of the American Educational Research Association, Denver, CO, May.

Vagle, M. D. (2010b). Re-framing Schön's call for a phenomenology of practice: A post-intentional approach. *Reflective Practice, 11*(3), 393–407.

Vagle, M. D. (2013). Grafting the intentional relation of hermeneutics and phenomenology in linguisticality. *Qualitative Inquiry, 19*(9), 725-735.

van Manen, M. (1991). *The tact of teaching: The meaning of pedagogical thoughtfulness.* Albany, NY: State University of New York Press.

van Manen, M. (1997). *Researching lived experience: Human science for an action sensitive pedagogy.* London, ON, Canada: Althouse.

Ziemba, J. (2007). *Heidegger and phenomenology.* Retrieved from http://erleb nis.wordpress.com/2007/10/10/heidegger-and-phenomenology/

Ethnographic Research for Social Justice: Critical Engagement with Homelessness in a Public Park

Jeff Rose

Uhhghh. Today's not the day for low motivation. It's too early. It's too cold, it's too wet, and today's northwest winds mean moisture off the lake and no pretty landscape views. The Hillside will be muddy, but only in the places where it's not snowy. I really don't want to head out there today. I'll see the same people doing the same things they always do. And then, of course, after I'm wet and frozen to the bone after being out there all day, comes the writing; lots of writing! There's always more writing: more details, more descriptions, more narratives. Just when I think I've written enough, there's more to do.

Eating my morning cereal improves my initial internal feelings of low motivation. Maybe it won't be that cold on the steep, windswept terrain, I try to encourage myself. Also, I'm curious to see if Keith has moved to his new spot like he said he would. Will the "new" folks from yesterday have made it comfortably through the night? Perhaps there is hope: yesterday some of the early spring grasses were just starting to poke their new shoots through the crust of the stale, melting, sun-baked snow. My emerging curiosities about the day begin to trump my early misgivings about heading out to the Hillside this morning. Besides, I'm not just trying to find out what's happening on the Hillside: If I can't convince the local gravel company to delay or postpone their proposed upcoming blasting, the Hillside residents won't have anywhere to go. They'll effectively be kicked out their homes, even if their "homes" are heavily used tents and tarps and plastic coverings. In fact, this process I go through every day on the Hillside feels a lot less like research and a lot more like advocacy. Who am *I* to take the day off? The Hillside residents aren't taking this cold, wet day off from homelessness.

Corey W. Johnson and Diana C. Parry, editors, "Ethnographic Research for Social Justice: Critical Engagement with Homelessness in a Public Park" in *Fostering Social Justice Through Qualitative Research: A Methodological Guide,* pp. 129-160. © 2015 Left Coast Press, Inc. All rights reserved.

Consciously considering the privileges and comforts of my heated home, I put on my old faded-brown Carhartt work pants and tattered fleece jacket that used to be green. I pull my fleece hat low over my forehead, covering my ears and neck. I grab my always-ready notebook and digital recorder and head out, locking the door behind me, effectively securing my private space, yet another unacknowledged luxury that this research has forced me to now acknowledge. Time to start my "loop." I walk uphill to the nearby road, hop the concrete barricade, and then carefully, but quickly, cross the busy commuter corridor. The Hillside emerges into view, with a faint human/game trail that leads high above the surrounding landscape, into the areas where the residents live. From this vantage, it's easy to ascertain the number of tents [12] on the Hillside. High above the Hillside's living locations, this now familiar trail contours across the Hillside, maintaining a consistent elevation. Moving north, the path intersects with a cobbled, overgrown track that was once used by trucks to access the gravel quarry. On most days it's easy to continue up the steep unkempt quarry path to access the Lake, the Kiln, and the Cave, all toponyms coined by the Hillside residents. These areas of the Hillside are more distant and have fewer residents, but they are extensions of my loop. The loop itself switchbacks down the quarry access road before plummeting sharply downhill until it ends in a rudimentary parking lot adjacent to the busy commuter road. The loop crosses the road again, concluding along the park's concrete paths to the springs before heading southward, eventually returning me back home.

My loop is never simple, as if it were just a route to traverse as part of my daily chores. Instead, it's my way of entering the "field." Developed over time, the loop is how I access the people and the ecology of the Hillside. And by this point in my ethnographic process, people know me and engage with me as if I belong. I'm expected around here. Max will gladly accept the Diet Pepsi I bring him every day. After he wakes up in the late morning, Simon will want to discuss metaphysical philosophy. Most important, all of the residents will want to know about my phone calls yesterday to the gravel company, the health department, and the local police; each of these institutions threatens to displace the Hillside residents from the place they call home. That's what this ethnography has become: rather than just trying to *understand* the people and the place of the Hillside, I've moved to *seeking justice*, through advocacy but also through an experientially informed critique of the social, political, and economic systems that continually reinscribe injustices that the Hillside residents face. The goal of my research is to live, interact, and better understand a group of individuals who live in and around the margins of an urban municipal park, as well as to "humanize" a classification of people that are often dehumanized through discursive and material practices.

We are all ethnographers. Ethnography, etymologically, simply means to write about people. More specifically, ethnography is a suite of methods engaged by a researcher to better understand particular cultural phenomena. This often means trying to understand the lived experiences of a particular group of people or people engaging with a specific place. An ethnographer typically employs the data collection methods of participation observation, interviewing, and artifact analysis as he or she lives in and across a culturally bound "field." In ethnographies, data collection strategies and levels of researcher immersion can be designed and modified to facilitate relationships that enable more personal and in-depth portraits of individuals and their communities. In these processes, researchers attempt to understand "social meanings and ordinary activities" in a sociocultural group's "naturally occurring settings" (Brewer, 2000, p. 10). What constitutes "ordinary" and "natural" in ethnographic research is a point that has gained steady academic attention, and ethnographers' responses to these questions reveal much about epistemological orientations, preferred strategies for inquiry, interpretation of results, and researchers' (intended and actual) outcomes for the ethnography.

In academic settings, research leverages data and enmeshes it with current or developing theories in the hopes of constructing new knowledges and new understandings of the world. Ethnographers generally have two goals: to describe a culture of interest in the context of a particular theoretical outlook, and to contribute to ongoing development of an applicable theory. Critical ethnographers, however, have goals above and beyond these traditional academic trajectories, making ethnography more than a method: in their hands, ethnography becomes a tool for social justice.

As exemplified in the opening narrative, I engaged in a critical ethnography that serves as the backdrop for this chapter and illuminates ethnography's potential contributions to social justice movements. Slowly and incompletely[1] I inserted myself into the "Hillside" community for over a year. The theoretical framework for this project was a tenuous mix of Marxist critical theory and poststructural affiliations to the productions of power that flow throughout social interactions. These epistemological fabrics helped transition my research from ethnography to critical ethnography, enabling me to ask broad research questions: How does a marginalized group negotiate everyday tensions between public and private space and between nature and society (J. Rose, 2014)? Therefore, this project required a methodology that promoted and enabled an "embedded researcher" while also appreciating and valuing the sensitive nature of the Hillside residents' everyday lived experiences. I needed methods that enabled me to be well acquainted and involved with the participants to gain, value, and appropriately represent their various knowledges and experiences. Ethnography demands that by "focusing on human agency and its production and negotiation of neoliberal urban landscapes, we forge *ethnographic* conceptual linkages between site-specific phenomena and the structural forces that explain their existence and survival" (Fairbanks & Lloyd, 2011, p. 7, original emphasis).

Neoliberalism is a political economic philosophy associated with a decreased role of government intervention in markets, regulation, and trade; government's primary purpose is providing for common defense, enforcing private property rights, and maintaining order and social stability. Critical theorists across disciplines have incorporated neoliberalism as a way of seeing into a variety of social, political, cultural, and environmental relationships, seeing multiple deleterious effects of contemporary neoliberal governance. See Harvey (2005).

In this chapter, I unpack various ethnographic research practices, and particularly the ways in which ethnography can work toward a more just world. To accomplish this endeavor, I use this chapter to examine ethnography's historical roots, strategies for collecting data, analysis of the data, and important considerations for how ethnography can help promote a critical, justice-oriented agenda.

Historical and Disciplinary Roots

Ethnographic research methods have been employed across a range of different academic disciplines. Anthropologists are regularly credited as being the first ethnographers, followed by efforts in sociology (Bernard, 2006) and related disciplines. A history of ethnography is one that is rooted in an effort to systematically understand those who are different and/or those who are "Othered." In anthropology, during the first half of the twentieth century, these efforts often took the form of ethnographers traveling to distant lands to study a foreign culture, where behaviors, languages, and religious activities were often portrayed as simplistic, inferior, or savage. Although Franz Boas is often considered the originator of U.S. ethnography, Margaret Mead is perhaps the most famous ethnographer for her work in Samoa (1928), where she examined sexuality and gender differentiation in Pacific

Islander culture.[2] Other prominent anthropological studies of distant cultures from this time period include the work of Malinowski (1922), Bateson (1936), Douglas (1963), and Lee (1976). These texts sought to understand the "Other," often with an explicit or implied reflection upon Western culture, or to "modernize" or "enlighten" these poorly understood cultures; both of these rationales are problematic, highly colonialized research perspectives for contemporary social justice scholars.

Beyond this anthropological lineage, another major ethnographic epoch of the twentieth century involved sociological understandings of human behavior, particularly behaviors that were perceived as outside of "normal." Chicago School sociologists used ethnographic techniques to create accountings of supposedly deviant and subversive groups, providing important trajectories for ethnographers studying those at the margins of society. Thrasher's (1927) study of gangs, Shaw's (1930) case study of the jack-roller, Cressey's (1932) work on taxi dance halls, and Anderson's (1923) research on homelessness all developed through this tradition. Their decree, as early sociological ethnographers, was to study social life in situ, examining groups in their native socioenvironmental habitats. As opposed to anthropologists traveling to distant places to study seemingly foreign cultures, Chicago School sociologists turned the gaze closer to home, developing important theories of urban behavior and life in burgeoning U.S. cities. This line of scholarship in many ways set the stage for researchers seeking embedded, nuanced, and critical understandings of groups systemically marginalized by politics, race, class, gender, or other sociopolitical markers.

Researching the "Other" through ethnographic methods—whether in distant lands or in a researcher's own backyard—generally takes a substantial amount of time. While the time required to ethnographically engage with a culture varies significantly (by academic discipline, cultural complexity, researcher comfort with immersion, methodological complexity, or otherwise), long-term commitments generally produce stronger, more nuanced texts than do brief encounters (Borneman & Hammoudi, 2009). Consider, for example, the work of French anthropologist Pierre Clastres (1998), who spent two years with the so-called "savage" tribes of indigenous groups in Paraguay in the 1960s. He acknowledged that even "being there" with his research participants did not break down considerable barriers of communication and cross-referenced understandings. Despite prolonged engagement, he found it difficult to fully understand the mythologies, embodiments, and social practices which lay at the heart of the very existences of the Guayaki Indians. Ethnographers need to acknowledge just how complex and difficult it is to navigate relationships and create understandings with the complicated existences of others. This relationship between ethnographers and groups under examination is undoubtedly mediated by important power differentials, providing opportunities to do both great harm and/or great good.

Today, ethnography has evolved substantially from its early beginnings in anthropology and sociology, and largely "rejects the more positivist, objectivistic, and scientist hegemony of its quantitative brethren" (Adler & Adler, 1998, p. xii). In this epistemic paradigm, "new" forms of ethnography have developed and are developing, including performance ethnography (understanding cultures through their performance practices), autoethnography (an exploration of the self, where one's own experiences and thoughts are data), duoethnography (two or more researchers examine themselves and their relationships in a particular setting), and virtual ethnography (using an online medium to explore groups, interactions, or settings), in addition to the many progressive hybridizations that inventive social scientists craft every day. These ethnographic variations all contain elements of participant observation as a form of data collection, and all can employ a critical orientation. Ethnography examines particular processes in particular places to address how and what forms of power and history combine to create subjective but patterned realities for people. The critical ethnography advanced here uses many of the elements of "traditional" ethnographies, but with an explicit advocacy for changing systemic inequities. Ethnographic inquiry of all sorts uncovers social structures and political and economic constraints, expressed materially and symbolically, through long-term, intimate contact with people in their everyday environments (Low, 2014).

Data Collection Strategies

Gaining Access to the Field

In ethnography, gaining access to a community is a significant undertaking. Issues of researcher reflexivity, sociocultural awareness, and sensitivities to differences are paramount dispositions throughout the ethnographic process. Further, when social justice outcomes are an intentional trajectory of the research process (see "Placing the Critical in Ethnography"), the social, cultural, political, economic, ethnic, racial, gender, and other differences existing between researcher(s) and the field requires more attention. Gaining access to a community of interest is less of an either/or than traditional researchers might prefer. Instead, access is often partial, mediated, temperamental, and conditional, and rarely follows a linear format of ever-increasing levels and depths of access. Ethnographers constantly navigate complex sociopolitical environments and adjust the level of access to a particular culture. Because access to a community of interest is gradually gained, ethnographers must carefully represent those experiences in ways that are sensitive, appropriate, and critical, maintaining and nurturing the levels of access already sought. Further, the "field" is not often a static geographic location, but a dynamic set of social relationships that may center on a particular culture, place, set of experiences, or some other (loosely) unifying theme. This "field," far from being monolithic, further complicates the notion of varying levels of access; ethnographers may have deep access to some parts of a field and less access to others.

Gaining Access to the Hillside

Gaining access to the residents of the Hillside was not a single event, but a process with both challenges and rewards, lasting over months of interaction. The approach was to embed myself—spatially, corporeally, materially, etc.—into the community. I walked, sat, and wandered around the park and the open space nearby so that my presence became normalized and less threatening over time. While my ethnographic experience with Hillside residents likely began the first day I experienced the park, my ethnography formally began during a series of observations for a graduate ethnography class. Soon after, I engaged in small conversations with individuals who were living there at that time.

During early dialogues, I was reticent to disclose that I was working on an academic project. I feared that the residents might recoil from "officials" (like me) who negatively judged them and their lives, losing any trust that I had built. In these initial interactions, I never lied about my position, but was also hesitant to fully disclose. I simply told them I was curious about the park and the folks who use it. Most residents took that explanation at face value, never questioning it much further. As my time in the field increased, my relationships with individual Hillside residents intensified, and I was comfortable disclosing my position as a scholar. To my surprise, most were curious about my intentions and seemed to appreciate my interest. Over time we developed mutual trust and I disclosed more about myself and my academic endeavors, and formed solid friendships with many of them. As a result of this mutual trust, I continue to be cautious about the potential to identify those living on the Hillside, or revealing their location to police, health department officials, or other institutions of control.

My positions vis-à-vis the Hillside residents were inconsistent and always evolving. Time on the Hillside and my relationships with folks living there was complicated. Some Hillside residents never accepted my presence, and the ones who did certainly did so conditionally and partially. Over the course of the study, I moved from a complete outsider who "didn't belong" to a consistent participant in the community, where my opinions and experiences were sought after and frequently validated. I was an outsider, insider, observer, participant, advocate, and friend.[3]

Prior to gaining access, and especially once access is achieved, ethnographers' framings of individuals have important ramifications for the research. Traditional ethnographic terms such as *informant* (Spradley, 1980), *participant* (Wolcott, 1999), and *subject* (Bernard, 2006) all lack a necessary implication of researcher solidarity commensurate with critical researcher positionality. Madison (2007) suggests "co-performative witnessing" as a way to "live and spend time in the borderlands of contested identities where you speak 'with' not 'to' others and where you (and their) ethnographic interlocutors are as co-temporal in the report and on stage as they were in the field" (p. 828). Whatever term is used, critical ethnographers should carefully consider the implicit and explicit meanings and power inferences associated with term(s).

Collecting Ethnographic Data

Ethnography is not a singular method, but a multi-instrument suite of techniques that enables researchers to better know a particular culture, place, or social setting, almost always through participant observation, regardless of disciplinary or epistemological background that might encourage additional techniques (Bernard, 2006; Spradley, 1980; Wolcott, 1999).

Goodall (2000) suggests general informal practices for a new ethnographer:

- Hanging out with others in their local contexts
- Engaging in verbal exchanges with them
- Sharing and learning about their everyday practices
- Digging back into our own—and their own—memories for likely antecedents to current practices
- Jotting down notes, or tape-recording interviews, when possible

- Returning to our offices/homes/rented rooms to write our representations of field experiences
- Engaging in armchair, after-the-fact self-reflection, analysis, and editing of the fieldnotes into a narrative (pp. 84–85)

Participant observation provides a way to understand worldviews and ways of life of people from the inside, in the context of their everyday lives. However, ethnographers complement participant observation with other data-collection techniques, which I elaborate upon later in this chapter. I engaged in techniques of participant observation, ethnographic interviewing, semistructured interviewing, and photography for data collection. Ethnographic fieldnotes, interview transcripts, archival support, photographic documentation, and the production of maps were data that were co-generated[4] from these techniques.

Participant Observation

Participant observation requires that researchers engage with a community to different degrees, a challenging and dynamic prospect. Spradley (1980) advocates a range of participatory positionalities for ethnographic researchers from nonparticipation to complete immersion (Figure 5.1). Nonparticipation, passive participation, moderate participation, active participation, and complete participation form benchmarks of the spectrum.

FIGURE 5.1. Spradley's (1980) Types of Participation. Redrawn from Spradley (1980, p. 58).

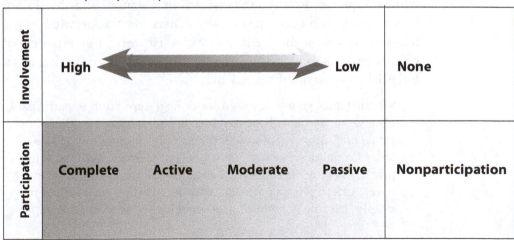

Nonparticipation points the ethnographer toward no involvement with the people or activities studied, while active participation involves full immersion into what other people are doing to more fully learn the cultural rules for behavior. Complete participation, on the other end of this spectrum, is best used for situations where the ethnographer is already an "ordinary participant" (Spradley, 1980, p. 61). Spradley's definition of nonparticipation likely does not resonate with the work of social justice ethnographers.

In contrast to the participation side of participant observation, the researcher-as-observer side of the equation deserves exploration. Observation is a contested data collection method within ethnographic research, as observation infers a clinical, removed, distant, scientifically objective stance. "It might be useful to shift from a concentration on observation as a 'method' per se to a perspective that emphasizes observation as a context for interaction among those involved in the research collaboration" (Angrosino, 2008, p. 165). While a pure observer might have very little interaction with the culture being studied, there is an inevitable presence of the researcher, regardless of how subtle s/he attempts to be. For this reason, and as discussed earlier, critical ethnographers should enter into a community carefully, thoughtfully, and respectfully.

Participant observation is difficult to describe systematically due to its elusive nature (Adler & Adler, 1994), its breadth (Bryman, 1984), and the fact that it remains "ill-defined and…tainted with mysticism" (Evans, 1988, p. 197). This mysticism stems from the few systematic outlines of participant observation. Ethnographers recognize the situated meanings of the sociocultural situation at hand, and simultaneously appreciate the researcher's essential immersion and participation in the creation of these meanings. The politics of ethnographic research and the research itself cannot and should not be separated, and social justice researchers must acknowledge and faithfully represent these entanglements. However, this experiential morass emerges as something more than a side effect; it exists as an essential component of the research itself.

> Working through my various roles along the spectrum of participant observation at the Hillside required difficult ethical considerations. I tried diligently to gain insider status in the community, but also knew I could never actually become a full member, as the various privileges of my life could not be readily dismissed. Since I generally have access to private property (a home, an office, etc.), I could not simply "become homeless," as those private spaces would always

be available. Having the knowledge that I could "quit" being home-less at any point never allowed me to be a full participant; I entered into this research from a position of privilege, with access to daily resources that many of the Hillside residents lack: housing, access to restrooms, and the ability to procure and cook food. I have a place to just *be*, spatially, materially, legally, and socially. Through the privi-leges of my own health, I do not have substance addictions or men-tal illness. Ultimately, I am not homeless, and so to present myself as anything to the contrary would be to engage in an act of deception. However, I wanted to understand the lived experiences of the Hillside residents and I wanted to understand how the process of homeless-ness—of living in public nature—is enacted and how it feels for these individuals. Beyond mere understanding, I also sought to enact a more just and available alternative to injustices encountered by those facing homelessness. Given some of these basic discrepancies be-tween me and the Hillside residents, negotiating the trust required to obtain semi-insider status required extensive relationship building. As an advocate for social justice, I hoped these relationships were useful to engage community resistance to current policies, and form-ative in proactively seeking social justice. With this caveat in place, I worked diligently to try to see, hear, feel, and understand Hillside residents' realities.

Duration and frequency of my research interactions at the Hill-side and beyond were important for the ethnography's integrity. I spent hundreds of hours "in the field," meaning directly and inten-tionally observing and interacting on the Hillside. I also spent count-less hours with some Hillside residents at local shelters, clinics, food provision agencies, social service provision agencies, gas stations, and libraries, all of which constituted part of the "field" of research. During these times, I talked with, observed, and listened to Hillside residents' experiences. Some of my experiences at the Hillside in-cluded spending nights in the field and into the next day. Some of my shorter experiences amounted to pure observation (e.g., when folks were asleep inside their tents), while other times felt more like pure participation (e.g., when I was cooking dinner with them over a fire). Some weeks, during periods of high activity or perceived threats of displacement, I was on the Hillside for days. Other weeks, when fewer residents lived on the Hillside, my engagement was more spor-adic. I charted my observations, recording the dates, times, duration, weather, the number of tents erected on the Hillside, the spatial lo-cations of sleeping spots and tents, and general interpretations. This ongoing record enabled me to locate and identify patterns, gaps, or oversights in my research, as I tried to vary the days of the week and the times of day when I was on the Hillside.

Ethnographic Interviews

Ethnographic interviewing (Spradley, 1979, 1980) is a series of informal, casual conversations during participant observation where researchers politely try to understand participants' perspectives. Many researchers seek frequent and extensive ethnographic interviews throughout the research process. Ethnographers also try to use ethnographic interviews to support or refute specific observations made in situ or, perhaps, observations that are better understood after rereading fieldnotes. Ethnographic interviews should not feel like "interviews" for participants but like spontaneous conversations of topics of mutual interest. Ethnographic interviews are often open-ended, unstructured friendly conversations (Spradley, 1979). Three broad types of ethnographic interview questions are: 1) explicit purpose questions, where the ethnographer clearly states the research objective; 2) ethnographic explanations, where the ethnographer explains questions to facilitate the process of the participant as a learner in the ethnographic process; and 3) ethnographic questions, a variety of types of questions, including descriptive questions, structural questions, and contrast questions that are employed by the ethnographer over a number of interviews (Spradley, 1979).

An example of an ethnographic interview from my research revolved around an issue of safety, health, and cleanliness on the Hillside:

> *Jeff:* Wait, you said they don't think this place is safe? What do you mean?
>
> *Keith:* Yep, they came up here yesterday and said we were a public nuisance, and we were causing "health problems" [used his fingers to make air quotes]. Going to the bathroom, taking dumps, leaving trash, that kind of stuff.
>
> *Jeff:* How'd you respond?
>
> *Keith:* Well, you can imagine what I said, it wasn't too polite, and I probably went overboard with it as always. [Pause] I just don't see why the damn Health Department comes up here [at] the same time they want to get the quarry running again. We're not causing problems. Our place is clean…

Semistructured Interviews

Semistructured interviews allow participants the space to describe and respond to political, social, and economic forces that affect their everyday lives (Fontana & Frey, 2008). As part of an ethnographic research design, these purposeful conversations can be helpful in further understanding another person's thoughts, feelings, and experiences in their own words. Careful questioning and listening enables learning and understanding beyond what researchers could not see or readily understand. They also provide spaces to explore other understandings or explanations of information that researchers felt they already understood. More formalized than ethnographic interviews, semistructured interviews are planned in advance with some predetermined questions. Further, having a semistructured interview protocol—a basic but flexible list of questions—provides consistency in asking questions across multiple individuals, groups, or settings.

> I conducted semistructured interviews with six Hillside residents (Max, Wayne, Keith, Ralph, Ray, and Louis), men who know the Hillside well and could fully attest to their lived experiences there. They were conducted relatively late in the ethnography, after substantial relationships had been formed and I was mostly clear on themes I wanted to further develop. The interviews enabled me to better understand the Hillside experience, as well as a clearer, first-person context for the ways in which the residents engage in everyday life.
>
> The time, place, and implementation of the semistructured interviews were important for both the substance and the quality of the information. The interviews were conducted in places that were comfortable for them, ranging from inside a tent on the Hillside to the library. Given the vulnerability of this population, knowing that they understandably shy away from "officially" using their names, I only sought verbal consent and repeatedly assured them of their confidentiality. I took scrupulous notes during the interviews. For instance, I kept track of Max's tone of voice when referencing the police, Wayne's frustrated facial expressions when referring to the downtown shelter, and even of my own thoughts or reactions. The interviews were rarely planned; most times when I scheduled an interview, the individual did not show at the agreed-upon time. Instead, I learned to always carry my digital recorder and interview protocol so that if someone agreed to participate, I was prepared. My basic interview protocol became a dynamic document that morphed as the research process unfolded and I became more aware of different issues and intriguing questions.
>
> *Jeff:* How did you get introduced to this place?
>
> *Louis:* Huh? What do you mean?
>
> *Jeff:* Well, tell me about the first time you came to the Hillside.
>
> *Louis:* I don't know, I guess it was when Keith was talking about it a while back at the Feed Bag, saying he found a great place to sleep one night. But that was probably five or six years ago when I was working construction…

Photography

While descriptive fieldnotes illustrate a researcher's understandings and interpretations of a culture or place, photographic documentation can serve as data for an ethnographic project. Ethnographic photography is the use of photographs for the recording and understanding of cultures and/or places (Scherer, 1995). A photograph is not ethnographic due to the intention of its production, but rather in how it is used to inform viewers ethnographically. Specifically, photographs elucidate particular situations and are compared over space and time to better understand various lived contexts. Photography is also helpful in supporting the intent or purpose of the photographer, or as pieces of documentation that give depth or detail to ethnographic subjects. Photography is a visual method (G. Rose, 2001) that may be particularly helpful in documenting physical environmental changes as well as culture members themselves. As all ethnographic photography has an intended audience (Scherer, 1995), ethnographers hope that photographs viscerally support and augment descriptions of place experiences and daily living. However, social justice researchers should always carefully consider and prioritize vulnerable populations' privacy, desires, and overall wellbeing.

Ethical uncertainties associated with photography provide opportunities to do more harm than good, because photographs tend to capture a snapshot open for viewers' interpretation rather than engaging in the process of writing thorough description. For this reason, the analysis may not be as fully formed, and the interpretation relies more upon the author and less upon the reader and/or viewer. Though photography often ironically *removes* authors' interpretations, the benefit of its visceral nature and orientation to the place might outweigh the losses of authorial authority.

> Max's tent seems to always look good: taut, meticulously erected, well cared for, and symmetrical (Figure 5.2). In many ways, he's quite fastidious, which contrasts to many other aspects of his personality. His tent today almost blended in to the surrounding late-May verdant landscape. Considering last night's storm, his site looked really good this morning, probably because he shifts the orientation of the tent depending on the direction of the incoming winds. Given the gravel substrate underneath the tent, I bet he's pretty dry in there. I was especially happy to see his tent today because this is one that Tom gave me to bring out here, to give to whomever on the Hillside wanted it. Who knows, maybe I'm helping make a difference out here? Max wasn't home when I stopped by, meaning he probably walked to work today. One of his cats was outside, as were both of his bikes and a cooler.

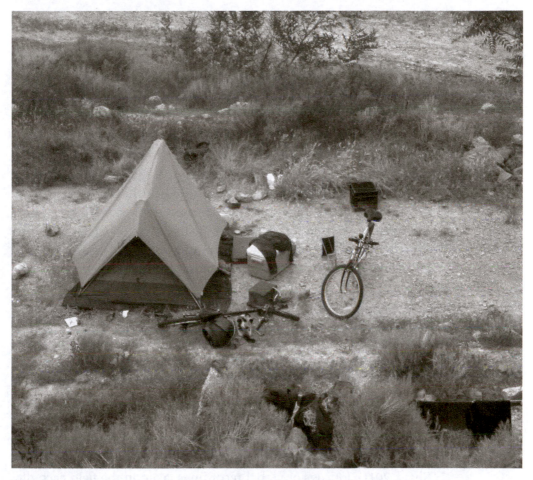

FIGURE 5.2. Max's home on the 2nd tier of the Hillside. Photo by the author.

In this section I briefly review aspects of participant observation, ethnographic interviews, semistructured interviews, and photography as I put them to use in an ethnographic project. Obviously, these are not the only tools in an ethnographer's belt to be put to use. Surveys, secondary research, document analysis, mapping, social network analysis, and more structured archival explorations might also be helpful, again depending on one's epistemological orientations and disciplinary affiliations. Researchers should acknowledge intertextuality in various practices of ethnographic data collection, noting the influential roles we play in the shaping of our research, while at the same time seeking to listen to the voices of the Others who serve as our co-investigators. The texts that result from such encounters are complex dialogues, indicating that sophisticated analysis is necessary to critically represent the experiences and the data collected during ethnographies.

Strategies of Data Analysis

Ethnography is not only a suite of data collection methods, but it is also a series of analytical tools that help make sense of data. In ethnography, data analysis is not a separate, discreet event that occurs after data are collected. Instead, ethnography requires an iterative analytical process in which collected data informs analysis that then (re)informs subsequent data collection. Analytical processes invite new perspectives, differentially focused questions, and continual introspection on the part of the researcher. Social justice researchers can use the analytical process as a way to further interrogate how the sociocultural situations of which they are a part either support or oppose dominant social orders. In this section, I bring forward fieldnotes, ethnographic data transformation, and discourse analysis as means of analyzing ethnographic experiences.

Fieldnotes

Documentation of participant observation experiences is critical to the depth and insight of an ethnographic research project. Fieldnotes record observations, encounters, and interactions in a rigorous and often systematic manner. The fieldnotes produced during ethnographies and beyond serve as a written record of observations, experiences, feelings, reactions, and reflections, ultimately serving as the primary data source for ethnographic research (Emerson, Fretz, & Shaw, 2011). Jottings or verbal recordings taken in the field each day (or as soon as reasonably possible) are transformed into fieldnotes, serving not only as a descriptive log of what happened, but also the researcher's feelings and reactions to those happenings (Emerson, Fretz, & Shaw, 2011). Jottings should be as specific as possible, with the realization that it is impossible to fully capture a scene or experience with only the written word. It is helpful to also write down verbatim quotes from individuals when possible. However, sometimes taking notes might be an impediment to relationships; during these times, ethnographers might choose to keep notebooks away, sacrificing informational detail in favor of one's own experience in that moment and whatever closeness could be gained with participants. The resulting fieldnotes are almost always more comprehensive, complex, and detailed than in-the-field jottings, and these notes serve as a written record of what researchers saw, heard, smelled, felt, tasted, and emoted during the ethnographic experience and beyond. However, fieldnotes that ethnographers produce serve as a systematic, cumulative, descriptive written record of their research experiences, and as a subjective representation of participants' experiences in a particular cultural context. Practically, fieldnotes and jottings do not necessarily have to be actual written notes, as many ethnographers use data recorders to note in-the-moment "verbal jottings" that can then be transcribed and transformed into more systematic fieldnotes at a more convenient time.

For my research, a primary purpose of my fieldnotes was to describe the Hillside and the culture of the individuals living there to the best of my ability. Sometimes I focused on physical characteristics of the environment, and other times I tried to make sense of the political–economic intertwinement of the urban setting. These rich descriptions allow readers to better understand the cultural setting of the Hillside, and they are not without subjectivity, as my perceptions and interpretations as a researcher helped navigate the descriptions (Emerson, Fretz, & Shaw, 2011).

Ethnographic Data Transformation

The goal of the data transformation process is to make sense of the ethnographic social, cultural, economic, political, and/or spatial settings. Data transformation, and its subsequent representation in an ethnographic form, rarely follows a set of static criteria. Rather, it is an iterative process that facilitates organizing and understanding information learned throughout the creation of an ethnography (Bernard, 2006). Data collection, analysis, and transformation are not discrete portions of the ethnographic research experience (Spradley, 1980), but constantly invite re-visits and re-theorizations. As ethnographers' experiences evolve, more is understood about the behaviors and the cultures being researched; subsequently, the units of analysis, and the research questions themselves; the overall direction(s) of the research also evolve alongside our ethnographic experiences (Madison, 2012). Fieldnotes from early stages of the ethnographic process might look and feel quite different from fieldnotes taken near the conclusion of the participant observation (Emerson, Fretz, & Shaw, 2011). Throughout data transformation processes, researchers must remain aware of the ethnographic imperative to describe, analyze, and interpret the experiences and the data (Wolcott, 1999).

Data analysis is a helpful process used to identify patterns of thought, behavior, relationships, and important events in the fieldnotes. Analysis of my data was an iterative process that was collaboratively co-constructed with colleagues I had involved in my work. During weekly meetings, we worked through recent sections of fieldnotes, identifying events of interest, questioning underlying assumptions in my writing process, and asking broad, open-ended questions. Themes were explored and negotiated and connected back to concepts and/ or theories. I consulted the Hillside residents about emerging themes to see how my explanations matched their everyday experiences. The analytic process consisted of organizing the data, immersing myself into the data, generating categories and themes, coding the data, interpreting findings, considering alternative understandings, and reporting the findings (Saldana, 2013). The excerpt below illustrates the transformation of participant observation data from fieldnotes to analyzed text; note the combined use of description, analysis, and interpretation.

> Max was also really excited to see his cat. He mentioned his cat three separate times before we saw her. It's funny. When I was at the 2nd Tier probably 45 minutes before, I searched for the cat and called for it to no avail (no surprise given most cats' temperaments). Then, when Max came into the area, the cat immediately emerged from some rocks above the 2nd Tier and came to him. Max picked up the cat, stroked its tabby fur softly, talked in a high-pitched voice, and held it close to his face. She looked like she was almost stuffed under the bill of his trucker's hat. I remember being struck by the juxtaposition of his wrinkled, sun-damaged cheek next to her soft fur. He then found a bag of food, carefully pouring some into a frying pan, before spending some time thinking aloud about how he would transport the fidgety cat up to [another place on the Hillside where he was moving]. He then wondered out loud how he would get her to figure out where her new home is, and ultimately, to stay up there. Max said he was a little concerned because he would now have to take water up there for her, since he wouldn't have the water seep at the 2nd Tier, complete with its well-cared-for pool of clear, collected water below. The cat's current home, and her connection to Max, was upended by the Health Department's efforts to "clean up" this supposedly detrimental environmental situation.

Although there are many ways to "analyze" data for ethnography (Saldana, 2013; Wolcott, 1999), coding is one technique. After determining several themes, ethnographers can then compare past fieldnotes to identify support for proposed themes. For some themes, ethnographers can make notes to return to this topic in future conversations or experiences. Other times, when a thematic topic has become "saturated" in researchers' notes and experiences, it is not necessary to return to it ethnographically.

Interpretation involves coming to more full understanding about both the space and the culture of the ethnographic setting. During the interpretive process, it is important to raise questions or associations that might produce new awareness, new understanding, and perhaps new knowledge. Taking data from the ethnographic experience and aligning them with already established theories creates a rigorous and thorough process. Interpretations surrounding the ethnographic culture are based upon details, categories, and connections that are developed in narrative descriptions and continually informed by the ongoing processes of analysis. In this way, description, analysis, and interpretation are mutually reinforcing and constitutive processes. However, interpretation is where connecting data to theory provides a platform to promote greater social justice. These processes allow ethnographic researchers to create—rather than discover—theory (Emerson, Fretz, & Shaw, 2011).

Discourse Analysis

Discourse, and its subsequent analysis, owes much of its academic development to Michel Foucault, who considered how "historically and culturally located systems of power/knowledge construct subjects and their worlds." He viewed discourse as "socially reflexive, both constitutive and meaningfully descriptive of the world and its subjects" (Holstein & Gubrium, 2008, p. 183). Foucault was particularly interested in the social locations or institutional sites that serve as the practical operation of discourses. This perspective links the discourses of particular subjectivities with the construction of people's lived experiences. Discourses are complex webs of both subtle and explicit communication providing information about a particular subject. Discourses "are not a mere intersection of things and words: an obscure web of things, and a manifest, visible, colored chain of words.... [They are] practices that systematically form the objects [and subjects] of which they speak" (Foucault, 1972, pp. 48–49).

As a result, discourse analysis helps to understand many of the unseen, unspoken, and unannounced practices and happenings by critically orienting the ways in which talk, conversation, and other communicative processes are used to make meaning (Holstein & Gubrium, 2008; G. Rose, 2001). Foucauldian critique of power differentials embedded within oppressive discourses is helpful, but critical ethnographies give substance and proactivity to the situation. Consistent with the goals of social justice, critical ethnographers often try to advocate, support, and defend perspectives that not only humanize communities of interest, but contribute to changing current oppressive systems that result in inequalities. Critical discourse analysis is a primary result of extended, immersed, ethnographic time in the field, where direct engagement helps to better understand (and represent) their experiences (Chambers, 2003).

Discourse analysis contributed to the overall understanding of spaces and individuals of the Hillside, providing a larger *gestalt* of subtle and less-than-subtle discursive productions taking place on the Hillside. Through discourse analysis I arrived at how constructs, such as public space and nature, are ultimately defined not only by their material characteristics, but often more so by their discursive production. Critical discourse analysis of the site and the context of this situation helped decode the inherent power discrepancies involved (Perakyla, 2008). This discourse analysis involved reading the signs (G. Rose, 2001) and landscapes (Mitchell, 2002) of the Hillside.

> The newly erected reflective sign simply said "Park Closed 11pm to 6am," and the other one announced a local no-littering ordinance for the city. But to the Hillside residents, the message was clear: **You're not wanted here**. Wayne told me that it's not what the signs say, but where the signs are located. "Why don't they have them down there near the soccer field or the picnic tables? Cause that's where the families and shit are. They just put the signs up here, near us, to tell us to 'move on' [using air quotes]. This place ain't for us!" He was right. As public spaces are increasingly "cleaned up" for commodified, consumable urban experiences, these signs seemed explicitly directed at the Hillside residents.

While fieldnotes, data transformation, and discourse analysis are presented here, there is further analytic work to be done while working through an ethnography, including various coding schemes, memo writing, and others (compare with Saldana, 2013). Ethnographic analysis requires a continual visitation to research questions, methods of data collection, and questioning of one's own positionality vis-à-vis the entire research process. For critical ethnographers interested in social justice concerns, it remains paramount for one's analysis to align theoretically, methodologically, and empirically with the other concurrent aspects of the research process. Further, ethnographers should consider the crisis of representation that accompanies situated, nuanced, subjective accounts of people's lived experiences and perspectives.

Considerations Related to Social Justice

It should now be clear that ethnography has the potential to be much more than a methodology. What if it was more than a systematic way of collecting and analyzing data about a particular culture of interest? What if, as ethnographers, we sought more than a sympathetic understanding of the Other? What if our incoming perspectives include recognizing that institutions tend to be either in support of or opposition to dominant social orders? What if ethnography included specific goals of making this world a better place; not just for ourselves, but for those who have suffered at the hands of dominant social, cultural, political, and economic institutions? What if ethnographic inquiry, like other critical qualitative research methods, was envisaged as a process of researchers sending forth in the name of justice? This space of possibility is where critical ethnography emerges as a combined methodology and worldview that demands of researchers a focus on engagement/ entanglement with research participants, thereby explicitly questioning systems of injustice, being an ally and advocate for the dispossessed, and relentlessly striving toward a more just world.

Placing the Critical in Ethnography

While a more contemporary and nuanced view of ethnography is that it is "a way of working, a way of entering the world every day, which privileges asking questions about others in cultural contexts constructed and understood by a self whose presence is very much in the text" (Goodall, 2000, p. 21), critical ethnography has the potential to do even more. What separates ethnography from critical ethnography is the latter's engagement with various institutionalized *systems* that perpetuate injustices, rather than blaming proximate and local forces. These systems are power laden rather than politically inert, enabling critical ethnographers to take an explicitly normative approach rather than one that claims the objectivity of disinterest (Robbins, 2012). Being critical requires that research and scholarship is political, as opposed to being apolitical. If politics are understood as plays of power in the distribution and negotiation of various resources, then politics are, in fact, everywhere. In this sense, a critical ethnography is both a set of research tools and an intervention. Low (2014) refers to criticality as an *engaged* process, where there is a commitment to participants and communities through an ethnographer's values-based stance in promoting rights and equity. Critical ethnography, then, contributes not only to enriching our collective knowledge about ourselves and our world, but also to the constructive ways of envisioning and enacting a just future. In such cases, ethnographers address issues of inequity based upon race, class, gender, orientation, ability, patriarchy, consumption, political economy, and/or ideology, among many others. In my critical ethnography, the systems requiring critique were multifaceted and overlapping: the privileging of private space; the lived oppression under neoliberal capitalism; the institutionalization of severe poverty; the patriarchal defiance of the welfare state; and the rampant objectification of nature.

Madison (2012) defines the methods of *critical* ethnography as "always a meeting of multiple sides in an encounter with and among others, one in which there is negotiation and dialogue toward substantial and viable meanings that make a difference in the others' worlds" (p. 10). Contemporary critical theory is an amalgamation of a variety of social theories over the past century that view action and behavior as being either in support of or opposition to a dominant social order (Giroux, 1983). From the Frankfurt School of the early twentieth century to contemporary critical race and participatory action scholars, these theorists often led the charge for engaged, reflexive, and political critique. Building off of Marxist critiques of power discrepancies and injustices of dominant social, political, and economic relations, critical scholars engage in research that is explicitly oriented toward progressive change, toward liberation and emancipation of the systemically marginalized and the oppressed. Critical political ecologists expanded Marx's critique of dominant social relations to also include various exploitations and dominations found in relationships between nature and society (Robbins, 2012).

Ethnographic research began incorporating these critical perspectives into participant observation studies, combining the rigor of understanding lived experiences with politicized perspectives concerning power, dominance, and justice. Critical ethnography insists upon an explicitly politicized stance against injustices found throughout social power inequities.

> Critical ethnography begins with an ethical responsibility to address processes of unfairness or injustice within a particular lived domain…. It means she will use the resources, skills, and privileges available to her to make accessible—to penetrate the borders and break through the confines in defense of—the voices and experiences of subjects whose stories are otherwise restrained and out of reach. This means the critical ethnographer contributes to emancipatory knowledge and discourses of social justice. (Madison, 2012, pp. 5–6)

Both practically and epistemologically, critical ethnography serves a different purpose and role than more standard cultural ethnographies that traditionally come from anthropological inquiries. Critical ethnography suggests a level of political engagement by the researcher that extends beyond many traditional roles. While the incorporation of Marxist critical stances is vital to critical ethnography, there is also a subtlety of action that is required of the researcher. Critical political action must be balanced with an insider's knowledge of community norms, values, and material realities. The role of the researcher is not merely somewhere along the participant observation spectrum. The

TABLE 5.1. Critical Ethnographic Perspectives

Perspective	Ethnographic	Critical	Critical Ethnographic
Purpose of research	Describe/expose (oppression within) a culture	Justice and emancipation from systemic inequities	Descriptive, lived critique; liberation
Nature of reality	Participatory/experiential perspective; multiple realities	Dominant reality; power imbalance	Multiple realities exist, but dominant realities create power imbalances
Roles of researcher	Participant observer (along a spectrum)	Activist; liberator	Co-performative witness; informed advocate

ethnographer becomes an advocate, supporter, and champion of a culture, in defiance of oppressions within a culture or oppressions toward the entire culture more generally. Proposed critical ethnographic perspectives are summarized in Table 5.1. This table is not meant to be a complete picture of critical ethnographic understanding, but rather key points concerning the purpose of the research, the nature of reality, and the roles of the researcher.

In contrast to critical approaches, traditional social science research, through claims of value neutrality, often serves the ideological function of justifying the positions and interests of the always-already powerful. Ethnographic methods work well with critical and post-structural approaches; specifically, research questions that address processes at "the community, neighborhood, and urban scales—quite often at the edges of formal institutions and legality—render ethnographic methods particularly germane" (Fairbanks & Lloyd, 2011, p. 6). Critical ethnography is explicitly political and has the potential to produce texts that emerge collaboratively from the lives of the researcher and the researched and is centrally about praxis—the application and embodiment of theory—and a political commitment to the struggle for liberation and in defense of human rights (Barton, 2001). Angrosino (2008) advocates that the following criteria should be used in critical participant observation methods:

> First, the researcher should be directly connected to the poor and marginalized.... The middle-class researcher who chooses to live with the poor and otherwise marginalized in our society (or with entire societies that are poor and marginalized vis-à-vis larger global powers) is, of course, in a very different position compared with residents of such communities who have no choice in the matter.... Second, the researcher should...ask questions based on our experience of life among the poor and marginalized rather than on our

experience of what others have written or said about them…. Third, the researcher should become an advocate. (pp. 174–175)

Marginality can be understood as a state of human being that is partially "outside" mainstream institutions, cultures, practices, beliefs, and spaces, and it is the job of critical ethnographers to recover and centralize these systemically marginalized voices and experiences. A question that critical ethnographers must constantly ask and re-ask is: How do we access and research the social worlds of the systemically marginalized? We must do this in the context of knowing that our understandings of these situations, no matter how contextualized or how immersed in the community of interest, remain partial and contingent upon the situation at hand.

> Examples of my own critical engagement/entanglement with the Hillside community are fewer than I hoped. However, I was able to support many of the individual residents with sleeping bags, tents, and clothes from my part-time employer. I refuted an article published in the local newspaper disparaging the health conditions in "homeless camps." During times of crisis or displacement, I engaged with officials from the mining company, the health department, the police, and local clinics, attempting to advocate on behalf of the Hillside residents. For the Hillside residents themselves, I supported and advocated for them during times of threatened displacement, I funneled resources to the Hillside in numerous ways, and I've drawn (academic and political) attention to the injustices commonly associated with homelessness. I also used my teaching as a platform for activism against irresponsible stereotypes and unhelpful constructions of homelessness. Foucault might argue that attempting to critically "humanize" the Hillside residents is actually just another technique of further controlling or surveilling a group. From this perspective, presenting the Hillside residents as "just like anyone else" disciplines away their unique singularities, bringing them further in line with mainstream, normative perspectives. I've presented a nuanced account of individuals that are largely misunderstood and misrepresented, and I've done so in a way that implicates problematic aspects of a sociopolitical system focused on unfettered capitalist accumulation.

Researcher Positionality

Researcher positionality, as Madison (2012) states, is "vital because it forces us to acknowledge our own power, privilege, and biases just as we are denouncing the power structures that surround our subjects" (p. 8). This perspective is particularly relevant for critical ethnographers, who should seek to *make naked* our own incoming thoughts, feelings, perspectives, and histories, providing relevant context for how these parts of ourselves interact with our research processes and participants.

> [P]ositionality requires that we direct our attention beyond our individual or subjective selves. Instead, we attend to how our subjectivity in relation to others informs and is informed by our engagement and representation of others. We are not simply subjects but we are subjects in dialogue with others. (Madison, 2012, p. 10)

Positionality interrogates an often-false dichotomy between personal life and professional life (Johnson, 2009), as if these two entities are somehow easily separable. In my research, this blurring or interpenetration occurred constantly. While positionality is clearly important, this research was not primarily about me. It was about a community of individuals living at the intersections of the problematic dichotomies of public and private, human and nature. However, one of the potential paths forward in this dilemma is for individuals coming from a place of greater privilege to recognize and perhaps eschew some of those privileges, so as not to discount the possibilities that come with researcher reflexivity. As much as possible, the ethnographic narratives in this research resist "the trap of gratuitous self-centeredness" (Madison, 2012, p. 9). My interests were in learning about these individuals' experiences through participant observation and interviewing; I also learned much about myself (Fontana & Frey, 2008), creating a situation that is hopefully mutually beneficial for all parties involved (i.e., Delgado-Gaitan, 1993). Self-exploration enables social justice researchers to see the myriad ways in which we, ourselves, are also often implicated in the systems of injustice that we critique.

> Throughout the ethnographic process, I tried to maintain a careful perspective on my own positionality. In addition to chronicling the events and interactions on the Hillside, I also attempted to explore and explain my own feelings and perspectives, with particular attention to how I changed through the ethnographic research process.[5] I not only used my fieldnotes as a space to say "what happened" on the Hillside, I also used it as a space to uncover and inspect any preconceived notions that I brought into the ethnographic experience. The goal, in this case, was not to reduce or eliminate bias, but to acknowledge my incoming positionalities as ever-present lenses through which I view my encounters with the Hillside community and my encounters with the world at large.
>
> Any ethnographic inquiry ultimately reflects the views of the researcher, requiring forthright and proactive disclosure. Given the context of my ethnographic immersion, I also took into consideration

my personal welfare throughout this research, not only for safety purposes, but also for data consistency and trustworthiness (Nilan, 2002). That said, over the more than a year that I was "in the field," I was certainly in physically, socially, psychologically, and legally uncomfortable positions from time to time; positions that I now relish for their richness and their insight. "If ethnography is about anything it is about putting your body on the line. It is about being in a particular space for a particular period of time.... You can't do ethnography without embodied attention to the symbols and practices of a lived space". (Madison, 2006, p. 401)

Further Social Justice Implications

In ethnographies, various dimensions of method, theory, politics, and meaning become interwoven with the day-to-day practices of ethnographic field research. These daily practices can have vast ramifications for the improvement of people's lives by addressing the systemic inequities that exist throughout our social, political, economic, and environmental lives. Forms of activism or social justice for people involved in ethnographic research processes are often significant. Critical engagement in the form of political activism receives most attention when it focuses on large-scale, publicly visible forms of social justice advocacy. These efforts are obviously very important, but large-scale political change can ignore or neglect daily aspects of research processes as being potentially transformative encounters. Ethnographic research processes can serve as a series of transformative encounters for everyone involved in the process (researcher, participants, readers, audience, etc.), making it possible for ethnography to be inextricably linked to social justice.

While ethnography was historically and somewhat recently wedded to scientist necessities of objectivity, instrumentality, and the discovery of the "native other," contemporary ethnographies are much more likely to eschew their possibilities as a value-neutral, polititically uncharged methodology that is disinterested in advancing the welfare of those facing oppression at the hands of unjust systems and institutions. In this sense, social justice has interwoven itself not just into the aims of ethnographic inquiry, but into the actual data collection processes and analyses that have become part of the entire methodological process, from the beginning to its ongoing engagements. For instance, today, it is much more likely in ethnographies that research questions are developed with social justice concerns in mind; that researcher positionality is appropriately acknowledged, embraced, and implicated; that interactions, observations, and engagements with participants are more aware and sympathetic toward institutionalized inequities; that analytical processes are undertaken with specific aims toward participants' material and discursive emancipation; and that the ethnographic product(s), the various forms of representation of the data, have specifically political ends that seek to address injustices in many of their multifaceted and often hidden formulations.

Critical ethnographies such as those that confront sociopolitical issues of marginalization, oppression, and opposition are vitally important for academia and the public at large, but such relationships between researchers and research subjects/participants should not be taken lightly. Transforming the life experiences of those facing homelessness (for instance) into descriptive and analytic narratives can both educate and entertain readers (consumers). In this sense, ethnographies, like all methodologies in the social sciences, exploit research subjects as socioeconomic capital, and this relationship should be more explicitly acknowledged and critiqued. Ethnographers often produce products (narratives of marginalization, poverty, oppression, criminality, etc.) for people (consumers) who have never closely encountered such situations, except in the most removed and sensationalized manners. This ethnographic product is sold to them, either literally in the form of journal articles, books, or book chapters, or less directly in other forms of knowledge transfer. Selling the (often painful) experiences that other people face on a regular basis has the added benefits of providing academics and writers with accolades, job offers, professional promotion, and perhaps income from a grant or book sales. Researchers regularly gain professional benefit from their fieldwork and from the in-the-field cooperation of research subjects by way of presentations, published articles, books (including the words on these pages), and other prerequisites of academic career advancement.

Some of my work with the Hillside residents has benefitted some residents more than others, but in the end, I am the one who will likely most benefit from my experiences. I am certainly not the only academic to benefit from relationships with research participants, but researchers (and ethnographers) should leverage their forums and positionalities to address these undertheorized relationships. In a powerful reminder concerning ethnographies of criminality, Bourgois (1996) notes that "college-educated intellectuals are usually too elitist or too frightened to be capable of treating unemployed, drug-addicted, violent criminals with the respect and humanity that ethnographic methods require for meaningful dialogue to occur" (p. 249).

Ethnographers, like other critically reflexive methodologists, must ask difficult questions of themselves and the research products that emerge from our experiences. How am I implicated in the very systems of privilege and oppression that I seek to critique, and how is this implication represented in my ethnographic product(s)? What is the image of the individuals I create in my ethnographic narratives? Will I, perhaps unintentionally, (re)create stereotypical, objectified characters? Will I remain neutral, offering some facts about their lives, but concealing others? Will I share the political implications of the research? How will I present their sometimes awful behaviors for public consumption? Some of the Hillside residents have committed serious crimes, escaped prosecution, and now evade incarceration for these crimes. In my ethnography, do I transform these particular individuals into contemptible people, or create images of them as victims of institutionalized poverty, structural inequalities, and neoliberal revanchism? Balancing these extremes is difficult and tenuous. Ethnographers must make certain that readers understand the dilemmas and shortcomings, and are conscious of the tensions between different styles of research. Ethnographers can (perhaps unwittingly) become embroiled within (and reproduce) the very processes that they often seek to critique.

Researcher involvement is of particular interest in critical ethnographies. In critical ethnographic research, the researcher's intrusiveness in the setting is not an issue, but the manner in which they intrude is paramount. I tried diligently to do so in a way that was respectful, compassionate, and thoughtful. While I always intended to "do no harm" in my research, I also sought justice. My presence in the place and in the lives of the Hillside residents was undeniable, and this embedded sense informs my ethnographic descriptions, analysis, and interpretations. My interviewing and ethnographic experience designated my role as both the inquirer and the respondent, destabilizing classic notions of researcher–subject dualisms. Such a level of reflexivity removes the imagined neutrality that comes with much academic research, and it supports political involvement, a positive and sought-after outcome for critically informed academic perspectives. Ethnography, in its many forms, remains a powerful tool for many researchers; it becomes imperative, then, to use this methodological tool in ways that advance dignity, rights, equity, and justice.

Ethnography, previously just another social science method trying to understand the "other," is steadily transforming into its more critical form. Ethnographic inquiry into marginalized individuals and communities requires that researchers not only understand, but advocate for and advance the rights of participants. An early ethnographic interview with Max illustrated this point:

Max: What is it that you want me to tell you here?

Jeff: I don't know. I just want to understand your experience through life, you know? See where I can be a support or whatever.

Max: Well, I don't guess I got anything to say about that, 'cause it's all right here. Ain't nothing to hide. I don't gotta tell you nothing; you just gotta be out here and do it, live it like we live it. Then you'll understand. Then you'll see why we are who we are. You'll see why we get pissed off about things…. See if *you* don't want to change things after you've been out here with us a while.

NOTES

1. I never fully immersed myself into the culture of the Hillside. In addition to cultural factors, my various privileges prevented me from "pretending to be homeless" or "going native," as my existing support systems could not be dismissed.

2. Mead's pioneering anthropological work was posthumously and controversially criticized for its objectification, simplification, and basic inaccuracies regarding Samoan culture. Scholarship suggests that some of Mead's interactions with her research participants were elaborate hoaxes or jokes on the part of some of the Samoans. For critiques of Mead, see Freeman (1983, 1999).

3. It is possible that my relationship with individuals living on the Hillside was less than positive. Perhaps I was seen as a threatening outsider or even an agent who could expose them to authority figures. While I do not think that I was perceived in this manner, it is important to acknowledge this possibility.

4. Critical ethnographers often use the "co-generation" concept to acknowledge the agency and importance of not only the research participants, but also the authors of archival material and maps. This epistemological positioning further reinforces the disavowal of neutrality throughout the research process.

5. Critical ethnographies should consider including epistemological, experiential, and sociodemographic places from which researchers come, but also illustrate the ways in which some of these stances morph over ongoing ethnographic experience.

REFERENCES

Adler, P., & Adler, P. (1994). Observational techniques. In N. Denzin & Y. Lincoln (Eds.), *Handbook of qualitative research* (pp. 377–392). Thousand Oaks, CA: Sage.

Adler, P., & Adler, P. (1998). Forward: Moving backward. In J. Ferrell & M. Hamm (Eds.), *Ethnography at the edge: Crime, deviance, and field research* (pp. xii–xvi). Boston, MA: Northeastern University Press.

Anderson, N. (1923). *The hobo: The sociology of the homeless man*. Chicago, IL: University of Chicago Press.

Angrosino, M. (2008). Recontextualizing observation: Ethnography, pedagogy, and the prospects for a progressive political agenda. In N. Denzin & Y. Lincoln (Eds.), *Collecting and interpreting qualitative materials* (pp. 161–184). Thousand Oaks, CA: Sage.

Barton, A. C. (2001). Science education in urban settings: Seeking new ways of praxis through critical ethnography. *Journal of Research in Science Teaching, 28*(8), 899–917.

Bateson, G. (1936). *Naven: A survey of the problems suggested by a composite picture of the culture of a New Guinea tribe drawn from three points of view*. Palo Alto, CA: Stanford University Press.

Bernard, H. R. (2006). *Research methods in anthropology: Qualitative and quantitative approaches*, (4th edition). Lanham, MD: AltaMira Press.

Borneman, J., & Hammoudi, A. (Eds.) (2009). *Being there: The fieldwork encounter and the making of truth*. Berkeley, CA: University of California Press.

Bourgois, P. (1996). Confronting anthropology, education, and inner-city apartheid. *American Anthropologist, 98*, 249–258.

Brewer, J. (2000). *Ethnography*. Philadelphia, PA: Open University Press.

Bryman, A. (1984). The debate about quantitative and qualitative research: A question of method or epistemology? *The British Journal of Sociology, 35*, 75–92.

Chambers, E. (2003). Applied ethnography. In N. Denzin & Y. Lincoln. (Eds.), *Collecting and interpreting qualitative materials* (pp. 389–418). Thousand Oaks, CA: Sage.

Clastres, P. (1998). *Chronicle of the Guayaki Indians*. (P. Auster, Translator). London, UK: Faber and Faber.

Cressey, P. (1932). *The Taxi Dance Hall*. Chicago, IL: University of Chicago Press.

Delgado-Gaitan, C. (1993). Researching change and changing the researcher. *Harvard Educational Review, 63*(4), 389–411.

Douglas, M. (1963). *The Lele of the Kasai*. London, UK: Oxford University Press.

Emerson, R., Fretz, R., & Shaw, L. (2011). *Writing ethnographic fieldnotes* (2nd Ed.). Chicago, IL: University of Chicago Press.

Evans, M. (1988). Participant observation: The researcher as research tool. In J. Eyles & D. M. Smith (Eds.), *Qualitative methods in human geography* (pp. 197–218). Cambridge, MA: Polity Press.

Fairbanks, R., & Lloyd, R. (2011). Critical ethnography and the neoliberal city: The US example. *Ethnography, 12*(1), 3–11.

Fontana, A., & Frey, J. (2008). The interview: From neutral stance to political involvement. In N. Denzin & Y. Lincoln (Eds.), *Collecting and interpreting qualitative materials* (3rd ed.) (pp. 115–159). Thousand Oaks, CA: Sage.

Foucault, M. (1972). *The archaeology of knowledge*. New York, NY: Pantheon.

Freeman, D. (1983). *Margaret Mead and Samoa*. Cambridge, MA: Harvard University Press.

Freeman, D. (1999). *The fateful hoaxing of Margaret Mead: A historical analysis of her Samoan research*. Boulder, CO: Westview Press.

Giroux, H. (1983). *Critical theory and educational practice*. Melbourne, Australia: Deakin University Press.

Goodall, H. L. (2000). *Writing the new ethnography*. Lanham, MD: AltaMira Press.

Harvey, D. (2005). *A brief history of neoliberalism*. New York: Oxford University Press.

Holstein, J., & Gubrium, J. (2008). Interpretive practice and social action. In N. Denzin & Y. Lincoln (Eds.), *Strategies of qualitative inquiry* (3rd ed.) (pp. 173–202). Thousand Oaks, CA: Sage.

Johnson, C. W. (2009). Writing ourselves at risk: Using self-narrative in working for social justice. *Leisure Sciences, 31*(5), 483–489.

Lee, R. (1976). *Kalahari hunter-gatherers: Studies of the !Kung San and their neighbors*. Cambridge, MA: Harvard University Press.

Low, S. (2014). *Spatializing culture: An engaged anthropological approach to space and places*. New York: Routledge.

Madison, D. S. (2006). Staging fieldwork/Performing human rights. In D. S. Madison & J. Hamera (Eds.), *The Sage handbook for performance studies* (pp. 397–418). Thousand Oaks, CA: Sage.

Madison, D. S. (2007). Co-performative witnessing. *Cultural Studies, 21*(6), 826–831.

Madison, D. S. (2012). *Critical ethnography: Methods, ethics, and performance* (2nd ed.). Thousand Oaks, CA: Sage.

Malinowski, B. (1922). *Argonauts of the Western Pacific: An account of native enterprise and adventure in the Archipelagoes of Melanesian New Guinea*. London, UK: Routledge and Kegan Paul.

Mead, M. (1928). *Coming of age in Samoa: A psychological study of primitive youth*. New York, NY: Penguin.

Mitchell, D. (2002). Cultural landscapes: The dialectical landscape—recent landscape research in human geography. *Progress in Human Geography, 26*(3), 381–389.

Nilan, P. (2002). "Dangerous fieldwork" re-examined: The question of researcher subject position. *Qualitative Research, 2*(3), 363–386.

Perakyla, A. (2008). Analyzing talk and text. In N. Denzin & Y. Lincoln (Eds.), *Collecting and interpreting qualitative materials* (3rd ed.) (pp. 351–374). Thousand Oaks, CA: Sage.

Robbins, P. (2012). *Political ecology: A critical introduction.* Malden, MA: Blackwell.

Rose, G. (2001). *Visual methodologies.* Thousand Oaks, CA: Sage.

Rose, J. (2014). Ontologies of socioenvironmental justice: Homelessness and the production of social natures. *Journal of Leisure Research, 46*(3), 252–271.

Saldana, J. (2013). *The coding manual for qualitative researchers* (2nd ed.). Thousand Oaks, CA: Sage.

Scherer, J. C. (1995). Ethnographic photography in anthropological research. In P. Hockings (Ed.), *Principles of visual anthropology* (2nd ed.) (pp. 201–216). New York: Mouton de Gruyer.

Shaw, C. (1930). *The jack roller.* Chicago, IL: University of Chicago Press.

Spradley, J. P. (1979). *The ethnographic interview.* New York: Holt, Rinehart, and Winston.

Spradley, J. P. (1980). *Participant observation.* New York: Holt, Rinehart, and Winston.

Thrasher, F. (1927). *The gang.* Chicago, IL: University of Chicago Press.

Wolcott, H. F. (1999). *Ethnography: A way of seeing.* Walnut Creek, CA: AltaMira Press.

One *Day* on *Earth*: Featuring Social Justice in Case Study Research

Brett D. Lashua

[T]he way to re-enchant the world…is to stick to the concrete. (Rorty, 1991, p. 175)

Consider one day. What is your day like and how does it unfold? Who is involved in your day, what might you do, and where might you go? Why? Is this day like any other, or exceptional? How so? Also, consider the day as a snapshot in time and space: What is the frame or boundary of your snapshot? For instance, does considering your day start with a routine (e.g., awakening, getting dressed, breakfast, etc.), or does it start with establishing a context (e.g., a place, a room, a house, a city, a region, or global context)? Pondering these questions begins to sketch out a day and requires that you also consider *how* you go about investigating a day. That is, what counts as noteworthy in your day: is it the routes, routines and movements you make, the settings, or the social relations you encounter and embody? On what basis do these "things" count; that is, *why* do they matter? In addition, how could you go about documenting your day: a blog, journal or diary, fieldnotes, photos, or videos? As an opening exercise, considering one day and how it is ordered evokes the complexities of a case. A seemingly simple line of inquiry opens into a kaleidoscope of questions of what counts and what to record, descriptions of how the case operates, and analysis of why it matters.

In this chapter I will return to the idea of "one day" as an exemplary case throughout, particularly later when exploring a global participatory documentary filmmaking project called *One Day on Earth*

Corey W. Johnson and Diana C. Parry, editors, "*One Day on Earth*: Featuring Social Justice in Case Study Research" in *Fostering Social Justice Through Qualitative Research: A Methodological Guide,* pp. 161-189. © 2015 Left Coast Press, Inc. All rights reserved.

(2012a). To start, I agree with the supposition that at some level most qualitative research is case study (i.e., bounded or framed by some unit of analysis): a study of an individual, group, social process, location, organization, program, institution, or event (Yin, 2009). Some of my own scholarship is characteristic of case studies; for instance, focused on a classroom (Lashua, 2007), a small group (Lashua, 2013a), a neighborhood (Lashua, 2011), and a single event (Lashua, 2013b). However, these topics only become case studies when considered within wider analytical frames that address questions concerned with how or why something happens. For Thomas, "[t]he heart of case research lies in the in-depth analysis of what happens" (2011, p. 34). "One day" in itself is not yet a case study, but becomes one when one asks *how* a day is structured and *why* people do the things they do (Wieviorka, 1992; Yin, 2009).

Already this chapter is beginning to shade in a rough definition by highlighting the uniqueness, rich description, multiple views and significance of context in case studies. As I further sketch out the possibilities of case study research, the chapter considers methodological questions (i.e., asking what kinds of "things" one can know through case study approaches), in concert with questions of methods or "how to" conduct a case study (i.e., the steps taken to carry out case study research). Both sets of questions are addressed in regard to pursuing possibilities for social justice through qualitative research practices (Denzin & Giardina, 2009). First, I develop definitions by tracing a line through the historical roots and disciplinary routes in the development of case study research. Next, I address strategies for data collection and analysis before finally delving further into questions of how qualitative case study research may change the world, grounded in the example of *One Day on Earth*.

Historical and Disciplinary Roots and Routes

By way of exploring the background of case study research, first I want to continue sketching out a rough definition. At a glance case study research appears so obvious—investigating a specific case—that it warrants little explanation. Yet for VanWynsberghe and Khan (2007, p. 80) the term *case study* is so often "irregularly, randomly, and poorly defined" or "used as a catch-all category" that it "loses its meaning." Similarly, Stake (2005) is concerned that "here and there, researchers will call anything they please a case study" (p. 445). Tight (2010, p. 329) appears exasperated when asking if case studies were "a method, a methodology, a strategy, a design, an approach, or what?"

while Gerring (2004, p. 342) laments the case study as "a definitional morass." For something so apparently simple, what's so complicated about case study research?

While academic literature offers multiple, flexible, and at times competing definitions (Lincoln & Guba, 1985), case study research does tend to share some characteristics. These include: (1) being an in-depth exploration of a real-life context, and (2) attempting to address questions of *how* or *why* a social context operates (Yin, 2009). In this regard, Stake agrees, offering that a "case study concentrates on experiential knowledge of the case and close attention to the influence of its social, political and other contexts" (2005, p. 444). Case study research is further characterized by small and clearly bounded samples or "units of analysis," such as a biography, a family, a neighborhood, or, as I mention above, one day. However, as Tight (2010) laments, case study scholars differ in their definitions and uses of the "case study" label. Most definitions tend to cleave between those that view case study as a method (Yin, 2009) or an object to be studied (Stake, 1995). That is, what constitutes a case? Considering one day: is your case the day itself, or is it the way you study your day? For Thomas (2011, p. 3), a case study is a "thing in itself," whereas for others a case study approach is a method that has overlapped and blurred with other approaches such as ethnographic fieldwork, participant observation, or life history research (Gomm, Hammersley, & Foster, 2000). The differences between these definitions are perhaps better understood as characteristic strengths and weaknesses rather than points of opposition. As I discuss later, these conceptualizations have some bearing on case study research design and data collection steps.

Whether method or object, and contrary to simplistic appearances, case study research "elevates a view of life in its complexity" (Thomas, 2011, p. ix), and aims to grapple with the intricacy of a context in all of its multifaceted and glorious details. For Stake, case study research involves engaging with the "particularity and complexity of a single case, coming to understand its activity within important circumstances" (1995, p. xi). Specifics, particulars, and minutiae matter: case study researchers should ground their cases and get "close to the action" in the concrete aspects of life that Rorty (channeling John Dewey) argues will "re-enchant the world" (1991, p. 175). To address questions of why and how such concrete details and particulars matter, it is important to understand the development of case study research within the social sciences.

Case study research is at least as old as the social sciences, if not older and broader. After all, detectives do "cases," as do lawyers, doctors, and counselors (Gomm, Hammersley, & Foster, 2000). Considering that many social science disciplines, including anthropology, sociology and psychology, are fairly "young," case study research has deep roots; case study approaches are sometimes called "case work" or "case history," for example, in Freud's ([1905] 1963) classic case studies of hysteria. Despite its position as "the first method of social science," case study research has a "neglected history" (Gerring 2007, p. x). Arguably this history is important in understanding how qualitative research has changed the world and has been part of critiques of the (inequitably) changing world.

For Johansson (2003), the first generation of case studies appeared around 1900 within the emerging discipline of anthropology, and extended through the fieldwork of scholars such as Franz Boas, Bronislaw Malinowski, and George H. Mead, each of whom sought to understand in rich detail the lived experiences of particular groups of people. Case study approaches also featured in pioneering sociological research. One notable early case study researcher was Frederic Le Play, a mining engineer and amateur sociologist who spent much of his time during the mid-nineteenth century living with working-class French families (Gerring, 2007; Porter, 2011; Thomas, 2011). His case studies of family life condemned the conditions of French workers and led to government social and economic reforms. Crucially, these early sociological and anthropological case studies ran counter to evolutionary biological science, which was gathering strength at the time. The scholarship of Le Play, Boas, and others who followed (e.g., symbolic interactionists) argued forcefully that human behaviors and cultural differences are produced through social relations, learning, and interaction, not by inherent biology and genetics. Therefore, it can be argued that early case study research was important not only in terms of challenging social injustice across a range of differences (e.g., explaining how class inequalities perpetuate poverty and debunking racialized differences of intelligence, for instance in Boas's [1899] work, based on social context instead of skull diameter!), but also for laying foundations for constructivist research.

This landmark case work, and the emerging constructivist-interpretivist theories and philosophies of science that underpin it, developed further via the scholarship in what became known as the Chicago School of sociology from the 1920s through the 1940s (Deegan, 2001). Perhaps best known of these studies is William Foote Whyte's ([1943] 1993) *Street Corner Society: The Social Structure of an Italian Slum*. Like Le Play, Whyte also lived with a local working-class family, and argued that it was context—in this case "the slum" of Boston's North End—that influenced whether young men succeeded as "college boys" or failed and became "corner boys" (p. 272). Interestingly, Whyte's work is more widely considered now as a classic case of ethnographic participant observation than "read as it was originally intended by the author: as a multiple-case study of boys' gangs" (Johansson, 2003, p. 6). In addition to gangs and families, case studies in the Chicago School were concerned with topics that are now hallmarks of case study approaches: life histories, schools, the church, and other community organizations. Exemplary studies in this tradition—including Robert Park's (1925) *The City*, Frederic Thrasher's (1927) *The Gang*, Louis Wirth's (1928) *The Ghetto*, and Harvey Warren Zorbaugh's (1929) *The Gold Coast and the Slum*—were extensive investigations of particular groups and specific settings (Bryman, 2004). These studies aimed to understand small social groups and local communities (e.g., Wirth's study of Chicago's Jewish ghetto around the Maxwell Street market) as microcosms of society: as *cases*. These cases were constructed concretely, through "everyday face to face interactions in specific locations" to offer insights into "dynamic processes of social change, especially disorganizing and rapid changes" (Deegan, 2001, p. 11). That is, Chicago School researchers used case study approaches to understand *how* and *why* specific foci operated as they did: trademarks that I hope are becoming clear indicators of qualitative case study research. Chicago School case studies were important in their emphasis on the construction of meaning by people through their everyday actions, locations, and social relations.

Chicago School case studies were not without their critics. As Long (2007, p. 99) noted, "[f]or all its celebrated status, Whyte's (1943) study has been criticized for ignoring women (particularly the role of the mother in the family) and the church, two central pillars in Italian-American communities of the time." Other criticisms have included an over-determining emphasis on social structure, with accompanying underemphasis on individual agency and too much focus on deviance and criminality. Case study was also disparaged for its perceived lack of generalizability (an issue addressed later in this chapter); because of its specificity and particularity of context, can any one case be compared with any other? If not, what is the value of case study in building theory? How many cases does it take to provide enough evidence of "scientific" fact? By the 1950s, when more sophisticated quantitative methods (with greater statistical generalizability) associated with scientific positivism emerged as the dominant paradigm in social research, case study research fell out of favor. Many critics viewed case study and qualitative approaches more generally as "the weak sibling among social science research methods. Investigators who do case studies are regarded as having downgraded their academic disciplines. Case studies have similarly been denigrated as having insufficient precision (i.e., quantification), objectivity or rigor" (Yin, 2003, p. xiii). Despite these criticisms, the studies that fall within the broad traditions of the Chicago School and its predecessors were widely influential because of their exemplary use of qualitative case studies (Platt, 1992).

In addition to anthropology and sociology, the legacy of Chicago School case study approaches can be traced through research that led to the development of cultural studies. Important texts in the foundation of British cultural studies include E. P. Thompson's (1963) *The Making of the English Working Class,* readily viewed as a historical case study of class formation (Gerring, 2004). Building upon work by Thompson, Raymond Williams, Richard Hoggart, and, from the 1960s through the mid-1980s, researchers from the Centre for Contemporary Cultural Studies (CCCS) at the University of Birmingham (often referred to as the Birmingham School) produced a series of works that established cultural studies as a critical force in academic thought. Although not always identified specifically as *cases,* many CCCS studies adopted the foci and ethnographic observation approaches that had characterized Chicago School case study research methods. Yet CCCS researchers shifted their analytical emphases away from place and criminality to matters of style, power, and resistance. The foci of many of these groundbreaking CCCS studies were indeed often cases: small groups of young people, including Teddy Boys (Jefferson, 1976); school-age students (Willis, 1977); "idle" youth (Corrigan, 1976); Mods and Rockers (Cohen, 1972); hippies, bikers, or skinheads (Brake, 1977; Clarke, 1976); punks (Hebdige, 1979); and teen girls (McRobbie & Garber, 1976). Like Whyte's (1943) research, CCCS studies are now more widely heralded for their ethnographic (and also semiotic) approaches to studying subcultural style, yet they may be read usefully as case studies that aimed to understand specific moments of the changing cultural and political landscape of postwar Britain.

Because of its attention to questions of culture, power, context and change, cultural studies scholarship is ideal terrain for case study research. Reflecting the development of the academic field, one later and outstanding example in cultural studies research is Du Gay, Hall, Janes, Mackay and Negus's (1997) case study of the Sony Walkman portable cassette player. Du Gay et al. (1997) explored the Walkman's popularity as a cultural artifact by investigating meaning making, and remaking, in people's use of the Walkman through their theory of the "circuit of culture" (the role of representation, identity, production, consumption, and regulation in the cultural value of the Walkman). As a case, the Walkman is an "ideal type" for cultural analysis, echoed in later work by Bull (2007) on the iPod. Overall, scholarship within now-established cultural studies traditions often exemplify case study research that is concrete, contextual, and critical, within clearly bounded frames of analysis: hallmarks of case study research, whether it is labeled as such or not.

Although out of favor in some academic circles in the 1950s and 1960s, case study methods experienced something of a renaissance—particularly in education research—in the 1970s and 1980s (Bassey, 1999). During this rebirth, case study approaches were part of a broader turn toward qualitative inquiry that Denzin and Lincoln described as "a quiet methodological revolution" (1994, p. ix). Writing at the time, Simons (1980, p. 1) noted that "the use of case study in education has been comparatively recent; its specific relevance to education has not been explored to the same degree" as in sociology, anthropology, psychology, political science, law, and medicine. Simons (2009) provides a thorough account of the adoption and development of case studies approaches in education. In sum, Simons argues that in the 1960s and 1970s, many scholars recognized that positivist, quasi-experimental, quantitative studies had failed to illustrate the complexity of participant's subjective views of events and social relations in the contexts of their own lives. As part of the push toward more effective evaluations of educational programs and policies, Simons (2009) argues that the turn toward qualitative case study research took place in education because of its aims to understand the *how* and *why* in concrete, situated detail. As such, case studies in education "represented a sea-change in how evaluation could be conceived to contribute to social and political action.... [I]t signified a more direct participatory, if not transformative, role for certain groups in society" (Simons, 2009, p, 18).

Such a shift is evident, for example, in one recognized "classic" case study in education, Colin Lacey's (1970) *Hightown Grammar: The School as a Social System*. In his explorations of the issues that shape the experiences of students at the school, Lacey engaged with troubling questions of social inequality in education. Like case studies in the Chicago School tradition (e.g., Whyte, 1943) and CCCS (e.g., Corrigan, 1976; Willis, 1977) Lacey treated the Hightown Grammar School as a microcosm of wider society in seeking to understand the poor performance of working-class boys at school. Lacey noted how the school's process of differentiation between streams of high, middle, and low achievers made students in the lowest streams feel like failures, which reinforced their sense of class inferiority. By the same token, the social construction and abjection of their working-class identities reinforced their low-achieving performance.

Lacey's work is mirrored, and in some ways extended, by Herb Childress's (2000) study of a California high school, *Landscapes of Betrayal, Landscapes of Joy: Curtisville in the Lives of its Teenagers*. Bearing all of the classic hallmarks of critical, in-depth case study research, Childress spent a year hanging out with a small group of students in and around a high school. Through his attention to how schooling operates in the context of these young people's everyday lives, Childress reported that the education system is a "betrayal" of young people when schools are no longer the creative and joyful places they could be. Beyond the microcosm of each school, both Lacey's and Childress's accounts analyzed the social construction of students' life chances, vividly illustrated through in-depth case studies of schools; both case studies have challenged understandings of education, social class, and the power of place (Ellis, 2004). These are only two examples of case study research in education. Since the 1980s—particularly following the publication of Yin's (1984) *Case Study Research: Design and Methods*—case studies have flourished in education studies.

Case study approaches remain popular throughout the social sciences and beyond. Many case studies echo the earlier work noted above, particularly as they highlight key foci: small groups of young people, neighborhoods, housing, curricula, public spaces, and qualitative research. This begs the question: Does the proliferation of case study research show how useful these approaches are, or does it indicate Tight's (2010, p. 329) critique that the generic phrase "a case study of" has become too easily tacked on to studies "with little or no reference to the existing social research literature on case study"? This question highlights debates over whether "case study" is an object of study or comprehensive method, a point I address further in the next sections of this chapter. In this section, I have traced a crooked line through only four moments in the development and application of case study research (plus a brief note on its enduring popularity). Given the variety, flexibility, and complexity of case study, I have used these moments also to highlight some key characteristics of case study research.

Doing Qualitative Case Study Research: Strategies of Data Collection

Although case study definitions are often unclear, strategies for data collection in case study research are succinctly summarized by Thomas: "Case study has broad and capacious arms: it loves all methods" (2011, p. 37). For Becker (1998), case study methods are all "fieldwork" and often draw from across the range and variety of qualitative methods and ethnographic approaches, such as interviews, observations, surveys, etc. For Punch (2005, p. 144), "[t]he basic idea is that one case (or perhaps a small number of cases) will be studied in detail, using whatever methods seem appropriate." However, these methods are not chosen capriciously, with merely "whatever" might work. Rather, methods should be selected with due care and consideration of which approach will best fit to explain the case and the issues that circumscribe the case. For example, in my case study of "vanished" social clubs in Liverpool's Toxteth neighborhood (Lashua, 2011), my collaborators and I chose oral history interviews with older adults because we wanted to understand *how* and *why* the area had changed. Although these changes had erased the physical presence of the social clubs, many local residents remembered them fondly, and as important neighborhood foci. An oral history approach provided richly textured accounts—memories—that other methods, such as a qualitative survey, might not have allowed, and also resonated with social justice perspectives (Janesick, 2007). While the social clubs once figured significantly at the center of Liverpool's Black diasporic communities, there was very little information about them in the city's "official" archives and records; they were a "hidden history." As such, although I visited these archives, an archival case study wasn't the best approach either. The focus of the case required careful selection of its method while also considering the issues that inscribed or characterized the case, such as postcolonial race relations in the United Kingdom. An oral history case study provided powerful, detailed narratives that addressed the *how* and *why* of neighborhood change (a frequent focus of case study research). In sum, my point here is that case study design invites thoughtful consideration of the methods chosen to investigate a specific, bounded case (in this example, a Liverpool neighborhood) in view of wider issues (racialized relations and urban change).

In this section I focus on case study research design—selecting and shaping a case study—rather than sifting through the range of qualitative methods that might be selected to explore a case. In both Yin's (2009) and Stake's (2005) books, "most of the guidance given is fairly generic in nature, and could readily be applied to other qualitative, and even some quantitative, forms of research…. [Both books are] essentially generic qualitative research guides" (Tight, 2010, p. 333). Furthermore, as case studies are widely employed across different research milieu, the academic literature is replete with a variety of examples of ethnographic case studies, biographical case studies, or historical or archival case studies ranging across disciplines of sociology, education, psychology, political science (e.g., Allison's [1971] account of the Cuban Missile Crisis is widely cited as a classic case study), and beyond (e.g., nursing; see Houghton, Casey, Shaw, & Murphy, 2013; and in education, see Bassey, 2000): far too much to cover here. Qualitative methods are also well documented in numerous, outstanding reference textbooks (Atkinson & Delamont, 2011; Blaxter, Hughes, & Tight, 2006; Denscombe, 1998; Denzin & Lincoln, 2005; Hammersley & Atkinson, 2007; Long, 2007; Silverman, 2005) as elsewhere in this volume. I begin by exploring design possibilities of case studies before discussing the importance of developing multifaceted approaches to data collection in case study research.

Designing a Case Study

As noted earlier, conceptual definitions of case study research are not always clear, and in practice there are affordances and constraints that result from different definitions. These tend to diverge between those that position case studies as *things* and those who approach case study as a *method* (Yin, 2009). At the level of research design, case study may be understood as *both* the topic of inquiry *and* the inquiry itself; a case study can be understood as a situation and an all-encompassing method to collect evidence to explain and understand a situation (Yin, 2009). For instance, Yin (2011) offers a useful three-step method to conducting case study research, which I follow loosely here. Others extend the definition even further to challenge taken-for-granted ideas about how the world is constructed and the assumptions that underlie these ideas; that is, case study as a paradigm. This view is "more akin to the kind of portrayal of the social world that is characteristic of novelists, short-story writers and even poets" (Gomm, Hammersley & Foster, 2000, p. 5): a view I engage also when considering case study via documentary filmmaking.

Along with documentary filmmaking, writing poetry, and novels, case study research is sometimes compared to investigative journalism. Like journalists (and detectives), case study researchers should start from a position of curiosity, wonder, and even speculation. Such an exploratory focus makes case study approaches exciting and engaging opportunities for researchers who are interested in developing rich understandings of specific "things," relations, processes, and contexts. That is to say, qualitative case study research cares most about building a quality *case*. Such a case should be characterized by careful consideration of the issues which inform and frame the case before building up the detail and "thick description" used to describe a case's concrete context, making appropriate interpretations and producing an analysis (as I discuss later in this chapter) (Thomas, 2011). With a particular and strong focus on issues in mind, according to Yin (2009) the first step of case study method is "binding" your case (what might also be called "freezing the frame"), or clarifying what is your instance, phenomenon, or unit of analysis for the case.

How does a researcher begin to bind a case study? Because case studies are opportunities for researchers to learn (Stake, 2005), it is critical to start by selecting a case that's interesting. What makes a particular case stand out? Are you somehow already (intrinsically) connected with it? Is it a "typical" or "common" case, or is it an exceptional one (i.e., an outlier)? What has drawn you to this case, and what are the issues involved? Perhaps the draw has something to do with questions of social justice? Stake (2005) argues that the central pivot of a case study must be issues: "The selection of key issues is crucial" (p. 448), as these form its conceptual core structure. Binding the case helps to ensure that the study does not become too broad, vague, or simply too ambitious. While the researcher considers a particular, sharply focused case from the outset, issue development should continue throughout the study as ongoing and concrete descriptive, interpretative, and reflective "brainwork" (Stake, 2005). For Stake, the "simplest rule for method in qualitative casework is this: 'Place your best intellect into the thick of what is going on'" (2005, p. 449). This kind of brainwork allows the case study researcher to move back and forth between specific detail of the clearly bounded case and the wider issues that frame and contextualize it. However, the initial decisions made about the focus of the case—binding the case—are critical also in determining the approach and kind of case study that will be developed.

Accordingly, Yin (2011) described selecting the type of design as "step 2" in the case study method, following binding the case. The types of case study have been well documented (Baxter & Jack, 2008; David, 2006; Stake, 2005; Tight, 2010; Yin, 2009); I highlight only some case study designs, which are by no means exhaustive or exclusive. Yin (2009) categorizes explanatory, exploratory, or descriptive case studies, while differentiating between single, holistic case studies and multiple-case studies. Stake (2005) identifies case studies as intrinsic, instrumental, or collective. In brief (adapted from Baxter & Jack, 2008, pp. 547–549), I present a few case types:

- *Explanatory* cases explain the presumed causal links in real-life interventions that are too complex for the survey or experimental strategies (Yin, 2003);

- *Exploratory* cases explore those situations in which the intervention being evaluated has no clear, single set of outcomes (Yin, 2003);
- *Descriptive* cases describe an intervention or phenomenon and the real-life context in which it occurred (Yin, 2003);
- *Intrinsic* case studies aim "to better understand the case…. The purpose is not to come to understand some abstract construct or generic phenomenon" (Stake, 2005, p. 445);
- *Instrumental* case studies provide insight into an issue or help to refine a theory. "The case is of secondary interest; it plays a supportive role, facilitating our understanding of something else" (Stake, 2005, p. 445);
- *Multiple* or *Collective* case studies are "a number of cases [that] may be studied jointly in order to investigate a phenomenon, population, or general condition…an instrumental study extended to several cases" (Stake, 2005, p. 445–446).

The type or design of a case study is important for selecting its methods. Again, using one day as a context, to understand one person's journey through her day, a researcher might be interested in a single, holistic case study, and might employ face-to-face interviews or diaries to gain thorough evidence that helps to convey how she understands and navigates her day. If interested in understanding how she engaged in attempts to change the world during her day, the researcher would be interested in an *instrumental* case study, and a participant-observation approach might be better suited. A collective case study approach might aim to understand the daily experiences of many people involved in a single organization or event, and would necessitate different methods. In this latter regard, my exploration of the crowdsourced (i.e., made up of voluntary contributions from many people) documentary film *One Day on Earth* is perhaps best considered a collective, multiple-case study. In sum, a case study of "one day" could involve any of these approaches, and there is a direct relationship between the selection of the case, the type of case study, and the methods used to gather evidence for the case.

Thomas (2011, p. 94) argues that any decision about the type of case is not "the beginning and end" of one's reasons for a case study. It is not surprising, given parallels to a detective's aim to "solve a case," that the central purpose of data collection in case study approaches, whatever the methods, is to gather evidence in support of an idea or supposition. How does a researcher develop case evidence and context? Case study research may draw from a range of sources to illustrate and "flesh out" the rich details of a specifically focused case. Data collection in case study research should generate evidence that allows a researcher to "paint" as complete as possible a picture to illustrate how and why the case operates or happens. Continuing with the consideration of one day as our unit of analysis, what data sources might be drawn upon to study it? No matter the type of case study, data collection should involve developing multiple points of view, trying to describe the case from as many various angles as possible. Instead of a flat, static, two-dimensional view (i.e., "triangulation"), Richardson and St. Pierre (2005, p. 963) refer to this process as "crystallization." Using a range of carefully selected data sources for a case study ensures the issue is explored through different angles of approach, each presenting different facets of the context. Along similar lines, Thomas (2011) encourages what Foucault (1981, p. 4) called developing "a polyhedron of intelligibility"; that is, a researcher may best come to know much about a case by examining it as an object with many different sides (i.e., a polyhedron) rather than adopting a singular one- or "flat" two-dimensional view. This means that many data sources offering multiple points of view are sought in conducting a case study; a mix of data collection and analysis methods also may be used.

As I note at the opening of this section, data-gathering tools and techniques are, of course, nearly as diverse as potential objects of case study research. What matters in case study research is selecting methods that are fit for the purpose and that offer the best means of engaging with the case. For instance, I recall a recent undergraduate dissertation that offered a case study of initiation rituals or "hazing" on a university sports team. Curiously, the student had chosen focus group interviews for data collection. However, would athletes openly discuss the dangers, risks, and potential humiliations of hazing while sitting among their teammates? Interestingly, as an athlete already on the team, the researcher also attended and observed a handful of initiation events as part of the dissertation project. As participant-observer, the researcher's field notes provided a richly textured and highly critical account of these initiation processes, and produced a fairly compelling case of how initiations worked to secure order, power, and hierarchy within this particular team. That is, the fieldnotes worked well to describe and contextualize the case. The focus group interviews, as anticipated, reported only superficial, unproblematic statements about the usefulness of initiation ceremonies to feel a part of the team. In this descriptive case study, individual interviews might not have worked either; because the researcher was a senior member of the team, it was unlikely that junior players would divulge any criticism to her. Although this was a particularly sensitive case, the point is that the chosen methods must work well to allow the researcher an in-depth exploration of the *how* and *why* of the case. This example also highlights the importance of developing multiple points of view to better understand the case. Arguably, this stands for any good research project and its chosen method(s), but in case study research perhaps it holds a bit more, because context matters so very much in developing one's analysis. It is important to re-emphasize, as Flyvbjerg also pointed out, "[c]ases exist in context" (2001, p. 136), and developing context is central in case study research. Context matters throughout: in binding the case, collecting detailed data within the case, and then carefully considering the issues that frame that case. Furthermore, the next step involves linking contextualized issues to theories. Indeed, for Yin (2011), "step 3" in the case study method involves using case analysis to build theory. Accordingly, I explore the critical links between theory and analysis in the next section.

Between the Concrete and the Concept: Data Analysis in Case Study Research

Returning once again to the early Chicago School case studies, Znaniecki (1934, p. 25) argued that theory development involved "a movement from concrete reality to abstract concepts and from abstract concepts back to concrete reality—a ceaseless pulsation which keeps science alive and forging ahead." This back-and-forth relationship, or *dialectic*, hints at central issues and debates in the analysis of case study research. If a case is so very specific, particular, and contextual, how can it be useful in knowing something about other cases and contexts? To what does the analysis of just one case contribute? These are essentially questions of the interpretation, generalizability, and transferability of case study research. As Tight (2010) and Thomas (2011) note, there is often little to differentiate case study methods from other kinds of qualitative methods, such as looking for patterns, themes, or "critical moments" within the in-depth detail of the case study. What is, however, significant about case study analysis revolves around matters of interpretation (i.e., "making sense" of the case) and then connecting the rich and highly specific description to broader contexts and theorizations. These concerns are central to concepts and critiques of "scientific research" when pondering the production and transferability of knowledge.

These matters return to the disciplinary roots and developmental routes of case study considered earlier in this chapter. It is important to note again that most qualitative case study research is underpinned by the constructivist-interpretivist paradigm. In terms of constructivism (i.e., "the social construction of reality"; see Berger & Luckmann, 1966), case study researchers do not pursue sweeping "universal truths" of natural "reality"; this also comes back to questions of defining and binding a case. For Alasuutari (1996, p. 371):

> Instead of assuming that any corner of social reality leads to the traces of some universals to be pointed out in the final analysis, in cultural studies a case study is understood to reveal a local and historically specific cultural or "bounded" system.

By the same token, case studies are not exercises in limited subjective analysis involving intensive but ultimately trivial thought. As indicated above, through its development in anthropology, sociology, cultural studies, and education, case study research is useful in developing deeper understanding of social relations, agency, and structure, and in addressing questions of power (inequality) and cultural formations. For instance, case studies have shown how inequality perpetuates poverty, have critiqued scientific racism, and have contributed, more broadly, to social justice by calling attention to covert, unseen, ignored, or otherwise hidden processes that oppress, marginalize, or disenfranchise individuals or groups (Charmaz, 2005). In this regard, Flyvbjerg refutes as "oversimplification" the notion that "[o]ne cannot generalize on the basis of an individual case: therefore, the case study cannot contribute to scientific development" (2006, p. 221). Flyvbjerg (2006) is adamant that case studies are useful to help support and build theoretical understandings regarding the issues that surround a case. Arguably, individual case studies can contribute to addressing social justice issues and inequities. This is why Stake, Yin, Thomas, and other case scholars (e.g., David, 2006; Ruddin, 2006) emphasize the importance of linking a specific case focus with the wider issues that subsume the case.

Furthermore, theories should be derived from a case, rather than in control of it. That is, theory is not imposed "from above" to make sense of the case; rather, the case should lead the researcher to seek theoretical understandings that help explain the case "from the ground upward" (see chapter 3 in this volume). This may involve developing new theories, ideas, or "ways of seeing" the world when needed. In this regard, case study research, like most social research, is an active intervention into people's lives; as such, it often invites people, including the researcher, to question existing social relations and structures. It can therefore be a powerful tool for change, like in Le Play's early case work (see Porter, 2011), that leads participants (and potentially broader publics) to see the "case" and its context in new ways.

Thus the interpretation, generalizability, and transferability of case studies are interwoven concerns. One criticism of the case study method is that the case under study may not be representative of a wider social setting, and some critics argue that the results of case study research cannot be used to make generalizations. Is your "typical" day actually comparable to anyone else's day? How so, or not? What is meant by *typical* (David, 2006)? On this issue some scholars are absolute, often stating in opposition: "you cannot generalize from a single case" (Thomas 2011, p. 3) versus "[y]ou can generalize, stupid!" (Ruddin, 2006, p. 797). On one hand, Innes (2001) argues that although case study research produces empirically rich data, it is not possible to comment on the resonance of the results beyond that case example. As such, any case remains only a small-scale study in wonderfully contextual but isolated detail. On the other hand, like Ruddin (2006), Gerring (2004) argues that case studies should indeed "aim to generalize across a larger set of units" (p. 341). Lincoln and Guba also assert "any information found in any part must be characteristic of the whole" (2000, p. 43), and cases can be illustrative examples of wider phenomena. For example, arguably there are similarities in many people's experience of "one day," and a multiple-case study approach could allow the researcher to explore *how* and *why* these similarities (and dissimilarities) exist and operate. However, this remains a matter of debate within the case study literature.

These debates mirror broader shifts in qualitative research. Reflecting on a career in case study research, Bassey (2000, p. 2) admits he once "argued there were no empirical generalizations of use to teachers. I have changed my mind." Bassey offers that his initial opinion, formed regarding his scientific research in chemistry, had shifted due to the kinds of "fuzzy" generalizations possible in different research paradigms (e.g., constructivism). Despite these contradictions, it seems clear enough that case study research is useful indeed to describe particular detailed case contexts and then move the detail forward through analysis to allow the development of wider theoretical understandings of the case's issues.

On this note, regarding the challenges of developing broader "understanding" from case research, it is clear from the literature (e.g., Ruddin, 2006; Thomas, 2011) that the relevance and generalizability of any case study ultimately comes down to the reader who may interpret and make sense (or not) of the case study report. As in detective work, the case researcher's analysis must produce a convincing and well-evidenced account. As evidence (whether as a written account such as an academic paper or a novel, or as a documentary film as discussed below), the case study must—as also argued by Zna-niecki (1934)—offer enough concrete detail to allow any reader (or viewer) to gain access and insight into the lived "world" of the case while also framing the issues that subsume the case with sufficient scope to show how the "nitty-gritty" of everyday life operates within wider social processes. Without this kind of back-and-forth movement between the concrete and the conceptual, case studies may be wonderfully descriptive, yet lack broader relevance.

Case Study Research To Change the World: *One Day on Earth*

Finally, in addressing questions of the relevance of case study research as a "way to re-enchant the world" by "stick[ing] to the concrete" (Rorty, 1991, p. 175), I turn to a more extensive example of my own case study research. In doing so, I also follow Sennett's (2009) advice to "show, don't tell" (see also Thomas, 2011). Building from my opening example, I again present the idea of "one day," but this time as a collective or multiple-case study produced as an extraordinary documentary film, *One Day on Earth* (2012a). *One Day on Earth* (*ODOE*) was a collaborative documentary project; contributions were made by tens of thousands of volunteers from all over the world, filming on the same day: October 10, 2010 (10.10.10).[1] The global day of filming aimed to capture and archive "a world that is greatly interconnected, enormous, perilous, and wonderful" (*ODOE*, 2012b).[2] Although it started out as a small-scale endeavor by a handful of filmmakers, by its premiere *ODOE* had been produced in collaboration with the United Nations and more than 60 global charities; it premiered in more than 160 countries on Earth Day 2012 (April 22), including a screening at United Nations headquarters in New York City.[3] Here I use *ODOE* as an exemplary case to sift through and assess the affordances and constraints of this approach when engaging with qualitative research to change the world.

As a case study, *ODOE*'s structure charts the events in a single day—10.10.10—on the planet. This is the "binding" of the case, evidenced most obviously in footage at daybreak and nightfall at the film's beginning and end; the case's unit of analysis is clearly defined as one day. In addition, during the bulk of the daytime "action," the film's primary case structure is augmented through standalone sections focused on footage related to specific themes; these are the "issues" that subsume the case. For example, one section of the film features topical footage related to water (potable water, pollution, swimming, surfing, drought and floods, etc.). Other sections are ordered around themes such as children and youth, commerce, food, sport, music, education, and transport. As such, each video contribution forms part of a themed case, which in the aggregate comprise a multiple case—they are cases within cases (Stake 2005, 2013), what Yin (2009) refers to as "embedded" or "nested" cases (Thomas, 2011)—within the documentary film. The themed sections are bookended by brief pauses in the rapid-fire presentation of video clips. During these pauses (at the start of each new theme or issue), a statistic is shown on a plain black background to introduce the coming section, such as the "youthfulness" on Earth ("On 10.10.10, 26.3% of the world's population was under age 14"), the scale of global commerce ("On 10.10.10, over 172 billion dollars were spent"), or availability of potable water ("On 10.10.10, 1.3 billion people did not have access to clean water"). One reviewer disparaged these as "a series of factoids designed to wow us with the sheer accumulation of, well, everything" (Schenk, 2012). However, the accumulation of glorious, specific detail is both the task and the promise (to borrow a phrase from Mills [1959]) of case study research. After each "factoid," a sequence of video clips are presented to offer concrete evidence from user-generated footage shot around the world.

As a complex, multiple, or collective case study (Stake, 2013), *ODOE* was assembled from more than 3,000 hours of video shot on 10.10.10 by 19,000 volunteer contributors. The digital video files created by participants were uploaded via a link from the project's homepage (www.onedayonearth.org), then compiled and edited by a production team[4] led by the film's director, Kyle Ruddick. This approach to documentary filmmaking—using volunteer contributors—can be seen as part of social media trends collectively referred to as *crowdsourcing* (Brabham, 2010; Howe, 2009; Seltzer & Mahmoudi, 2012).[5] According to Howe (2009, p. 134), "crowdsourcing is rooted in a fundamentally egalitarian principle: every individual possesses some knowledge or talent that some other individual will find valuable. In the broadest terms, crowdsourcing involves making a connection between the two." In an era of user-generated media and online file sharing, crowdsourcing enables large numbers of people to connect and participate in support of shared interests or causes. Miah (2011) refers to such public and participatory activities as "citizen media" and champions its democratic politics. Similarly, Allen (2013) refers to the democratic potential of "citizen witnessing" through mass, participatory journalism. However, for Brabham (2010, p. 1125) the power of crowdsourcing is sheer quantity rather than qualitative depth: "the crowd's strength lies in its composite or aggregate of ideas, rather than in a collaboration of ideas.... This 'wisdom of crowds' is derived not from averaging solutions, but from aggregating them." That is, as *ODOE* powerfully illustrates, crowdsourcing approaches are capable of drawing in a vast quantity of user-generated materials, but making some sense of these materials requires a coordinated effort to pull it together coherently, or not, as some critics commented. Even so, a *New York Times* reviewer celebrated *ODOE*'s crowdsourcing approach:

> The crowd-sourced global diary, a new kind of documentary in which thousands of videos shot around the world at the same time are assembled into a concise chronicle of a day in the life of the planet, is an astonishing technological and organizational achievement. (Gold, 2012)

Crowdsourcing has been adopted for other film projects. For its premiere, *ODOE* was promoted as "the first film made in every country of the world on the same day and the largest collaboration of media creation in the world's history" (*ODOE*, 2012b). This tag line was an attempt to differentiate *ODOE* from similar projects produced at the same time, most notably *Life in a Day* (2011). Dubbed "Hollywood's YouTube collaboration" for its partnership with renowned directors Ridley Scott and Kevin Macdonald, *Life in a Day* was also assembled from crowd-sourced footage created and uploaded to YouTube by volunteer filmmakers. The United Kingdom's *Daily Telegraph* newspaper commented on the two films:

> While the premise is the same as *Life in a Day*—to create a time capsule, capturing scenes and perspectives from people around the globe on the same day—[Executive Producer] Litman and Ruddick's documentary is more culturally and environmentally minded than Ridley Scott's offering. (*One day on Earth captured on film*, 2011)

In both films, massive voluntary participation was invited to try to document the huge variety of activity that took place across the globe in one day, and graphically illustrate the complexity of this case. Ruddick (*ODOE*, 2012b) stated he thought of the film "as the world's new media time capsule." A contained "time capsule" that documents a moment or snapshot in time is another way of saying that *ODOE* was "bound" as a case.

As a catalyst for social change, *ODOE* also aimed to foster a social movement and community online. Politically, social media has offered revolutionary and potentially democratic ways to connect and empower people in ways that were undreamt of until fairly recently

(Jenkins & Thorburn, 2004). *ODOE*'s use of crowdsourcing offers an eye-catching illustration of the participatory scale, immediacy, and interconnectivity of global social movements and media making. Within the case's parameters of one day, although much of the contributed footage is quotidian and often mundane (e.g., having a drink of water), it is also overtly political and touches upon matters of social justice, peace, the plight of refugees, human rights, education, poverty, and other global inequities. As a series of multiple, collective, and nested cases, its foci are imminently and readily connected to a kaleidoscopic range of issues and wider theoretical frames, such as theories of globalization, media, citizenship, and participatory politics, that surround the case. Returning again to my opening gambit— to consider one day—*ODOE* is an incredible, global case study that invited "everyone, everywhere" to do the same. The results, while obviously not receiving contributions from *everyone*, are staggering, insightful, and visually evocative of the rich tapestry of all the action in one day on Earth.

Case Study Research and Social Justice Inquiry

Although the case study examples outlined above offer links to social justice inquiry, these relationships can be made more explicit. As noted, within the social sciences case study research has usefully addressed scientific racism (e.g., Boas, 1899), class inequalities related to locality and neighborhood (e.g., Whyte, [1943] 1993), questions of youth and marginalization (e.g., Willis, 1977), and disadvantage in education (e.g., Lacey, 1970), among other pressing social concerns. My central example, the crowd-sourced documentary film *One Day on Earth* (2012a), showcases the everyday, often mundane, and sometimes extraordinary action on Earth on October, 10, 2010. In each instance, the selection of "a case" and the issues that bind it are a political act: the researcher (or filmmaker) has selected something or someone that she is interested in, somehow already (intrinsically) connected with, or stands out to her (Stake, 2005). In addition, case study research is driven by a researcher's attempt to address questions of *how* or *why* a social context operates (Yin, 2009). This means that case study researchers are concerned with addressing the controversies, issues, or problems that contextualize and frame the case. These issues offer ready links to social justice inquiry.

For example, in my experience of conducting oral history interviews to produce a documentary film about the "vanished" social clubs in Liverpool's "L8" neighborhood (Lashua, 2011), the case study provided a powerful counternarrative in line with social justice inquiry; the stories of these clubs and the people who frequented them are important but largely unrecognized and unsung within the broader "official" history of Liverpool. Janesick (2007, p. 116) describes the potential for oral history interviews as a social justice project:

> [W]hen a person sets out to interview another human being, there is a written record eventually, so that knowledge of the past can serve to refute myths, half truths, fabrications, and faulty perspectives. This, alone, marks oral history as a social justice activity when the outsiders and peripheral members of society are included in oral history research projects.

This view of social justice inquiry is echoed, more broadly, by Chapman and Schwartz (2012, p. 25), who argue that "social justice researchers focus on the experiences of historically underserved communities and view participants as important agents in effecting change." As part of developing the context that explains a case, an understanding of history empowers people not only by highlighting their present condition, but also by showing that things have changed, and as such *can be changed*. Although writing specifically about oral history research and social justice, Janesick's (2007, p. 117) words are applicable more broadly to qualitative case study research and projects such as *ODOE*:

> Stories from individuals who may have been overlooked in traditional projects may now have the opportunity to have a voice. Not only that, we may all learn from those outside the mainstream, and we may learn more about the human condition overall. By learning about the lives, ways of knowing, culture, speech, and behavior of those on the periphery of society, we stand to learn more about our society as a whole. In fact we may become more aware of social justice issues as we come to understand the perspectives of another.

As a piece of filmmaking, *ODOE* also invited viewers to consider many different perspectives; this also echoes documentary styles of filmmaking that are interactive and interventionist (Lashua, 2010; Nichols, 1991). Moreover, as a filmmaking process, *ODOE* called on people to contribute directly to the creation of the documentary, to share some aspects of their stories, relations, and contexts of their lives. Therefore, as a collective case study of the politics of everyday life, *ODOE* exemplifies many of the characteristics that underscore social justice inquiry. For example, Denzin and Giardina (2009) call for an approach to inquiry that "makes a difference in everyday lives by promoting human dignity and social justice" (p. 13). Furthermore, in tune with the kind of collaborative, participatory approaches involved in *ODOE* (e.g., crowdsourcing), Denzin and Giardina also call for active, participatory research: "we are no longer called to *interpret* the world…we are called to *change* the world and to change it in ways that resist injustice while celebrating freedom and full, inclusive, participatory democracy" (2009, p. 13). In its emphases on matters of global quality of life, diversity and equity, and participatory action, *ODOE* represents a collective case study with social justice ambitions.

Because case study research seeks to address *how* or *why* something happens, it is an ideal partner for social justice inquiry. Its marriage to social justice returns case study research to some of the more radical aspects of its roots, as discussed earlier in this chapter. In case study design, when the initial idea or step of binding the case begins with social justice in mind, the potential impacts of the research help to concentrate the researcher's attention on addressing the *how* and *why* of the case. Data collection is fueled by ambitions to understand the underlying conditions, circumstances, or causes of the injustice(s) that subsume the case. Unless these underlying issues are the central foci of the study, the case will remain inadequately explained or unanswered. Therefore, attention to social justice sharpens the relevance of case study research. As a mode of social justice inquiry, case study research aspires to help "solve" a problem; through its case study report (or, as in the case I have used throughout this chapter, a documentary film), it aims to publicize a problem, help mobilize people toward collective action, and begin to right a perceived wrong. Case study research can play a vital part in movements for social justice, diversity, and equity (e.g., Gorski & Porthini, 2014).

Conclusions: The Not-So-Mysterious Case of Case Study Research?

In this chapter I have produced a kind of case study of case study research. Although offered in as much detail and concrete specificity as possible, like any case study, I provide only a partial snapshot of the huge variety of its focus and scope of its issues. Despite these constraints, I also have tried to demystify case study research, if not in the step-by-step methods (which, as noted, are widely covered in qualitative research texts), then in the definitions, purpose, and rationale of case study research. In addition, much of the beauty of case study research is in its potential for detailed attention to context, which is in turn dependent upon a case's clear limits and the boundaries of what constitutes the case. The more carefully selected and clearly defined the case, the more powerfully and vividly the researcher will be able to offer detail within it. Furthermore, the links between a case and the broader issues that surround it are crucial. As the examples noted throughout the chapter point out, case study research is a powerful way to engage directly with critical contemporary issues and social problems. That is to say, case study research can be more overtly political—the researcher has strong reasons for choosing a case—than other approaches.

Case study research provides a means for academics to grapple with the concrete relations in people's everyday lived experiences. Case studies, particularly when engaged through ethnographic fieldwork, offer more in-depth and detailed accounts than many other kinds of methods afford. In this regard, case study methodologies have served as a critique of positivist, quantitative, and dispassionately "hard" sciences. Through education research since the 1970s, the development of case study research has followed the broader turn toward qualitative methods in the social sciences and humanities (Denzin & Lincoln, 1994).

I have offered a brief discussion of the documentary film *One Day on Earth* to illustrate many of the characteristics, affordances, and constraints of case study research. Through its voluntary, participatory crowdsourcing approach to documentary filmmaking, *ODOE* served to record the mundane aspect of everyday life and also provided a catalyst for involvement, activism, and promotion of a number of global social justice issues. Case study research is more than a way to document the world; case study research can *change* the world.

NOTES

1. According to its production notes (*ODOE*, 2012b), "Ruddick choose 10/10/10 as the shoot date, calling it a 'blank slate holiday,' as it is memorable and allowed participants to make it their own celebration. 'Nearly everyone looks for something special to do on a day like 10/10/10, but that special thing is different for everyone. It's this sense of participatory ownership that made it a great day to inspire people.'"

2. Individually shot digital video was uploaded to a central archive and assembled by an organizing team in Los Angeles at a later date. Organizers have been involved with *ODOE* documentary events since 2008, with the footage filmed on October 10, 2010 (10.10.10) released as a full-length feature film in 2012: its production forms the hub of this chapter. Additional days of global filming events have taken place on November 11, 2011 (11.11.11) and December 12, 2012 (12.12.12) as part of a trilogy of film projects. It is estimated that 34,000 people worldwide filmed on 12.12.12.

3.   The email announcement sent to *ODOE* community members for the premiere said: "On Sunday, April 22nd, with the help of our incredible community of inspired media creators and non-profit partners, we will screen the first *One Day on Earth* film in every country in the world. Working closely with World Heritage Sites and the United Nations, we have the pleasure to bring local communities together in celebration for a truly worldwide cinema experience. From the ancient walls of Baku, Azerbaijan, to Stone City in Zanzibar, we want you to join us wherever you are, to help make this event as big as possible" (personal communication, February 22, 2012).

4.   *ODOE*'s production team included no less than 14 various executive, associate, and assistant producers, and no fewer than 27 various editors, footage reviewers, and "other crew" involving 250 participant outreach coordinators, more than 70 translators, and 1,486 "contributing cinematographers" (IMDB, 2013). The film's credits run more than eight minutes.

5.   Like the voluntary crowdsourced video contributions, financing for the editing and post-production on *ODOE* was "crowdfunded" using Kickstarter (www.kickstarter.com). Kickstarter is a funding platform for arts, film, music, design, and technology that allows individual backers to donate to projects that they deem worthwhile. The *ODOE* production team raised $44,637 (surpassing a $25,000 goal) from 1,083 individual backers.

REFERENCES

Alasuutari, P. (1996). Theorizing in qualitative research: A cultural studies approach. *Qualitative Inquiry, 2*(4), 371–384.

Allen, S. (2013). *Citizen witnessing: Revisioning journalism in times of crisis*. Cambridge, UK: Polity Press.

Allison, G. (1971). *Essence of decision: Explaining the Cuban missile crisis*. Boston: Little, Brown.

Atkinson, P., & Delamont, S. (2011). *Sage qualitative research methods*. London, UK: Sage.

Bassey, M. (1999). *Case study research in educational settings*. Buckingham, UK: Open University Press.

Bassey, M. (2000). Fuzzy generalizations and best estimates of trustworthiness: A step towards transforming research knowledge about learning into effective teaching practice. Retrieved from http://www.tlrp.org/pub/acadpub/Bassey2000.pdf

Baxter, P., & Jack, S. (2008). Qualitative case study methodology: Study design and implementation for novice researchers. *The Qualitative Report, 13*(4), 544–559.

Becker, H. S. (1998). *Tricks of the trade: How to think about your research while you're doing it.* Chicago, IL: University of Chicago Press.

Berger, P. L., & Luckmann, T. (1966). *The social construction of reality: A treatise in the sociology of knowledge.* New York: Anchor Books.

Blaxter, L., Hughes, C., & Tight, M. (2006). *How to research.* Maidenhead, UK: Open University Press.

Boas, F. (1899). Some recent criticisms of physical anthropology. *American Anthropologist, 1*(1), 98–106.

Brabham, D. C. (2010). Moving the crowd at Threadless. *Information, Communication and Society, 13*(8), 1122–1145.

Brake, M. (1977). *Hippies and skinheads–Sociological aspects of youth cultures.* Ph.D. Thesis. London, UK: London School of Economics.

Bryman, A. (2004). *Social research methods* (2nd Ed.). Oxford, UK: Oxford University Press.

Bull, M. (2007). *Sound moves: iPod culture and urban experience.* London, UK: Routledge.

Chapman, S., & Schwartz, J. P. (2012). Rejecting the null: Research and social justice means asking different questions. *Counseling and Values, 57*(1), 24–30.

Charmaz, K. (2005). Grounded theory in the 21st century. In N. K. Denzin & Y. S. Lincoln (Eds.), *The Sage handbook of qualitative research* (pp. 507–535). London, UK: Sage Publications.

Childress, H. (2000). *Landscapes of betrayal, landscapes of joy: Curtisville in the lives of its teenagers.* Albany, NY: State University of New York Press.

Clarke, J. (1976). The Skinheads and the magical recovery of community. In S. Hall & T. Jefferson (Eds.), *Resistance through rituals: Youth subcultures in post-war Britain* (pp. 80–83). London, UK: HarperCollins.

Cohen, S. (1972). *Folk devils and moral panics: The creation of the mods and the rockers.* Oxford, UK: Martin Robertson.

Corrigan, P. (1976). *The smash street kids.* London, UK: Paladin.

David, M. (2006). *Case study research.* London, UK: Sage.

Deegan, M. J. (2001). The Chicago school of ethnography. In P. A. Atkinson, A. Coffey, S. Delamont, J. Lofland, & L. Lofland (Eds.), *The handbook of ethnography* (pp. 11–25). London, UK: Sage.

Denscombe, M. (1998). *The good research guide: For small scale social research projects.* Buckingham, UK: Open University.

Denzin, N. K., & Giardina, M.D. (2009). *Qualitative inquiry and social justice.* Walnut Creek, CA: Left Coast Press.

Denzin, N. K., & Lincoln, Y. S. (Eds.). (1994). *Handbook of qualitative research.* London, UK: Sage.

Denzin, N. K., & Lincoln, Y. S. (Eds.). (2005). *The Sage handbook of qualitative research* (3rd ed.). Thousand Oaks, CA: Sage.

Du Gay, P., Hall, S., Janes, L., Mackay, H., & Negus, K. (1997). *Doing cultural studies: The story of the Sony Walkman*. London, UK: Sage.

Ellis, J. (2004). The significance of place in the curriculum of children's everyday lives. *Taboo: The Journal of Culture and Education, 8*(1), 23–42.

Flyvbjerg, B. (2001). *Making social science matter: Why social inquiry fails and how it can succeed again* (trans. Steven Sampson). Cambridge, UK: Cambridge University Press.

Flyvbjerg, B. (2006). Five misunderstandings about case-study research. *Qualitative Inquiry, 12*(2), 219–245.

Foucault, M. (1981). The order of discourse (trans. I. McLeod). In Young, R. (Ed.) *Untying the text: A poststructuralist reader* (pp. 48–78). London, UK: Routledge.

Freud, S. B. ([1905] 1963). *Dora: An analysis of a case of hysteria*. New York: Scribner.

Gerring, J. (2004). What is a case study and what is it good for? *American Political Science Review, 98*(2), 341–354.

Gerring, J. (2007). *Case study research: Principles and practices*. Cambridge, UK: Cambridge University Press.

Gold, D. M. (2012, June 1). Movie review: Flashes of a day in 2010, all over the world. The *New York Times*. Retrieved from http://movies.nytimes.com/2012/06/01/movies/one-day-on-earth-directed-by-kyle-ruddick.html?_r=1&

Gomm, R., Hammersley, M., & Foster, P. (Eds.). (2000). *Case study method: Key issues, key texts*. London, UK: Sage.

Gorski, P. C., & Porthini, S. G. (2014). *Case studies on diversity and social justice education*. New York: Routledge.

Hammersley, M., & Atkinson, P. (2007). *Ethnography: principles in practice* (3rd ed.). London, UK: Routledge.

Hebdige, D. (1979). *Subculture: The meaning of style*. London, UK: Methuen.

Houghton, C., Casey, D., Shaw, D., & Murphy, K. (2013). Rigour in qualitative case-study research. *Nurse Researcher, 20*(4), 12–17.

Howe, J. (2009). *Crowdsourcing: Why the power of the crowd is driving the future of business*. New York: Three Rivers Press.

Innes, M. (2001). Exemplar: Investigating the investigators—studying detective work. In N. Gilbert (Ed.), *Researching social life* (2nd ed.) (pp. 211–223). London, UK: Sage.

Internet Movie Database (IMDB). (2013). *One Day on Earth*. Retrieved from http://www.imdb.com/title/tt1900946/fullcredits?ref_=ttspec_sa_1

Janesick, V. J. (2007). Oral history as a social justice project: Issues for the qualitative researcher. *Qualitative Report, 12*(1), 111–121.

Jefferson, T. (1976). Cultural responses to the Teds: The defence of space and status. In S. Hall & T. Jefferson (Eds.), *Resistance through rituals: Youth Subcultures in Post-War Britain* (pp. 81–86). London: Hutchinson University Library.

Jenkins, H., & Thorburn, D. (2004). *Democracy and New Media*. Cambridge, MA: MIT Press.

Johansson, R. (2003). Case study methodology. In *Methodologies in housing research*. Stockholm: Royal Institute of Technology, International Association of People–Environment Studies (IAPS), pp. 1–14. Retrieved from http://www.infra.kth.se/BBA/IAPS%20PDF/paper%20Rolf%20Johansson%20ver%202.pdf

Lacey, C. (1970). *Hightown grammar: The school as a social system*. Manchester, UK: Manchester University Press.

Lashua, B. D. (2007). Making an album: Rap performance and a CD track listing as performance writing in The Beat of Boyle Street music programme. *Leisure Studies, 26*(4), 429–445.

Lashua, B. D. (2010). Crossing the line: Addressing youth leisure, violence and socio-geographic exclusion through documentary filmmaking. *Leisure Studies, 29*(2), 193–206.

Lashua, B. D. (2011). Popular music memoryscapes of Liverpool 8. *Media Fields Journal*, 3. Retrieved from http://www.mediafieldsjournal.org/popular-music-memories-of-live/

Lashua, B. D. (2013a). Community music and urban leisure: The Liverpool One Project. *International Journal of Community Music, 6*(2), 235–251.

Lashua, B. D. (2013b). Pop up cinema and place-shaping at Marshall's Mill: Urban cultural heritage and community. *Journal of Policy Research in Tourism, Leisure and Events, 5*(2), 123–138.

Life in a Day [DVD]. (2011). Directed by Kevin Macdonald. Washington, DC: National Geographic Films.

Lincoln, Y. S., & Guba, E. G. (1985). *Naturalistic inquiry*. London, UK: Sage.

Lincoln, Y. S., & Guba, E. G. (2000). The only generalization is: There is no generalization. In R. Gomm, M. Hammersley, & Foster, P. (Eds.) *Case study method: Key issues, key texts* (pp. 28–44). London, UK: Sage.

Long, J. (2007). *Researching sport, leisure and tourism*. London, UK: Sage.

McRobbie, A., & Garber, J. (1976). Girls and subcultures: An exploration. In S. Hall & T. Jefferson (Eds.), *Resistance through rituals: Youth subcultures in post-war Britain* (pp. 209–222). London, UK: Hutchinson University Library.

Miah, A. (2011) Towards Web 3.0: Mashing up work and leisure. In P. Bramham & S. Wagg (Eds.), *The new politics of leisure and pleasure* (pp. 136–152). Basingstoke, UK: Palgrave Macmillan.

Mills, C. W. (1959). *The sociological imagination*. Oxford, UK: Oxford University Press.

Nichols, B. (1991). *Representing reality: Issues and concepts in documentary*. Bloomington, IN: Indiana University Press.

One Day on Earth [DVD]. (2012a). Directed by Kyle Ruddick. Los Angeles: One Day on Earth, LLC.

One Day on Earth. (2012b). *One Day on Earth: Production notes.* Retrieved from http://www.onedayonearth.org/productionnotes

One day on Earth captured on film. (2011, 5 August). *Daily Telegraph.* Retrieved from http://www.telegraph.co.uk/culture/film/film-news/8683239/One-day-on-Earth-captured-on-film.html

Park, R. E. ([1925] 1974). The city: Suggestions for the investigation of human behavior in the urban environment. In R. E. Park, E. W. Burgess, & R. D. McKenzie (Eds.), *The City* (pp. 1–46). Chicago, IL: The University of Chicago Press.

Platt, J. (1992). "Case study" in American methodological thought. *Current Sociology, 40*(1), 17–48.

Porter, T. M. (2011). Reforming vision: The engineer Le Play learns to observe society sagely. In L. Daston & E. Lunbeck (Eds.), *Histories of scientific observation* (pp. 281–302). Chicago, IL: The University of Chicago Press.

Punch, K. (2005). *Introduction to social research: Quantitative and qualitative approaches* (2nd ed.). London, UK: Sage.

Richardson, L., & St. Pierre, E. (2005). Writing: A method of inquiry. In N. K. Denzin & Y. S. Lincoln (Eds.), *The Sage handbook of qualitative research* (pp. 959–978), London, UK: Sage Publications.

Rorty, R. (1991). *Philosophical papers.* Cambridge, UK: Cambridge University Press.

Ruddin, L. P. (2006). You can generalize stupid! Social scientists, Bent Flyvbjerg, and case study methodology. *Qualitative Methodology, 12*(4), 797–812.

Schenk, F. (2012, June 4). One Day on Earth: Film review. *The Hollywood Reporter.* Retrieved from http://www.hollywoodreporter.com/review/one-day-on-earth-fiilm-review-332672

Seltzer, E., & Mahmoudi, D. (2012). Citizen participation, open innovation, and crowdsourcing: Challenges and opportunities for planning. *Journal of Planning Literature, 28*(1), 3–18.

Sennett, R. (2009). *The craftsman.* London, UK: Penguin.

Silverman, D. (2005). *Doing qualitative research.* London, UK: Sage Publishing.

Simons, H. (1980). *Towards a science of the singular: Essays about case study in educational research and evaluation.* Norwich, UK: University of East Anglia, Centre for Applied Research in Education.

Simons, H. (2009). *Case study research in practice.* London, UK: Sage.

Stake, R. E. (1995). *The art of case study research.* Thousand Oaks, CA: Sage.

Stake, R. E. (2005). Qualitative case studies. In N. K. Denzin & Y. S. Lincoln (Eds.), *The Sage handbook of qualitative research* (3rd Ed.) (pp. 433–466). Thousand Oaks, CA: Sage.

Stake, R. E. (2013). *Multiple case study analysis*. New York: Guildford Press.

Thomas, G. (2011). *How to do your case study: A guide for students and researchers*. London, UK: Sage.

Thompson, E. P. (1963). *The making of the English working class*. London, UK: Victor Gollancz.

Thrasher, F. (1927). *The gang: A study of 1,313 gangs in Chicago*. Chicago, IL: The University of Chicago Press.

Tight, M. (2010). The curious case of case study: A viewpoint. *International Journal of Social Research Methodology, 13*(4), 329–339.

VanWynsberghe, R., & Khan, S. (2007). Redefining case study. *International Journal of Qualitative Methods, 6*(2), 80–94.

Whyte, W. F. ([1943] 1993). *Street corner society: The social structure of an Italian slum* (4th Ed.). Chicago, IL: The University of Chicago Press.

Wieviorka, M. (1992). Case studies: History or sociology? In C. C. Ragin & H. S. Becker (Eds.), *What is a case? Exploring the foundations of social inquiry*. Cambridge, UK: Cambridge University Press.

Willis, P. E. (1977). *Learning to labour: How working class kids get working class jobs*. Farnborough, UK: Saxon House.

Wirth, L. (1928). *The ghetto*. Chicago, IL: The University of Chicago Press.

Yin, R. K. (1984). *Case study research: Design and methods* (1st ed.). Thousand Oaks, CA: Sage.

Yin, R. K. (2003). *Case study research: Design and methods* (3rd ed.). Thousand Oaks, CA: Sage.

Yin, R. K. (2009). *Case study research: Design and methods* (4th ed.). London, UK: Sage.

Yin, R. K. (2011). *Applications of case study research*. London, UK: Sage.

Znaniecki, F. (1934). *The method of sociology*. New York: Farrar & Rinehart.

Zorbaugh, H. W. (1929). *The gold coast and the slum*. Chicago, IL: University of Chicago Press.

Moving Forward, Looking Back: Historical Inquiry for Social Justice

Tracy Penny Light

On May 14, 2013, an op-ed appeared in The *New York Times* detailing Angelina Jolie's "medical choice" to have her breasts removed via a double mastectomy. She explained that she carries "a 'faulty' gene, BRCA1, which sharply increases [her] risk of developing breast cancer and ovarian cancer" (Jolie, 2013). She told her readers that her "doctors estimated [she] had an 87 percent risk of breast cancer and a 50 percent risk of ovarian cancer, although the risk is different in the case of each woman" (Jolie, 2013). For this reason, because her mother and aunt both died of breast cancer, and her own desire to mother her children, she decided on the radical course of treatment. I say radical because as she herself noted, "only a fraction of breast cancers result from an inherited gene mutation. Those with a defect in BRCA1 have a 65 percent risk of getting it, on average" (Jolie, 2013). Yet these numbers may be misleading; according to the National Cancer Institute at the National Institutes of Health in the United States:

> Risk estimates that are based on families with many affected members may not accurately reflect the levels of risk for BRCA1 and BRCA2 mutation carriers in the general population. In addition, no data are available from long-term studies of the general population comparing cancer risk in women who have harmful BRCA1 or BRCA2 mutations with women who do not have such mutations. Therefore, the percentages given are estimates that may change as more data become available. (Landsman, 2013; National Cancer Institute, 2014)

Jolie's experience reflects a wider medical discourse that deals with shifting definitions of health, increasing agency of patients in determining their own role in health and how to prevent disease, and the ways that medical knowledge is translated from experts to the community. Understanding how to critique these issues in the contemporary context is important, but to do so effectively, we need to understand where ideas about, in this case, cancer treatment, the body, and cosmetic surgery, come from. Of course, we can make the same argument about really any issue we encounter today: everything has a history.

Cosmetic Surgery

Here I have used the term *cosmetic surgery* to describe Jolie's mastectomy because it was a procedure performed in the absence of disease as a proactive measure, whereas *plastic surgery* is generally viewed as a practice to treat abnormal or unhealthy/diseased bodies.

Historical inquiry can help us to explore the genealogy of ideas to document shifts in discourses and make more educated decisions about everything. We might not think, at first, that the case of Angelina Jolie's mastectomy is a social justice issue. As a medical historian, however, I see many potential challenges for citizens. For instance, at a basic level there are potential inequities in medical practice: Jolie is a Hollywood star with access to many doctors and procedures and does not face the challenges that many citizens in North America might encounter in terms of the cost of professionals and treatments. What does her story mean for the "average" citizen who might not have such access? Are patients without her means being oppressed by the telling of her story, or does it potentially liberate patients by providing them with a role model for their own experiences? By examining more closely the contemporary medical and popular discourses at play, it becomes evident that Jolie's experience is inextricably linked to current ideas about health and the body that promote the idea that we should alter ourselves to adhere to specific societal and cultural constructions of what it means to be healthy. Are these new constructions, or have doctors and society always viewed surgery this way? Have there always been social inequalities embedded in these discourses? To answer these questions, we need studies that pay close attention to the roots of these ideas and trace where they come from to understand how and when social inequalities and oppression existed in the past. In this chapter, I draw on this example of cosmetic surgery and health as well as others to argue that historical forms of inquiry allow us to identify the ways that injustice has come to be embedded in different social, historical, and cultural contexts. Employing the process of historical thinking can help us to trace the roots of marginalization to critique the ways that these injustices continue to remain unaddressed in our contemporary world. I begin by tracing the roots and methods of historical inquiry and then provide strategies for data collection and analysis to provide a foundation for using this approach to address social justice issues. This method allows us to bring to the surface "previously silenced histories" (Rossiter & Clarkson, 2013, p. 26) to ensure a more just society for all by fostering change today and in the future.

Historical and Disciplinary Roots

Why History?

In his 1946 book *The Idea of History*, R. G. Collingwood suggests that history is for "human self-knowledge" and that "the value of history…is that it teaches us what man has done and thus what man is (p. 10). Peter Stearns (1998) notes that, "history should be studied because it is essential to individuals and to society, and because it harbors beauty" (p. 1). These two statements, taken together, suggest that the merit of historical inquiry is that it can provide insight into the ways in which we have come to know or understand the world, and that it allows us to uncover why we believe what we do. Of course, the authors are separated by fifty years and we can see instantly that the way in which each historian conceived of history was quite different, despite some inherent similarities. For Collingwood, writing at the end of World War II, history was about men and the important role they played in the world. Today, we might find this sentiment offensive, particularly if we adhere to a feminist positionality. If this is the case, we might prefer Stearns' notion that history is important not only for individuals, but also for society, as it implies that we all have a role to play as historical actors. Part of the challenge for those who are learning to think historically is to develop the ability to situate perspectives within the time and place in which they were conceived. We also need to learn to move beyond simply exploring the causes of historical events toward a consideration of "…the [complex] interplay of causal factors ranging from the focused influence of the choices made by historical actors to the broad influence of prevailing social, political, cultural, and economic conditions" (Seixas & Morton, 2013, p. 104). In other words, Angelina Jolie's decision to have a double mastectomy is not only about her discovery that she carries the BRCA1 gene, but rather is connected to wider influences, including the history of her family's experience with cancer, the trust that society places in medical science and doctors, her ability to afford health care and a variety of procedures, the influences of her doctors' beliefs about medicine and science, and so on. While historians can never understand every factor in the web of causality (nor do they seek to), they do employ a critical approach to determine which factors will allow them to best understand historical events and to situate those events in a wider context, paying attention to—and having empathy for—actors whose viewpoints might be different from ours today. In other words, historical inquiry focuses on the interpretation of events, which is shaped by the various documents and perspectives explored by the researcher and the process of historical thinking they employ.

Causality

Causality is an interesting concept in history. While it may have been considered the goal in histories of the past, today most historians would argue that it is impossible to trace direct causes for events because of the multiple perspectives and the impossibility of tracing each one to certainty.

My definition of historical thinking is most closely embodied in what van Drie and van Boxtel (2008) describe as "historical reasoning." For them, historical reasoning is most focused on "activity and knowledge use" and is "in line with socio-constructivist and socio-cultural theories of learning which argue that knowledge is actively constructed, rather than transmitted or passively received" (p. 88). They argue that much of the research related to historical thinking focuses on one activity (typically the use of evidence) when, in reality, historical reasoning involves a "whole range of more or less related activities" (p. 88). This approach to historical thinking takes into account what Seixas and Morton (2013) call "the big six historical thinking concepts": historical significance, evidence, continuity and change, cause and consequence, historical perspectives, and ethical dimensions. Defining and practicing historical thinking allows researchers to arrive at their interpretation and to explain how they got there. Unpacking the web of factors can help to illuminate ways that the past helps us to understand our contemporary world. In this, there is a logical connection to social justice because history allows us to clarify inequities and systems of oppression rooted in the past and explore the ways that these shift and change over time, thereby enabling us to make different decisions in the future. For instance, in the case of Angelina Jolie's mastectomy, we need to consider the ways that cancer was diagnosed and treated before the discovery of the BRCA1 and BRCA2 genes, and how this relatively new discovery has shifted both the understanding and treatments of cancer in women. While we might approach historical thinking this way today, the practice and products of history have not always been viewed in this manner.

History of Historical Thinking

History, like other disciplines, has its own past. Traditional historical inquiry, before the linguistic turn, tended to be rooted in either relativism or narrative.

Relativism

It might seem simplistic to say, "it's all relative," but in terms of historical inquiry, that basically says it all. More traditional relativists looked for the various factors that might influence historical actors: for Marx, economics provided the lens through which to understand why historical actors behaved the way they did. Since the linguistic turn, relativism has come to mean that there is no "truth" to be uncovered in history; rather, everything is an interpretation based on the evidence the researcher draws on to come to that interpretation.

Narrative

Traditionally, narratives (or grand narratives) were overarching stories about important events (like wars) and/or historical actors (great men) that historians viewed as pivotal in shaping the past. Today, while some histories might appear to take a narrative form and structure (they tell a story), they are more likely to be nuanced, with the historian aiming to talk about a variety of historical actors and perspectives that might have shaped events in the past.

Relativistic historians view the artifacts of the past as having histories of their own; those historical actors who left evidence were shaped by the time and place that they lived and that context was translated into those texts. For example, in his book *What Is History?*, E. H. Carr suggests that history is shaped by the people who write it, and that those people are "products of their own times, bringing particular ideas and ideologies to bear on the past" (Carr, 1961; Evans, 1999, p. 2). A relativistic approach to the Angelina Jolie case would explore the ways that doctors understand cancer and cancer treatment today, and where that understanding comes from. The other traditional form of historical inquiry privileged historical narrative, which, at its core, focused on political events and often the "great men" of history. In contrast to Carr's take on the nature of history and historical study, G. R. Elton's (1967) book *The Practice of History* defends the idea that history and historical study can be objective and therefore lead us to the "truth" about what happened in the past. According to Elton, the core of historical study should be political events, and information about these events should be drawn from documentary evidence. In other words, he argues that the documents themselves tell the story of the past, and the historian's job is simply to read and record what the documents say. If applied to the example of the treatment of breast cancer, this approach suggests that simply reading the scientific documents related to the BRCA1 and BRCA2 genes would tell us all that we need to know about how these genes affect cancer treatment. However, we know that even the National Cancer Institute has suggested that the quantitative data about those genes are currently inconclusive. As such, a strictly narrative approach to understanding the past seems overly simplistic and even somewhat naive today. Yet, even with the emergence of new social and quantitative approaches to history in the 1970s and 1980s that emphasized the importance of social history and the need to understand all aspects of society, these traditional viewpoints underpinned historical thinking and the resulting historiography.

Historiography

Historiography is, at the most basic level, the history of history writing. Historians and other scholars examine particular topics in history (for instance, historiography of medicine in Canada) to trace where ideas, methodologies, and approaches to the study and writing of history come from. In fact, the study of the historiography on a topic is as important as the topics of inquiry themselves. Implicit in the study of historiography is an examination of the scholars who write history, who they are, where they were trained, how they were influenced, and their theoretical approaches to understanding a topic. We can trace, through historiography, shifts and changes in the writing of a topic to better understand how knowledge on a topic has evolved.

However, since the 1980s, all of the various approaches mentioned above have been in question. The linguistic turn called into question the ability of some historians to reconcile the idea that language itself is a construction, suggesting that we can never truly know the "truth" about the past, and it has led some historians to claim that history is dead.[1] Other historians, however, undaunted by the idea that there is no objective past to be uncovered, have taken the opportunity to employ new approaches to their studies, opening up more opportunities for understanding how ideas of the past can be relevant today.

Historical forms of inquiry enable researchers to ask critical questions not only of the past, but also of the world around us to understand contemporary issues; this is at the heart of historical inquiry for social change. The ways in which historical inquiry is employed is essential for pursuing such studies.

Employing Historical Thinking

Once the decision is made to conduct historical research, using historical thinking is necessary to ensure a credible interpretation. Seixas and Morton's (2013) six steps of historical thinking can be used to explore the differences between approaches to historical study.[2] Regardless of the variation in methodological approach, these steps should always be applied in some manner. The ways in which different approaches deal with the six steps are covered in more detail here.

Historical Significance The issue of determining historical significance is important for researchers because it affects how we identify topics worthy of further study. Paying close attention to social justice issues often leads us to explore topics that have previously been unexplored or even deemed unworthy of study. For instance, lack of attention to inequities in health care systems might mean that we take at face value the hype around Angelina Jolie's surgery rather than asking critical questions about whether her experience can be more broadly generalized to cancer treatment for other women. In this example, I consider her writing on the topic and public support for preemptive surgery significant because her status as a celebrity means that her experience is linked to broader issues that are important because they have had (or will have) some kind of impact on society. Those engaged in historical forms of inquiry then might consider particular historical actors (i.e., Jolie, her doctors, etc.) and their role in influencing the past, specific events, or broader developments that have shaped the way we understand the world today. These people, events, or developments might have significance for us because of their ability to affect particular ideas, ideologies, worldviews. For example, how many women will decide to have the preemptive surgery (if it is an option) because Jolie did so? The determination of historical significance often varies in different times and places (Seixas & Morton, 2013; Wineburg, 2001). In other words, things that may be historically significant for us today in North America may not be of interest to academics in the Global South. Similarly, they may not have been of interest at all to researchers in other time periods. In a historical study, context is everything; it shapes not only the questions we ask, but also how we understand and interpret the evidence that we find in light of social justice, among other goals.

Evidence Determining the historical significance shapes the research question and, by association, the evidence consulted to form an interpretation that answers it. Evidence (or data) can be qualitative and/or quantitative in nature and must be systematically and rigorously analyzed to suit the methodology used to construct a plausible interpretation of the past. The types of evidence consulted are an important consideration for researchers because the evidence itself influences the interpretation. For instance, examining medical literature written for doctors will provide a much different picture of cancer treatment than literature produced for popular consumption.

Continuity and Change Just as the types of evidence consulted will affect the interpretation, so too will paying close attention to when there were shifts/changes in the past with different topics of study. Effective historical inquiry projects seek to understand continuities and changes to situate the topic of study within broader social and cultural contexts. At times, society changed rapidly, or not at all: for instance, one might argue that the women's liberation movement fostered significant changes for women in North America that created more equitable social conditions. However, we might also argue that, despite political, social and educational advances, the expectations for women or prescriptions for femininity have not been altered significantly (Penny Light, 2013). As Seixas and Morton (2013) argue, one of the keys to continuity and change is to look for change where common sense suggests that there has been none and, similarly, to look for continuities where we assumed that there was change. To do this, we may compare different aspects of the past and present or examine a particular time period (for instance, interwar Canada).

Cause and Consequence The examination of cause and consequence in history is rooted in understanding the ways that historical actors were affected and influenced by the past, and even how they resisted the ways events unfolded in the past. Understanding why people behaved a certain way in other periods, the context in which they acted, and the variety of influences that played on their motivations are all important considerations when doing history. The theoretical perspective and methodological approach of the historian, together with the types of evidence explored, often leads to differences in how causes and consequences are interpreted and understood.

Historical Perspectives It is important not to impose our contemporary sensibilities on a reading of the past. We might think about this aspect of historical thinking as empathy. People living in the past were shaped by and understood the world differently than we do. Consider people living during World War I: their access to information was quite different than it is for us today. Since they did not (and could not) receive immediate updates on the home front about what was happening on the front lines, their perspectives and understanding of the war were different than our understanding of contemporary wars because we are shaped by our ability to access information almost whenever and wherever we want. It might be difficult to understand how citizens living on the home front understood war in 1914 because our experiences are so different. Empathy in historical inquiry emphasizes the need for the researcher to strive not only to understand what people did in a different time period, but also to attempt to get at why they did what they did given their own beliefs, customs, and values. Regardless of our own positionality, we must privilege the historical context in which actors moved through the world. To do this, we need to situate historical inquiry within the context in which historical actors lived. Paying attention to diverse perspectives is as important as being careful not to take for granted previous interpretations of the past. Since history is all about interpretation, we need to situate our own perspectives in the present and work to understand the important differences between the historical context we are studying and the one in which we live.

Ethical Dimensions The ethical dimension of historical inquiry is of paramount interest to those of us undertaking historical analysis for social justice. Considering the ways that society has been oppressive and unjust for certain members in the past can help us to make different decisions in our contemporary context and lead us to consider our responsibilities as citizens in decision-making today. At the same time, we need to appreciate and take into account that our ethical stance today may be different than those who acted in the past. This does not mean, however, that we need to remain neutral about historical events: in the case of Angelina Jolie's choice, for instance, historical inquiry allows us to contextualize her decision-making based on the evolving understanding of cancer prevention and treatment, to come to an opinion that takes into account the various stakeholders in such practices. Another example is that today many people view eugenics, the practice of connecting social problems to biological causes and attempting to breed out such problems through controls such as marriage restrictions, segregation, and even the sterilization of those who were viewed to be "unfit," as unjust (McLaren, 1990).

Eugenics

Eugenics was developed by Francis Galton (a cousin of Charles Darwin) in 1883 and is the belief and practice of connecting social problems to biological causes. At the root of eugenics is the idea that the genetic quality of the human race can be improved by promoting reproduction by those people who exhibit desirable traits and limiting (or even preventing) the reproduction of those deemed undesirable.

Yet, in earlier periods (for instance, post–World War I Canada), these practices were believed to be part of a larger solution to the rebuilding of the race after the losses of the war. While we may not agree with such approaches, particularly in light of abuses of this type of thinking, as was the case in Nazi Germany, it is important not to impose our values on historical actors. Instead, we ought to aim to understand why and how they held such beliefs. This is particularly important if our aim is to avoid social injustices in the future.

Given the desire to act in a socially just way, there is another dimension of ethical thinking that should be attended to in historical inquiry. We need to be ethical in terms of the reporting of our findings. Here I am referring especially to the need to respect the privacy of historical actors and ensure that in constructing historical accounts we do not unintentionally cause harm to the actors themselves or their descendants. While this is often more of a concern with more contemporary historical studies in which the actors involved may provide accounts (for instance, through oral history), it is important to consider how readers might view our interpretations and ensure that efforts are made to be ethical in our reports.

Ethics

Ethics deals with questions of morality in that it seeks to determine what is right/wrong or just/unjust in practice. Ethics guides our actions, whether it is in living out our daily lives or in terms of how we conduct our research.

It also suggests that we have a duty to report findings that might have an impact on contemporary policymaking. A good example of this comes out of the work of Mosby (2013). While conducting doctoral research on the history of food during World War II, he uncovered evidence that the Canadian government performed unauthorized studies on human subjects in First Nations communities and residential schools. Upon publication of this research, attention has been turned to these practices and even led to a national day of protest by Canada's First Nations. What can be learned from this example is the need to pay attention to ethical issues that might arise in historical inquiry projects and plan for appropriate ways to disseminate those findings.

Variations (Narrative Inquiry, Oral History, Genealogy/Archaeology)

There are many variations in the practice and dissemination of historical inquiry that speak to the interests of the researcher and what they hope to uncover using this process. Each methodology employs the same six steps outlined above but, as we will see, with different interpretive goals in mind.

Narrative Inquiry

Narrative inquiry seeks to uncover the story behind events and the actors involved in them. The narrative provides an overview of the events as well as a structure within which readers of the story can understand it. "The narrative thus defines a boundary between members who share the common past and those who do not" (Seixas, 2006, p. 6). The linguistic turn has encouraged a shift in the type of historical narrative that historians employ in the twenty-first century. Rather than focusing only on major (usually political) events and the actors (usually white men) involved, historians today seek to situate their narratives within the broader social contexts that shaped history by paying attention to a variety of historical actors (women, children, the working class, different racial and ethnic groups, etc.) involved. For instance, the well-known historian and biographer Charlotte Gray seeks to present narratives of historical topics for everyday readers. In her latest book, *The Massey Murder* (2013a), she explores the murder trial of a domestic servant accused of shooting her wealthy master. Situating the events in their historical context, Gray seeks to engage a diversity of readers of history. She takes "a real event from our collective past, and shapes it into a narrative that will appeal to mystery lovers and history buffs" (Gray, 2013b). In doing so, she works to provide evidence of the context for her historical narratives, but they are narratives written for a popular audience.

In contrast, Rossiter and Clarkson (2013) explore the institutionalization of people with intellectual disabilities (ID). They use a wide variety of sources, such as policy documents and newspaper articles, to understand the institutional abuse that occurred when persons with ID were institutionalized in Ontario, Canada. However, their work is more academic in nature. In their article about the institutionalization of persons with ID in the past, they note that current knowledge of this injustice "lacks a comprehensive account of the social and historical context of institutionalized people with ID in Ontario" (Rossiter & Clarkson, 2013, p. 2). To address this challenge, they review the institutionalization of persons with ID, paying particular attention to the "historically-silenced narratives from people with ID about institutionalization…[and allow these] to emerge and be entered into public record" (pp. 1–2). What they discovered in trying to piece together the history of such abuse were "narrative gaps" about the residents that lived in the site of interest (Huronia Regional Centre) and, as such, needed to include "stories about residents at other institutions (including psychiatric facilities) because they provide important detail about the lives of residents of large-scale, government-run mental health facilities" (p. 4).

This example, rather than claiming to present one overarching narrative of this injustice, instead seeks to provide the beginning of a "cultural, historical, and social context to provide groundwork for these experiences to be understood" while also making the case for class action lawsuits on behalf of residents of Huronia and other institutions against the Province of Ontario for allowing such abuse to take place (p. 26).

Oral History

Part of the challenge with the Huronia example above is, as Rossiter and Clarkson note, the narrative gaps in the story. To address this, they use oral histories from other institutions and seek out former residents to collect their stories. This case, and the desire to sue the Province for ill treatment, points to the importance of collecting oral histories from those historical actors who were there. Oral history is both an approach and a methodology.

The opportunity to collect firsthand accounts of events from historical actors makes oral history appealing because it offers researchers a way to understand how those "who were there" experienced the event. However, researchers need to be cautious in their use of oral history. Oral histories are generally documented after an event has occurred and, as such, memories of the event shift and change with different historical contexts. Our memories change with our experiences and therefore how we remember an event is shaped by our hindsight and future experiences. When interpreting oral histories, we need to be critical about the time and place in which they are collected, who the historical actors being interviewed are, what experiences they may have had to shape their recollections, and so on.

Genealogy and Archaeology

Genealogical and archaeological approaches are closely related because they both seek to trace the origins of ideas. These can be considered in two ways. The first is to think about genealogy and archaeology in very traditional ways whereby genealogy is the tracing of historical roots (typically used when tracing family histories), and archaeology is the uncovering of artifacts of the past to understand from where we have come.

Michel Foucault (1969, 1976) applied these concepts to the philosophy of history to better understand where ideas (such as those about sexuality and power) come from. In terms of genealogy, Foucault was interested not in showing the progression of ideas, but rather in documenting the ways that different discourses (medicine, for instance) gained power in shaping our ideas. His work demonstrates that all truths are questionable and that we can trace where truths (such as the truth about sexuality) come from and who constructed them in different periods. In my own work (2003), for instance, this manifests itself in my desire to explore the ways that the medical profession had the power/knowledge to speak about abortion in different time periods. By using a Foucauldian approach, I trace the shifts and changes in the medical discourse on abortion in Canada and how doctors' discussions of abortion are rooted in the social and historical contexts in which they occurred. By uncovering the history (or genealogy) of the discourse, I am able to show how and why doctors shifted their views on the practice during the period of its illegality.

In *The Archaeology of Knowledge,* Foucault (1969) outlined an analytical method to demonstrate how systems of thought and knowledge are administered by rules (beyond those found in language) that operate in the consciousness of individuals. This method was Foucault's critique of narratives of the past, which he viewed as ways for researchers to impose their ideas on history. In tracing the archaeology of knowledge, Foucault was able to document the ways that discourses established the power to speak about certain aspects of society (sexuality and politics, for instance), but not others. Rather than look for continuities in the past, his method explored the discontinuities in ideas and how a complex interplay between discourses and institutions affected changes in thinking. In other words, his view was that shifts in the broader socio-historical and cultural contexts in which they occurred was too simplistic. Instead, he sought to complicate the ways in which we view the past. In her work on intersex people in American history, Elizabeth Reis (2009) explores the ways that ideas about intersex bodies shifted and changed over time and how the two-sex standard in thinking about the body evolved over centuries, with a variety of discourses seeking to shape the male–female binary in different periods.

Intersex

Intersex is a term used to describe individuals who are not easily classified as either male or female. The term often suggests that there are ambiguous genitalia, but this is not always the case, as chromosomal anomalies and other variations in sex characteristics may signify a person who is intersex (in some cases, intersex people have typical external genitalia but internally are the anatomy of the other sex).

Data Collection Strategies

Generally speaking, historians privilege primary data when conducting their analyses of the past. Accounts of events by historical actors created at the time can be quite varied, ranging from firsthand accounts such as those found in diaries, letters, or memoirs, to newspaper or magazine articles or advertisements, academic articles or debates, or even oral histories. As Tuchman (1994) notes, "finding and assessing primary historical data is an exercise in detective work. It involves logic, intuition, persistence, and common sense..." (p. 252). It also involves careful analysis and planning because the goal of the project often determines the types of data that need to be collected and analyzed. Given my own interest in tracing where ideas about the body come from in the past, I employ a form of discourse analysis. In the next section I discuss two projects to highlight different types of data collection that I have used to uncover shifts and changes in how the body is viewed in the past.

Medical Discourse on Abortion in Canada

In one of my projects, I examined the history of abortion in Canada. I was interested in learning more about the ways that the medical profession discussed the practice of abortion during the period of its illegality. Since I was influenced by the work of Michel Foucault on the power of discourse, the project looked for shifts and changes in the discourse on abortion over a long period of time (1850–1969). The focus of this project was the medical literature on the practice as found in the public medical press (medical journals containing articles written by members of the profession for their peers). The data collected was from the English Canadian medical journals in existence during the time period. Since the goal was to uncover the professional viewpoint (my research question sought to explore *how* the medical profession in Canada understood the practice of abortion in different time periods), I did not seek to find individual doctors' accounts or attempt to interview physicians to collect oral histories.

While the perspective of individual doctors is important (I was open to hearing their own accounts of abortion history), I was more fascinated by the role that professional status accorded doctors in shaping their views on abortion. To accomplish this, I used a set of keywords to find articles that related to abortion or abortion practices. All articles written in medical journals on *abortion, birth control, maternal mortality, maternal education,* and *the law* were consulted for the entire period (1850–1969). While paying close attention to articles that used this terminology, I was also open to finding articles that did not use these words; throughout the data collection I uncovered sources that did not at first appear to be about abortion practices. I used this strategy because I wanted to understand how doctors discussed the practice and how they defined and understood abortion throughout the period; being open to articles that "didn't fit" allowed me to find sources that I might otherwise have ignored or missed. By collecting a number of articles from various medical journals, I was able to trace the ways their discourse shifted and changed over time and to situate those changes within the wider social, cultural, political, and economical contexts of the period. For instance, it was evident that doctors understood the meaning of the word *abortion* differently in different time periods. In the mid- to late nineteenth century, *abortion* was the term used to denote what we would today refer to as *spontaneous miscarriage*. By the early decades of the twentieth century, the definition shifted to a meaning that denotes the intentional termination of a pregnancy. By privileging the reading of all articles I could find for the period of study over sampling articles, I was able to point to the moments when changes in the medical discourse happened.

Changes in the medical discourse are shaped by the historical context in which they occur. Therefore, it was important to examine the medical profession's discussions of the practice in light of other dominant discourses throughout the period. As such, the data collected also included evidence of the perception of other medical groups such as Canadian nurses and public health officials, medical textbooks and advice manuals for women and men dealing with sexuality, and the relevant legislation governing abortion as well as legislative documents, legal cases and decisions for the period under study, newspaper and magazine articles discussing the practice, and religious discussions of the practice such as those found in religious periodicals from the period.

Constructions of Femininity

A second project that is relevant to this chapter is my project on the constructions of femininity in medical and popular discourses. In this study, I was interested in learning more about the ways that the medical profession and consumer advertisers discussed femininity during the interwar period (1919–1939) in Canada. I used the medical discourse on abortion collected for previous research as a way to contextualize how doctors understood femininity in light of abortion and birth control practices and what this said about prescriptions for femininity. However, I wanted to explore whether the social views of femininity conformed to that of the medical view by exploring the ways that products were advertised to women. To do this, I chose a prominent Canadian popular magazine for women, *Chatelaine*, as well as an American women's magazine, *The Ladies' Home Journal*, which was also widely distributed in Canada.

Using these two magazine examples, I surveyed the various advertisement types first to gauge what types of products were advertised to women in that period. This allowed me to categorize the ads into groups such as food, beauty products, and appliances. Since I was exploring the connection between the medical discourse on femininity and that found in popular discourse, I decided to look only at ads that explicitly used some form of medical science to sell their products. Given the large number of ads (each magazine appeared monthly) and the number of years I wanted to survey, I decided to collect data by sampling. My data set consisted of every ad that incorporated medical science, regardless of product type. I collected ads from each magazine in January, May, and December of each year under study (1919–1939). This provided a large representative sample of different types of ads that were then analyzed for the messages they sent to women about expectations around how to perform their femininity.

Strategies of data collection are important to discern in any historical inquiry project because the interpretation is driven by the data. The examples above demonstrate that the strategy affects the type(s) of data collected and the need to think carefully about how different data can help answer a given research question. In the next section, I explore how different types of data can be analyzed.

Strategies of Data Analysis and Examples

Depending on the type of historical inquiry and the type of data, there are a variety of analysis strategies. Baptiste (2001) notes that while there are many strategies or ways to go about achieving our research goals when analyzing data, there are always four major phases of analysis: defining the analysis, classifying data, making connections between and among categories of data, and conveying the message/write-up (Baptiste, 2001, p. 2). He notes that these "...are iterative, interactive, and non-linear" (p. 2) rather than linear or sequential stages of analysis. For instance, imagine conducting an analysis of the history of mastectomy as cancer treatment in the twentieth century. To define the analysis, the researcher would want to identify how to uncover the history itself. The researcher might decide to define that history in terms of how the medical profession diagnosed the need for the procedure, how they discussed it, and how they performed it. To do so, she determines the best way to get at this history is to read the medical literature on the topic. She would likely not assume, though, in reading articles in medical journals on the topic, that this would give the full story on the history of the practice. The researcher would also need to identify the norms and values of physicians involved in any given period, and to interpret the ways these were translated in the articles themselves. In addition, knowing who the doctors authoring the studies were, as well as how and where they were trained, would help to understand their broader worldviews about cancer and surgery. Also of importance would be understanding the medical system in place. Was this type of surgery easily available and affordable to all patients? Did patients encounter prohibitive socioeconomic factors? The researcher could then situate patient perspectives within the wider social and cultural perspectives on women's bodies, health and illness, and medical science in a given time period. She might then look for evidence of the experience of the women who had such procedures and consider how their own perceptions of health and illness factored into the decision to have or not to have a surgical procedure (mastectomy). In short, the definition of the analysis would seek to contextualize the multitude of factors that affected the view of the medical profession on the performance of this procedure and would thus shape the ways that data was collected and analyzed. As Baptiste (2001) notes, "the decisions that analysts make concerning defining the analysis may be tacit or overt. However, decisions (to define the analysis) are always made. Good analysts, therefore, strive to make these decisions as transparent and defensible as possible" (p. 5). As with the other phases of data analysis, this first step is often iterative. As data are consulted to answer the research question, the researcher may find that new angles emerge that were not initially considered. For instance, there might be evidence in the medical literature that there were considerations regarding mastectomy linked to the socioeconomic status of patients. This realization might require additional data to properly contextualize this aspect of the research so that an adequate interpretation of the data collected can be provided.

As with initial defining of the data, the classifying of all of the evidence is also an iterative process. As they are collecting data, researchers can also tag and categorize data. This assists in sorting material that is relevant and, perhaps more important, data that are not relevant to the study at hand. As Baptiste (2001) argues, *tagging* is the process whereby the researcher selects "…from an amorphous body of material, bits and pieces that satisfy…[their] curiosity, and help support the purpose of the study" (p. 9).. For instance, in the study of mastectomy, the researcher may encounter articles that deal with breast reduction surgery. While important for a broader understanding of surgical practices on the body, this material is not directly relevant to a history of mastectomy for cancer. As such, a researcher may categorize this data in an "other" category. Once all the data is tagged and categorized (categories may be constructs, concepts, variables, or themes), it is easier for the researcher to determine how those various categories contribute to an understanding of the research topic (Baptiste, 2001).

Understanding the ways in which the various categories are related or talk to one another allows the researcher to make connections to come to an interpretation of the topic. Baptiste describes this process as developing a "broader/deeper" understanding of the topic. For historical researchers, the interest is always in providing a new interpretation by presenting a narrative or theory about the topic under study. This is often one of the most challenging things for new historical researchers because they learn in their elementary and secondary classrooms that there is just one narrative of the past, a "right" answer to explain the way things were. Of course, this is not the case; historical research allows scholars to ask critical questions of the past and to interrogate new and different sources to make connections between the various data sources that have been collected. For inquiry with a social justice focus, this is particularly important. For instance, we may not initially think about the ways in which socioeconomic status might affect viewpoints on mastectomy, but oral histories of the experiences of patients who had the procedure might shine a different light on the ways that patients' living conditions might influence their ability to access the procedure, whether they believe it is necessary, how they understand their physicians' perspectives, and so on. Similarly, we may discover that physicians trained at a particular medical school have different views than others on the procedure. In other words, the connections that the researcher makes between the various data sources allow them to posit "…a parsimonious, integrated set of associations and relationships between and among the various concepts they have formulated—relationships that were previously undocumented, obscure, or unknown" (Baptiste, 2001, p.11). This (and the last phase of communication of the results) is particularly important for social justice work because historical research can shed new light on systems of oppression and their origins, the ways that certain individuals or groups have been marginalized in society, or the ways that dominant discourses shape our understanding of our world. The work of Rossiter and Clarkson (2013) and Mosby (2013) mentioned earlier are good examples of this. In the next section I present two examples of the ways that I categorized research to address the different phases mentioned above.

Medical Discourse on Abortion in Canada

As mentioned earlier in this chapter, the data collection for this project involved careful reading of all of the medical journals published in English Canada[3] during the period under investigation. Since I was looking to uncover any shifts/changes in the medical discourse over a long period of time, I defined the data as all the articles on the topic of abortion and related topics (birth control, maternal mortality, etc.) that existed in the professional medical literature (Canadian medical journals) for the period under study. However, I was also interested in how the medical discourse fit into the wider socio-cultural context of abortion and therefore also looked at a variety of other sources (advice literature, other dominant discourses such as religion and the law, etc.). The process of classifying the data from all sources was similar.

At first I tagged data as relevant or not for the study at hand. Once that was accomplished, I identified themes within the data and tagged sources related to chronology (when did a particular perspective emerge), views of women and abortion, views of doctors and abortion, connection to other practices (specifically, birth control), etc. By categorizing the data, I was able to uncover connections between themes. For instance, I noticed that data on abortion from 1850 to 1919 was connected to the regulation of the medical profession that occurred at that time. Similarly, it became clear that discussions of abortion in the interwar period (1919–1939) were connected to wider discussions of maternal mortality and women's welfare. These connections allowed me to make sense of the data and to develop an interpretation of the history of abortion in Canada that differed from other studies. Rather than viewing doctors as oppressors of women through the medicalization of women's bodies, my study provided a more nuanced view of the role the medical profession played in shaping abortion practices in Canada during its illegality. For me, understanding the role that physicians play in these practices is an important social justice issue, as it demonstrates the need to understand the perspectives of all historical actors in shaping health care practices, broadly speaking. This is the message that I was able to convey to my readers.

Constructions of Femininity

As in the study of abortion, I defined the data carefully to ensure that I was analyzing material that would allow me to better understand the ways that medical science converged or diverged from the popular ideas about femininity conveyed to women in popular discourse, specifically those found in advertisements in women's magazines. As in the abortion study, I classified the data by focusing on key themes that emerged from my analysis of the data—advertisements that focused on beauty, mothering, household work, family development, and maintenance—and the ways that these themes reinforced a particular expectation for women: they were "made to be mothers" (Penny Light, 2013, p. 46). By classifying the data this way, I noticed important connections between the messages in the advertisements and the prescriptions for women found in the medical discourse. Importantly, while there were many aspects of the popular discourse that converged with the medical discourse, there were also areas where they diverged. By connecting these two different discourses to a theme (femininity), I uncovered an instance where the power of medical science was used to promote a particular role for women at a time when doctors themselves were questioning whether every woman ought to be held up to that prescription because it might be damaging to her health.

Considerations Related to Social Justice

So how does historical inquiry add meaning to social justice work? At the beginning of this chapter I suggest that historical forms of inquiry help us explore where ideas come from and to document shifts and changes in contexts and discourses to identify systems of oppression. Understanding where ideas come from and how they have changed or been repurposed is important for grasping how we deal with these issues in the present. In advocating for historical inquiry, I am really arguing that we need, as citizens, to develop our historical consciousness. Indeed, other theorists have similarly argued that the value of developing historical consciousness is that we can acquire a fuller awareness of the historicity of everything we encounter in the present and the relativity of all opinions on all subjects. This allows us to at least be more critical of traditions, even if it does not allow us to break them altogether (Gadamer, 1987, pp. 89–90; Seixas & Peck, 2004). The work of historian Elise Chenier embodies this. For instance, she created a website devoted to exploring the topic of "interracial intimacies" that aims to teach visitors how to think like a historian as well as to elucidate the publication process for historical research. In presenting the thinking behind her research, she hopes to promote empathy and empowerment. She notes that "having empathy means trying to understand both the victims of racism and sexism, and those whose actions were racist and/or sexist. It is not enough to say something was right or wrong, harmful or helpful. We must explain why people acted the way they did. To do so means moving past judgment toward understanding" (Chenier, 2014). Another of her projects is the Archive of Lesbian Oral Testimony (ALOT). In this project, she uses digital technologies to preserve oral histories of lesbians to facilitate future research as well as to teach people about oral interviewing methodologies. What is significant about the archive is that it makes the stories of lesbians available to the wider community. In both of these projects, it is clear that for her, understanding the past is the key to bringing about change; this is inherently about social justice. In a postmodern and increasingly globalized world, we need more than ever to develop this ability to think critically about what is happening today; part of that requires us to situate contemporary issues and problems within the broader context that has shaped them.

Globalization

The idea that we are living in a globalized world comes from the ubiquitous use of information and communication technologies that allow us to connect with other cultures and economies. It also refers to the ways that the world is connected through capital, the movement of people between countries, and, more broadly, the dissemination of knowledge between and among different parts of the world. For example, we think about issues such as consumer capitalism or climate change as global issues, rather than only as issues of importance to our own home country.

If we use the example of Angelina Jolie, historical inquiry and historical consciousness affords us the opportunity to situate how her decision to undergo a double mastectomy was influenced by both the medical and public discourses on this surgical practice (as well as cosmetic surgical practices given her desire to have her breasts rebuilt after the mastectomy) and the origins of those ideas. This should better enable us to make more educated decisions about our bodies when we are encouraged to alter ourselves to adhere to specific societal and cultural constructions of what it means to be healthy. It also points to the need to problematize how we understand what it means to be "healthy" and "normal" in our world, and raises questions about the ways in which the medical profession constructed gender and sexuality through their professional authority over the body in the past and what the implications of that history are in our contemporary context. As Metzl and Herzig (2007, p. 697) (among others) note, the complex role that doctors play as scientific authorities is increasingly challenging today when patients ask for particular drugs or treatments (like mastectomies) that allow them to "…occupy active positions as advocates, consumers, or even agents of change…" rather than being "passive victims of medicalization."

Medicalization

Medicalization refers to the process of broadening the purview of medicine to include not only the treatment of illness, but also myriad human conditions and problems. These issues have become the subject of medical study, even though they are sometimes not rooted in illness per se.

By exploring these constructions we can better understand the perspectives of both physicians/surgeons and patients in participating in such practices to move "…past judgment toward understanding" (Chenier, 2014). Indeed, exposing the ways in which the disciplinary power of medical science constructed normal, healthy bodies in the past (and the influence of other discourses on those constructions) may well provide us with the tools to effectively construct alternate discourses about health, particularly in light of consumer capitalist messages about what it means to be "healthy" today (Penny Light, 2015).

My own work to understand Angelina Jolie's "medical choice" is just one example of how we might begin to use historical inquiry to make change in the world by raising awareness of social justice issues. To do so, we have to work to get at the "inside" of past events to understand the perspectives of those involved, which is sometimes challenging depending on the evidence that those actors leave behind (or do not). Jolie's op-ed is helpful to us in that it provides us with her own account of her decision. Yet, we do not have all of her thoughts and feelings at our disposal. As I have already noted, we would need to gather much more evidence from her physicians, family members, advisors, etc., to begin to put together an interpretation of the event and to understand how she and others view her mastectomy as a just (or unjust) act. This often requires rethinking and rewriting narratives that did not take into account the ways injustice is embedded in different social, historical, and cultural contexts, and how those injustices continue to remain unaddressed in our contemporary world. Jolie herself likely does not view publicly disseminating her decision as potentially unjust: indeed, my reading of her words suggests that she was trying to help other women who carry the BRCA1 gene. Yet, as has already been noted, it is quite likely that some women have been or could be oppressed by her words and actions. In our information age, we have increased access to more information than ever before; this affords us new opportunities to explore the ways that individuals and groups have been marginalized. Historical forms of inquiry allow us to consider how we might address that marginalization by uncovering and bringing to the surface "previously silenced histories" (Rossiter & Clarkson, 2013, p. 26) and, in the case of Jolie, those that are privileged in contemporary discourses. In doing so, we may be able to ensure a more just society for all today and in the future.

NOTES

1.   Two famous accounts of the "killing of history" are Keith Windshuttle's *The Killing of History: How Literary Critics and Social Theorists are Murdering Our Past* (1994) and Jack Granatstein's *Who Killed Canadian History?* (1998).

2.   See also The Historical Thinking Project (http://historicalthinking.ca/).

3.   The focus for this study was narrowed to English Canada partly to reduce the amount of data collection but also to take into account cultural and political differences between English and French Canada in the period under study.

REFERENCES

Baptiste, I. (2001). Qualitative data analysis: Common phases, strategic differences. *Forum: Qualitative Social Research, 2,* 3. Retrieved from http://www.qualitative-research.net/index.php/fqs/article/view/917/2002

Carr, E.H. (1961). *What is History?* Cambridge, UK: Cambridge University Press.

Chenier, E. (2014). *Interracial intimacies: Sex and race in Toronto 1910 to 1950.* Retrieved from http://www.interracialintimacies.org/index.html

Collingwood, R. G. (1946). *The idea of history*. Oxford, UK: Oxford University Press.

Elton, G.R. (1967). *The practice of history*. New York: Thomas Y. Crowell Company.

Evans, R. J. (1999). *In defense of history*. New York: W.W. Norton & Company.

Foucault, M. (1969). *The archaeology of knowledge* (translated by A. M. Sheridan Smith). London, UK: Routledge.

Foucault, M. (1976). *The history of sexuality, Vol. 1*. New York: Penguin Books.

Gadamer, H.-G. (1987). The problem of historical consciousness. In P. Rabinow & W. M. Sullivan (Eds.), *Interpretive social science: A second look* (pp. 103-160). Berkeley, CA: University of California Press.

Granatstein, J. (1998). *Who killed Canadian history?* Toronto, Canada: Harper Collins.

Gray, C. (2013a). *The Massey Murder: A Maid, Her Master, and the Trial that Shocked a Nation*. Toronto: Harper Collins.

Gray, C. (2013b). A scandalous crime, a sensational trial, a surprise verdict—The true story of Carrie Davies, the maid who shot a Massey. Retrieved from http://www.charlottegray.ca/books.html

Jolie, A. (2013, May 14). My medical choice. The *New York Times*. Retrieved from http://www.nytimes.com/2013/05/14/opinion/my-medical-choice.html?_r=0

Landsman, J. (2013, May 17). Conventional medicine openly admits confusion over BRCA1 gene. *Natural Health 365*. Retrieved from http://www.naturalhealth365.com/natural_cures/brca1.html

McLaren, A. (1990). *Our own master race: Eugenics in Canada, 1885–1945*. Toronto, ON, Canada: McClelland & Stewart.

Metzl, J., & Herzig, R. (2007). Medicalization in the 21st century: An introduction. *The Lancet, 369*, 697.

Mosby, I. (2013). Administering colonial science: Nutrition research and human biomedical experimentation in aboriginal communities and residential schools, 1942–1952. *Histoire Sociale/Social History, 46*(91), 145–172.

National Cancer Institute (2014). *Fact sheet. BRCA1 and BRCA2: Cancer risk and genetic testing*. Retrieved from http://www.cancer.gov/cancertopics/factsheet/Risk/BRCA

Penny Light, T. (2003). *Shifting interests: The medical discourse on abortion in English Canada, 1850–1969*. Unpublished Ph.D. dissertation, University of Waterloo, Waterloo, ON, Canada.

Penny Light, T. (2013). Consumer culture and the medicalization of gender roles in interwar Canada. In C. Warsh & D. Malleck (Eds.) *Consuming modernity: Gendered behavior and consumerism before the Baby Boom* (pp. 34–54). Vancouver, BC, Canada: University of British Columbia Press.

Penny Light, T. (2015). From fixing to enhancing bodies: Shifting ideals of health and gender in the medical discourse on cosmetic surgery in twentieth century Canada. In T. Penny Light, B. Brookes, & W. Mitchinson (Eds.), *Bodily subjects: Essays on gender and health 1800–2000* (pp. 319–346). Montreal, QC, Canada: McGill-Queen's University Press.

Reis, E. (2009). *Bodies in doubt: An American history of intersex.* Baltimore, MD: The Johns Hopkins University Press.

Rossiter, K., & Clarkson, A. (2013). Opening Ontario's "saddest chapter": A social history of Huronia Regional Centre. *Canadian Journal of Disability Studies, 2,* 3. Retrieved from http://cjds.uwaterloo.ca/index.php/cjds/article/view/99

Seixas, P. (Ed.) (2006). *Theorizing historical consciousness.* Toronto, ON, Canada: University of Toronto Press.

Seixas, P., & Morton, T. (2013). Thinking about cause and consequence. In P. Seixas, T. Morton, J. Colyer, & S. Fornazzari, *The big six: Historical thinking concepts* (pp. 104-115). Toronto, ON, Canada: Nelson Education.

Seixas, P. & Peck, C. (2004). Teaching historical thinking. In A. Sears & I. Wright (Eds.), *Challenges and prospects for Canadian social studies* (pp. 109–117). Vancouver, BC, Canada: Pacific Educational Press.

Stearns, P.N. (1998). Why study history? *American Historical Association.* Retrieved from http://www.historians.org/about-aha-and-membership/aha-history-and-archives/archives/why-study-history-(1998)

Tuchman, G. (1994) Historical social science: Methodologies, methods, and interpretations. In N. Denzin & Y. Lincoln (Eds.), *The handbook of qualitative research* (pp. 306-323). Newbury Park, CA: Sage.

van Drie, J., & van Boxtel, C. (2008). Historical reasoning: Towards a framework for analyzing students' reasoning about the past. *Educational Psychology Review, 20*(2), 87–110.

Windshuttle, K. (1994). *The killing of history: How literary critics and social theorists are murdering our past.* Sydney, Australia: Macleay Press.

Wineburg, S. (2001). *Historical thinking and other unnatural acts: Charting the future of teaching the past.* Philadelphia, PA: Temple University Press.

Participatory Action Research: Democratizing Knowledge for Social Justice

Bryan S. R. Grimwood

I think of it as a moment of beautiful disruption: that liminal space where the circumstances of doing research seem to take on a life of their own. As researchers, these moments jar aspirations for control and expertise, repeatedly inscribed upon us through academic discourse, by shifting authority over knowledge and its production into the realm of the commons. One such instance occurred in November 2012 when I met with representatives of the Lutsel K'e Dene First Nation, a community situated on the east arm of Great Slave Lake in Canada's Northwest Territories. As a non-northerner of Euro-Canadian descent, I was visiting Lutsel K'e to share qualitative and visual data derived from my work with tourists and Inuit inhabitants of the Thelon River watershed (Grimwood, 2011a), a place deemed sacred within Dene ancestral territory. A secondary objective was to explore possibilities for collaborating on a new and related project. During an informal workshop with community representatives, research products such as photographs, narratives, and maps were circulated for inspection and discussion. Emphasis was very much on dialogue, storytelling, and co-learning. Midway through the workshop, representatives politely—albeit firmly—requested that I leave the meeting so that they could deliberate in confidence and determine the path forward. The decision to include Dene participation in the Thelon River study was very much out of my hands. When I returned to the meeting, I listened intently as representatives shared rationale, processes, and expectations for adapting the study to their local context.

Corey W. Johnson and Diana C. Parry, editors, "Participatory Action Research: Democratizing Knowledge for Social Justice" in *Fostering Social Justice Through Qualitative Research: A Methodological Guide*, pp. 217-250.

In this chapter I focus on participatory action research (PAR), an orientation to inquiry distinguished by values and features that give rise to the kinds of moments described above. The chapter begins with a description of PAR, followed by a survey of its historical and disciplinary roots and an introduction to the methodological variation within PAR. Strategies of data collection and data analysis are then presented, followed by a section that highlights considerations related to social justice. Throughout this chapter, I draw on my own experiences and understandings of social science research in Arctic Canada, a place laden with hopes and tensions, and certainly ripe for social justice inquiry. These exemplars contextualize processes discussed and strategies for negotiating the opportunities and challenges of PAR.

What Is PAR?

Participatory action research is a process that "involves researchers and participants working together to examine a problematic situation or action to change it for the better" (Kindon, Pain, & Kesby, 2007a, p. 1). Conceived in such broad terms, PAR often represents a variety of different participatory and action-oriented approaches to research. Kemmis and McTaggart (2000) illustrate this, describing a range of approaches including participatory research, critical action research, classroom action research, action learning, action science, soft systems approach, and industrial action research. Included are approaches with clear social justice mandates, and others emphasizing the enhancement of educational practices or organizational efficiency and development (Kemmis & McTaggart, 2000).

Despite the variability under its banner, PAR is associated with some underlying and unifying values and features (see "Values and Features of PAR"). One of the most crucial is the characterization of PAR as an *orientation to inquiry*, rather than as a stringent methodological framework with prescribed data collection and analysis protocols (Kindon, Pain, & Kesby, 2007b). Priority is placed on collaboration between researchers and members of communities or organizations for studying or transforming circumstances relevant to, and determined by, those members (Greenwood, Whyte, & Harkavy, 1993). The aim here is to establish "a more democratic research process, which respects and builds co-researchers' capacity and generates more rich, diverse, and appropriate knowledge for community change" (Kindon, 2005, p. 207). Unlike conventional modes of research in which participants are treated as passive subjects by "professional expert" researchers, PAR envisions active community/organizational engagement in the quest for understanding and transformation (Whyte, Greenwood, & Lazes, 1989). This requires researchers willing to shed the veil of expertise and take on a facilitative role that is alert and responsive to the voices and knowledge embedded within study contexts. Partnerships *with* community members become the basis for identifying issues of importance, designing ways of studying them, collecting and interpreting data, and taking action on the resulting knowledge (Smith, Bratini, Chambers, Jensen, & Romero, 2010). In effect, research is done *with* and *by* participants, rather than *on* or *for* them.

Values and Features of PAR

PAR has multiple meanings and applications, which result from its roots in several disciplines and complex social circumstances. However, when regarded as an orientation to inquiry, PAR consists of agreed-upon values and features. Smith et al. (2010), for instance, identify three value-oriented commitments:

1. That there exists, at an ontological level, the possibility of a popular or public science in which knowledge creation doesn't simply reproduce worldviews and interests of dominant social groups;

2. That infusing power-sharing and reciprocity into knowledge production processes can transform conventional and oppressive relationships between research/researched or research subject/object;

3. That privileging local voices, cultures, and wisdom throughout the different stages of research engenders autonomy and identity within the collective process.

Consistent with these values-led guideposts are several distinguishing features of PAR. These include:

- Iterative and responsive processes of planning-acting-reflecting for change;
- Attention to power relations, ethics, and issues of representation;
- Collaboration between professional and community/ organization researchers in all stages of research;
- Reciprocity in terms of research benefits;
- Eclectic methods tailored to specific circumstances;

- Theoretical and applied outcomes that bind the knowledge-action nexus;
- Emergent project dimensions and depth (e.g., degrees of participation); and
- Criterion of success based on participant/community understanding, change, and transformation.

As the "PAR and Social Justice" box highlights, the promotion of social justice is, and always has been, of central concern to many PAR researchers. Accordingly, PAR is an explicitly political stance reflecting a researcher's own disposition, values, and attitudes. As PAR practitioners focus "on empowering disenfranchised and marginalized groups to take action to transform their lives" (Cornwall & Jewkes, 1995, p. 1671), they confront head-on the challenge of intertwining knowledge generation and the demand for action, something historically avoided in research (Whyte et al., 1989). Most adherents recognize this as an ideal process of shared learning based on trusting and respectful partnerships and with the potential to fuel emancipatory social change at diverse scales (Dupuis et al., 2011; Smith et al., 2010). Research is thus engaged as midwife to partnership, trust, capacity, participation, and dialogue—what Freire (1970) might name the seeds of social transformation—just as much as it is for advancing understanding, knowledge, or immediate action. In other words, the processes of doing research are valued just as much as the products, and the success of a given project is determined not strictly by the quality of information generated, but in association with the extent of skills, knowledge, and capacities participants and communities contribute or develop in relation to the research (Kindon, 2005).

PAR and Social Justice

One of the earliest voices in PAR, Orlando Fals-Borda, articulated the process as driven by social justice agendas. In an excerpt cited by Kindon (2005), Fals-Borda and Rahman define PAR as "an experiential methodology for the acquisition of serious and reliable knowledge upon which to construct power, or counterveiling power, for the poor, oppressed and exploited groups and social classes—the grassroots—and for their…organizations and movements. Its purpose is to enable oppressed groups and classes to acquire sufficient creative and transforming leverage as expressed in specific projects, acts and struggles to achieve goals of social transformation" (p. 207–208).

Historical and Disciplinary Roots

The variation associated with PAR makes it difficult to trace definitive historical or disciplinary roots of the process. Indeed, as Brydon-Miller et al. (2011) indicate, PAR may best be viewed as having varied origins. Some of these foundations rest in fields of adult education, international development, and social sciences (Khanlou & Peter, 2005), with sociology and anthropology noted as the disciplinary nucleus of the latter (Fals Borda, 2006). These scholarly arenas were attuned to the shifting social and political circumstances of the mid-twentieth century. Hearing the march of diverse campaigns promoting participatory and democratic solutions to social problems—for example, labor movements, women's movements, human rights and peace movements, and rethinking international development assistance (Brydon-Miller et al., 2011)—researchers in these areas were inclined to reformulate their practices. With growing recognition of feminist and African-American voices, for example, they sought "to create new forms of inquiry deeply connected to collective action for social justice" (Brydon-Miller et al., 2011, p. 388). This was tied to broader critiques of positivist social science that identified with knowledge not as objective and generalizable, but as always value-laden, partial, and effectual. In geography, my own disciplinary orientation, PAR emerged alongside such shifts as a tangible way of putting the aims of critical geographical perspectives into practice. Mirroring inclinations of other social scientists to "be of use," geographers began viewing PAR as an approach to addressing the racism, ableism, sexism, heterosexism, and imperialism that manifest in "people's unequal access to, and control over, resources, or in their positions within inequitable social relationships" (Kindon, 2005, p. 214–215). PAR's evolution was thus grounded in social realities; it arose along with challenges to other structures of power existing beyond the institutional walls of universities (Brydon-Miller et al., 2011).

Most would agree that these sort of academic and social trajectories crystallized into the genesis of PAR at some point in the early 1970s. On occasion, this development has been linked to affluent Western countries (Cornwall & Jewkes, 1995; Pain, 2004) where applied research into practical social settings was being adapted to enable participants to assume roles typically occupied by researchers from outside the study setting (Kemmis & McTaggart, 2000). As a case in point, the field of organizational behavior prompted the emergence of PAR as a means to resist assumed authority of survey research and quantitative modeling (Whyte et al., 1989). PAR also offered the pragmatic benefit of improved organizational effectiveness and efficiency over the long term, a result of involving members in decision-making and yielding a greater sense of member ownership and commitment (Cornwall & Jewkes, 1995).

Much of PAR's early development did, however, occur beyond the persuasions of Western Europe and North America. Fals Borda (2006) maintains that PAR's "first wave" originated in the Third World during the 1970s, specifically in the pioneering work of scholars from the global south. At this time, Fals Borda and other Latin American sociologists began describing their work as *investigation yaccion*, which translates directly to "participatory action research" (Brydon-Miller et al., 2011). Motives driving this intellectual movement centered on promoting values-engaged scholarship and social justice; or, to quote Fals Borda (2006) directly: "to protest against the sterile and futile university routine, colonized by western Euro-American culture, and so subordinating as to impede us from discovering or valuing our own realities" and "to right wrongs, so as to improve the form and foundation of our crisis-ridden societies by fighting against their injustices and trying to eradicate poverty and other socio-economic afflictions caused by the dominant systems" (p. 353).

Freire's (1970) work in adult education is another important contribution to PAR's development and its roots in global south social justice initiatives. Central to Freire's thinking and practice was the concept of *conscientization*, in which popular education enables socially dispossessed peoples to come to critical consciousness and challenge the oppressive status quo. Such an approach is particularly beneficial to marginalized populations for engaging their voices and unsettling circumstances based on dominance and oppression. As Cornwall and Jewkes (1995) explain, PAR has drawn from Freire the attentiveness to relations of power involved in doing research and the commitment to working with others confronted by inequalities produced by social differences. Much like Freire's pedagogy, PAR brings people into research by affirming the value of their own knowledge, regarding them as active agents of change rather than objects under investigation, and recognizing that they are most capable of analyzing their own situations and designing their own solutions (Cornwall & Jewkes, 1995).

Another, albeit intersecting way, of thinking about the roots of PAR has been to identify with the lineages of its component parts: action research and participatory research. The former has been likened to a "Northern tradition" and associated with the work of Kurt Lewin, a social psychologist in the United States who was concerned with developing methods to address critical issues like poverty, fascism, anti-Semitism, and marginalization (Khanlou & Peter, 2005). Lewin's initial formulation of action research involved a cyclical or spiralling sequence of planning, implementing, and evaluating action to solve problems and generate new knowledge. Its ideological basis was situated in clinical psychological and management theory, so much of the emphasis was placed on individual, interpersonal, and group-level analysis and efficiency (Khanlou & Peter, 2005). Over time, action research has evolved to take on new meanings, many of which maintain an explicit commitment to political, socially engaged, and democratic practice and incorporate participatory methods to add degrees of relevance and validity within local contexts (Brydon-Miller, Greenwood, & Maguire, 2003; Reason & Bradbury, 2008).

Participatory research, in contrast, is rooted in emancipatory movements associated with the "Southern tradition" (Khanlou & Peter, 2005). Its application dates back to Finnish social scientist Marja-Liis Swantz, who worked in Tanzania in the 1970s (Brydon-Miller et al., 2011). While no discipline is solely responsible for developing participatory research, its ideological basis draws mainly upon sociological, economic, and political science perspectives (Khanlou & Peter, 2005). Influenced by the cultural contexts of developing areas, participatory research seeks to mobilize people to 1) enhance awareness of their abilities and resources and 2) transform social structures that oppress and marginalize groups (Khanlou & Peter, 2005). It achieves this by involving "those conventionally 'researched' in some or all stages of research, from problem definition through to dissemination and action" (Pain, 2004, p. 652) and sharing ownership of the research process and outcomes with participants. Here again, in this decisively context-specific approach, we see the influence of Freire (1970). Participatory research forefronts situated, rich, and layered accounts of local conditions, experiences, and knowledge to actively interrogate social exclusion and difference (Pain, 2004).

Irrespective of these varied origins—or maybe even because of them—PAR's acceptance and legitimacy has increased dramatically in recent years. Its deployment and philosophy now extend into disciplines across the natural sciences, social sciences, and humanities (Fals Borda, 2006). Within the social sciences, the so-called "action turn" was detected near the beginning of the current millennium (Reason & Torbert, 2001). The first-edition publication of the *Handbook of Action Research* (Reason & Bradbury, 2001) played no small role in this concentrated shift as it brought together many participatory and action-oriented approaches under one banner (Dick, 2009). The base of scholarship has continued to thrive and grow ever since.

There have been no less than ten world congresses associated with PAR, most of them taking place at academic institutions (Fals Borda, 2006). A wide array of book-length volumes has been produced and several well-established journals devoted to the topic are in circulation. Special thematic issues related to PAR are not uncommon in major social science journals (see Dick, 2006, 2009).

Moreover, initial debates about the validity, scientific rigor, or theoretical and educational merits of PAR largely have been put to rest. It is estimated that PAR is now taught or practiced in more than 2,500 universities in more than sixty countries (Fals Borda, 2006). Major international initiatives have championed PAR approaches, from the 1989 United Nations Convention on the Rights of the Child, which prompted research communities to better recognize children's rights to participate in projects affecting them (Brydon-Miller et al., 2011) to, more recently, the 2007–2008 International Polar Year, which entailed a surge of internationally coordinated, interdisciplinary research activities with a clear mandate to engage Arctic communities via collaboration, education and training, and outreach (see Grimwood, Cuerrier, & Doubleday, 2012). In Canada, federal government agencies responsible for funding academic research include principles associated with PAR in their ethical guidelines for engaging Aboriginal communities (CIHR, NSERC, & SSHRC, 2010). Some authors caution that such widespread appeal reflects the "institutionalization" or "cooption" of PAR, which may enable governments, industry, and corporations to exert control over those on the margins (Fals Borda, 2006). In my view, the best response to this reality is not to discard PAR's principles and processes, but to think through them critically and reflexively, always asking, "Who benefits?" from the research.

Methodological Variation

Methodology in PAR is viewed less as a means to an end than it is as an end in itself. As a values-engaged and context-specific orientation to inquiry, PAR resists methodological dogmatism by engaging, adapting, innovating, and learning through methodologies to facilitate transformations called for by participants and their communities. PAR researchers are known to embrace a range of qualitative and quantitative techniques, determining methods in relation to issues facing communities and research questions they generate (Kindon et al., 2007b). But given PAR's focus on generating dialogue and knowledge through interaction, researchers often use methodological strategies with experiential or "hands-on" dimensions, especially when working with marginalized communities (Brydon-Miller et al., 2011; Kindon et al., 2007b). For example, recent research with Arctic communities includes on-the-land plant workshops with elders and youth (Cuerrier et al., 2012), postmodern dance training and performance (Barnett, 2012), and geographic information system (GIS) mapping of Inuit trails and sea ice use (Gearheard, Aporta, Aipellee, & O'Keefe, 2011). One rationale for interactive methods is that participants can develop skills, knowledge, and capacities through the research experience that are important to self-mobilizing change (Kindon et al., 2007b).

While PAR's inclinations toward nimble, dialogical, and experiential methodology may be messy, contributing perhaps to the blurred boundaries between the many varieties of participatory and action research (Dick, 2009), it is not the result of an unsophisticated theoretical basis. According to Brydon-Miller et al. (2003):

> There is a clear legacy of pragmatism and feminism that helps explain our penchant for messes. As a group, we seem unable to resist "embodied" intellectual practice. We never leave our corporeality; we are engaged in ongoing cycles of reflection and action in which our bodies and ourselves and those of our collaborators are not only present to us but essential to the very process of understanding messes. Pain, joy, fear, bravery, love, rage—all are present in our action research lives. (p. 21–22)

So, in contrast to modes of inquiry that demand adherence to firm protocols to achieve replicable, reliable, or objective outcomes, the methodological practices of PAR are tethered to researchers' situated epistemological and axiological orientations, and how these give shape to issues being addressed. In other words, methodological procedures are not strictly followed, but rather, methodological choices, informed by values and dialogue and circumstance, are consistently being made. In many ways, this boils down to a commitment to theorizing and interrogating power relations in processes of knowledge production, and practicing them anew to resist dominant social structures (Foucault, 1980).

Amid this values-engaged messiness, there are some useful conceptual tools for researchers trying to position their work. I highlight two general tools here. The first is to consider "participation" as something existing along a continuum. Participation is not a single variable, nor does it transpire homogenously across different projects or even within a single project. Rather, participation ranges from *shallow* or *passive*, where researchers control the entire process, to increasingly *deep* or *active* participation whereby researchers move towards relinquishing control and ownership of the process to community members (Cornwall & Jewkes, 1995; Kindon et al., 2007b). Kindon

(2005) positions various modes of participation along such a continuum. *Co-option*, for example, exists at the shallow end of the spectrum and characterizes conventional research driven by knowledge "experts." Participation deepens as movement is made towards the more collaborative and facilitative modes of *co-learning* and *collective action*. Yet participation within a given project may also fluctuate in relation to the perceptions of participation held by different actors, the number of people involved, and the various design, fieldwork, analysis, and reporting stages of research (Stewart & Draper, 2009). Theoretically speaking, PAR entails deep and wide participation in all research stages. But as Greenwood, Whyte, and Harkavy (1993) observe, the degree of participation achieved is a function of the character of the problems and environmental conditions under study, the aims and capacities of the research team, and the skills of the professional researcher. Participation is seldom full-blown at the outset of most projects, or ever fully achieved. Rather, it must be generated over time. From this perspective, PAR is not an "all or nothing" methodology, but an ideal or emergent process in which researchers continuously work at creating the necessary spaces, conditions, and actions that enable people to participate ever more fully in research processes (Greenwood et al., 1993).

The second general conceptualization reflects methodological choices as a function of researcher positionality relative to the communities in which they work. Herr and Anderson (2005) present a typology that locates PAR along a six-point continuum of action researcher positionalities ranging from insider to outsider. According to them, "the degree to which researchers position themselves as insiders or outsiders will determine how they frame epistemological, methodological, and ethical issues" (Herr & Anderson, 2005, p. 30) in the study. For instance, at the insider end of the continuum, researchers who investigate themselves for improved practice or professional transformation will take up traditions such as autobiography, narrative research, or autoethnography. The other extreme—the outsider studying insiders—reflects "extractive" approaches typical of university-based academic research *on* particular action research initiatives. Near the middle of the continuum is where Herr and Anderson (2005) situate PAR as an ideal process for insider–outsider teams focused on reciprocal collaboration and achieving equitable power relations. To be sure, one's position relative to the study setting can be difficult to define and can shift in relation to different project stages. Moreover, as researchers, we occupy multiple and intersecting positions based on gender, sexual identity, race, or social class, which invariably shape our worldviews, underpin our methodological choices and assumptions, and enter into our representations. Interrogating these multiple positionalities can yield nuanced understanding of the questions under investigation and illuminate blind spots in our thinking and practice (Herr & Anderson, 2005; Higgins-Desbiolles & Powys Whyte, 2013).

But ultimately, as I have implied earlier in this chapter, the methodological orientations and choices involved in PAR should arise in and through the relational contexts of a particular study. These circumstances include, but are not limited to, issues and questions relevant to communities; interactions between professional and participating researchers, as well as their respective histories and personalities; local and regional protocols, knowledge systems, and cultural values; and attention to the shifting effects of power both within local settings and broader social, cultural, and historical milieus. In the following paragraphs, I introduce four specific methodological frameworks that, from my perspective as an Arctic and Aboriginal community "outsider," are viewed as both timely and relevant to the Arctic Canadian contexts of my research. How these are applied elsewhere will certainly vary.

Engaged Acclimatization

The processes for initiating and nurturing the kinds of responsible research relationships inherent to PAR require careful, critical, and consistent consideration. *Engaged acclimatization* was inspired by the significance of preliminary fieldwork in orienting my doctoral thesis and conceptualized to represent the embodied and reflexive knowledge production occurring through immersive encounters with the material, political, cultural, and perceptual ecologies of Arctic communities (Grimwood, Doubleday, Ljubicic, Donaldson, & Blangy, 2012). Exploration, reflection, care, creativity, and interaction characterize these encounters, thereby challenging assumptions that research methods are best performed by those who bracket their experiences to stand apart from the messiness of context, and echoing various theoretical perspectives (e.g., feminism, critical theory) that create space for situated and positioned styles of inquiry. Four fundamental aspects are illuminated in our rendering of engaged acclimatization: *crafting relations, learning, immersion,* and *activism.* These are mapped, respectively, as an *intention, approach, practice,* and *effect* of engaged acclimatization. Conscientious application of these aspects can facilitate endogenous research by enacting research ethics as a lived experience, initiating and nurturing relationships as a central component of research, and centering methods on circumstances within participating communities. In reflecting critically upon my preliminary field research experiences, it was clear that these aspects invited a relational perception and intuition that informed subsequent research objectives, design, and procedures; how research was actually carried out; and later stages of analysis, writing, reporting, and future project identification (Grimwood, Doubleday, et al., 2012).

Appreciative Inquiry

Appreciative inquiry (AI) is an approach to action-oriented research that emphasizes the positive and productive possibilities of a situation or circumstance. Cooperrider and Whitney (2005) define AI as

> the cooperative, co-evolutionary search for the best in people, their organizations, and the world around them. It involves systematic discovery of what gives life to an organization or a community when it is most effective and most capable in economic, ecological, and human terms. (p. 8)

Conceptually speaking, AI works from social construction and critical theory positions that recognize the interconnections between language, knowledge, and action (Koster & Lemelin, 2009). By emphasizing dialogue about achievements, assets, innovations, traditions, opportunities, competencies, stories, and lived values, AI calls for a shift away from deficit- or problem-based theory and practice (Cooperrider & Whitney, 2005). Given the pervasiveness of vulnerability discourses relating to Arctic change—for instance, in terms of the impacts of climate change on cultural livelihoods (Ford & Smit, 2004) or tourism development (Lemelin, Dawson, Stewart, Maher, & Lück, 2010)—AI seems an important counterbalance. Empowering and engaging through positive messaging, community competencies, strengths, and successes, AI charts a path towards hopeful and collaborative futures. This has been demonstrated in relation to rural tourism (Koster & Lemelin, 2009), including work by Bennett and colleagues (2010) that involved exploring with Lutsel K'e the relationships between social-economy organizations, development, and a proposed protected area.

Indigenous Methodologies

Indigenous communities worldwide continue to express interest in academic research despite its difficult history and colonial legacies (Caine, Davison, & Stewart, 2009). Recent efforts across disciplines include work done *with* and *by* Indigenous peoples, which is one response to historical injustices Indigenous communities and scholars associate with much modernist research (Panelli, 2008; Smith, 1999).

This shift has enriched many Indigenous communities: they take owner-ship of research agendas, enable projects to follow local codes of con-duct, and honor Indigenous knowledge and worldviews (Wilson, 2008). Moreover, articulations of Indigenous methodologies—characterized by Louis (2007) to include relational accountability, respectful representa-tion, reciprocal appropriation, and endorsement of Indigenous rights and regulations—emphasize cyclical and dynamic research styles with the central intent of performing sympathetic, respectful, and ethical research from an Indigenous perspective. The politics of Indigenous methodol-ogies include instilling values into scholarship to challenge objectivity, universal abstractions, and generalized understandings (Panelli, 2008). It advocates styles of knowing, and approaches to producing knowledge, which are responsive to place (Johnson, 2010).

Community-based Participatory Research

Community-based participatory research (CBPR) is understood as a framework for research conducted by, for, or with the participation of a community (Markey, Halseth, & Mason, 2010). The practice of CBPR includes a range of action-oriented intentions, participation, and collaborative partnerships (Stewart & Draper, 2009; Markey et al., 2010). These goals have built awareness among researchers and community members of the capacity inherent in local knowledge systems, helping to substitute paternalistic and condescending prac-tices of research *on* communities. Accordingly, CBPR aims to: 1) balance research power relations by sharing control of research pro-cesses and outcomes; 2) foster trust through transparent, reciprocal, and interactive relationships; and 3) support community ownership of research priorities, decision-making, and knowledge generation (Castleden, Garvin, & Huu-ay-aht First Nation, 2008).

Caine et al. (2009) explained that, regardless of discipline, re-searchers working in Canada's north have been encouraged to mod-ify research priorities and methods to respond to the interests and agendas of Indigenous communities and their cultural traditions. Researchers will "often discover that communities are neither un-interested nor ignorant of the potential for research to benefit their communities and address deteriorating environmental conditions" (Caine et al., 2009, p. 490). Across Nunavut, for example, Inuit are well acquainted with research and with the practices of visiting re-searchers. This has fueled expectations for greater participation in all stages of research, including defining research priorities and methods, collecting data, and analyzing and disseminating results (ITK/NRI, 2007).

Researchers listening to such requests have welcomed opportunities for CBPR so that locally driven projects can contribute to the participants' quality of life and address local interests, priorities, and knowledge (Gearheard et al., 2011; ITK/NRI, 2007; Laidler & Elee, 2008; Stewart & Draper, 2009). These goals represent the high degree of research involvement desired and performed by Nunavut communities.

Data Collection Strategies

PAR embraces eclectic data collection strategies selected and adapted in relation to the context of the investigation. Figure 8.1 represents this diversity to include familiar qualitative methods (e.g., interviewing, participant observation), dialogical approaches (e.g., storytelling, community art and media), and active learning exercises (e.g., educational camps, exchange programs). While PAR's emphasis on processes of shared learning, communication, capacity building, and transformation is often more conducive to qualitative designs, quantitative approaches are not automatically dismissed. Rather, PAR researchers have incorporated quantitative methods when they are deemed useful to achieving the kinds of action outcomes desired by community collaborators and can occur in the context of reciprocal relationships (Kindon, 2005). The text box below describes one such example.

An Example of Integrating Quantitative Methods into PAR

The Panel Study on Homelessness evolved from partnerships between university researchers and a network of social service and nonprofit housing agencies committed to ending homelessness in Ottawa, Canada (Klodawsky, 2007). Cognisant of the evidence-based policy environment in which they were situated, the agencies sought information that they could use to inform bureaucrats' decision-making and support front-line workers. An extensive study of peoples' experiences of homelessness ensued, which included a survey instrument consisting of 157 closed-ended questions and standardized self-report measures. This methodological choice was directly tied to PAR goals of generating policy-relevant insights with respect to the multidimensional experiences of homelessness and the associated implications for program development and implementation (Klodawsky, 2007).

FIGURE 8.1. Common methods used in PAR (Kindon et al., 2007b, p. 17).

Surveys

Participant observation
data analysis

Secondary

Learning by doing

Dialogue

Political action

Group work and discussions

Interviewing

Storytelling

Mapping

Community art and media

Diagramming

Educational camps

Exchange programs

Ranking and scoring

Shared analysis, writing and presentations

In addition, recent reductions in technology costs have facilitated the increased popularity of arts, media-based, and visual data collection methods, trends that are reflected in northern (sub-Arctic and Arctic) North American research contexts. For instance, Lemelin et al. (2013) use *photohistory* as an active process to reclaim old photographs and prompt new research directions and partnerships, while Stewart, Jacobson, and Draper (2008) report on opportunities and challenges associated with implementing participatory GIS. Moving beyond conventional approaches to science outreach (public talks, school visits), Jensen (2012) uses various social media outlets (Facebook, Twitter, a blog) to engage with a broader learning community with interests in Alaskan archaeology.

Principles of PAR also support integrating multiple methods used across different projects and communities. Ljubicic's (formerly Laidler) collaborative research with three Inuit communities in Nunavut used semidirected interviews, experiential sea ice trips, and focus groups to develop baseline understanding of local sea ice conditions, processes, and features (Laidler, 2007). These data collection strategies sanctioned Inuktitut terminology and spatial delineations of localized sea ice dynamics. Such insights complemented coarser regional-scale studies to inform sea ice monitoring initiatives and to address community interests associated with adapting traveling and hunting practices in response to climatic change (Laidler et al., 2009).

Related research used participatory mapping exercises to document and represent Inuit use and occupancy of sea ice (Aporta, 2011). One aspect of this process involved Inuit elders and experienced hunters using maps to discuss and draw significant sea ice features and areas used today and relied upon in the past. These exercises were accompanied by several sea ice trips during which researchers and hunters documented ice-related features, trails, and activities with global positioning system (GPS) units, photographs, and video. Documentation was also facilitated by the development and testing of an innovative technological device for observing and monitoring the environment (Gearheard et al., 2011). Described as an integrated GPS/personal digital assistant (PDA)/mobile weather station, this device was created through the collaboration and ingenuity of Inuit hunters and geomatics engineering students (Gearheard et al., 2011). As Aporta (2011) explains, each of these techniques factor into a broader cybercartographic initiative that creates interactive online atlases available for public use, particularly for the partnering Inuit communities.

Within and beyond the Arctic, applications of participatory mapping have extended to depicting spatial scales other than landscapes and/or seascapes. Geographers, among others, have engaged participatory approaches to create detailed social maps on which facilities, services, or household attributes are marked, which in turn have led to mapping social stratification, the distribution of vulnerable groups, and assessments of health service uptake (Cornwall & Jewkes, 1995). The approach has also been adapted into body mapping, whereby participants produce drawings associated with the human body and helpful to project themes. Body mapping has been an especially useful "data" collection strategy for understanding health-related perceptions and vernacular of various communities (Kesby & Gwanzura-Ottemoler, 2007).

With respect to my research related to the Thelon River, data collection strategies have been significantly informed by my experience working with participatory and visual methods deployed by Nancy Doubleday's research team during the International Polar Year (Ip, Grimwood, Kushwaha, Doubleday, & Donaldson, 2008). As the lead social and community-based researcher of a large international scientific study of Arctic treeline dynamics, Doubleday partnered with the Inuit communities of Cape Dorset and Sanikiluaq (both in Nunavut) to facilitate two participatory processes. One involved university and community researchers traveling onto the land to identify and collect plant specimens for inclusion in a community-generated and -owned herbarium. Collected specimens were pressed, mounted, and labeled with Inuktitut and Latin names during subsequent community workshops with elders, youth, and other land users. The second technique, best described as *participatory repeat photography*, occurred in three stages.

First, community residents were invited to workshops to share photographs from personal collections that depicted some aspect of their respective environs and/or livelihoods. Second, the research team identified the locations of select photographs and returned to these to reframe the landscape in its present form. The third stage again involved community workshops, this time to display photographs and invite dialogue about the meanings and changes they represent. Data from all three stages were integrated as baseline "social observations" of environmental change and community wellbeing (Ip et al., 2008).

The first phase of my *Picturing the Thelon River* study (2008–2011) adapted these data collection strategies so that knowledge from river tourists and Inuit residents of Baker Lake, Nunavut, could be documented and used to foster dialogue about place-based responsibilities. Preliminary fieldwork included two consultative visits to Baker Lake, which were instrumental in building trust, clarifying and revising project objectives, familiarizing myself with community contexts, and identifying local research assistants (see also Caine et al., 2009). Consultations also occurred with a river tourism operator who later distributed study information to his clientele and invited me to participate in and observe one of his multi-day canoe expeditions. Formal data collection began in January 2009 and included three participatory modules.

The first module, photographic interviews, was structured as a form of photo-elicitation (Harper, 2002). Participants from tourist and Inuit communities were invited to select up to twelve Thelon River images from their personal photograph collections that reflected to them themes related to responsibility and nature-based experience (see Table 8.1). These photographs were subsequently used to direct individual, face-to-face conversational interviews concerning the participant's stories, meanings, and experiences in and of the Thelon. With participants' informed consent, photographs were copied and saved and interviews audio-recorded and later transcribed. Supplementary information was collected from canoe tourists via qualitative email questionnaires. The second module involved my participation as a researcher in experiential river journeys with Inuit hunters and canoe tourists from the Canadian south. This module included seven journeys by various modes of transportation over a range of distances, and lasting from half a day to ten days in length (see Table 8.2). Journeys were documented using ethnographic methods including participant observation, journaling, photography, and GPS tracking. The third research module entailed community workshops that emphasized knowledge sharing and translation as well as collective learning. More than a focus group, the participants at these workshops were invited to engage with the photographs and information derived from research modules 1 and 2, and to share their own knowledge, experiences, and meanings of the Thelon. As such, the workshops functioned simultaneously as a strategy for reporting results and for community interpretation of research, thereby contributing additional layers of riverscape knowledge while balancing out the expertise and power relations in doing research. Weaving throughout the implementation of these modules were my extensive observational and reflexive fieldnotes. As most PAR or qualitative practitioners would expect, this journaling proved to be an invaluable space not just for record keeping but also for clarifying method-level processes and reflecting on the decisions and justifications (be it rational or affective) underpinning these.

Strategies of Data Analysis

Consistent with its resistance to dogmatic methodological approaches, PAR does not prescribe specific strategies of data analysis. Again, the methodological choices involved in performing PAR are guided by the value orientations noted in this chapter and the particular contexts of the study. But as Pain (2004) suggests, the analysis of a PAR project prompts important questions about the interplay between academic researchers, community partners/participants, and the options available for disseminating findings. Pain observed that "some address this issue by asking participants to undertake data analysis or verification; others attempt to represent exactly what all participants said; some use mainstream modes of qualitative analysis arguing that transparency of procedures is important" (p. 658). Still others focus their analysis on knowledge translation and outreach with the intent of creating tangible products for participants and their communities (e.g., Pulsifer et al., 2012).

To date, the Thelon River research described here has integrated several different strategies of data analysis. The community workshops noted in the previous section represent a participatory approach to interpretation and, as implied, demonstrate the always fuzzy, or fluid, boundaries between the various stages of a PAR project. In Baker Lake, workshops were carried out with *Qillautimiut* (the community elders committee) and with young adults studying at the local branch of the Nunavut Arctic College. Research photographs—which were printed, labeled with the photographer's name, and laminated in advance—were circulated among workshop participants, who were invited to pull aside photographs that they found particularly interesting or curious. Participants used these images to deliberate the content and meaning of Thelon experience, communicate observations of change,

TABLE 8.1. Excerpt from instructions given to photographic interview participants.

From the photographs you have taken while traveling the Thelon River, please choose 12 pictures related to any one or more of the following "themes." You may choose any photograph from your Thelon River experiences, but please ensure that each theme is represented at least once. The themes are:

a.   A **positive** and/or **negative** encounter on the river

b.   Something that was **good** and/or **bad** about your river experience

c.   Something that was observed to be **fair** or **unfair** while on the river

d.   Something that **belongs** or **doesn't belong** on the river

e.   A **change** caused by **humans**

f.   A **change** that **just happens**

g.   Something **significant** about the river

h.   Something that tells you what to do or **how you should behave**

TABLE 8.2. Experiential journey descriptions.

Date (all 2010)	Mode of Transportation	Destination	Approximate Distance (km)	*Guide* and Participants
5/8	Snowmobile	Baker Lake to Halfway Hills	73	*Anautalik*
5/16	Walking	Baker Lake Blueberry Hill	7	N/A
7/10–7/20	Canoe	Thelon Wildlife Sanctuary	270	*Alex Hall* 8 clients
7/24	Motorboat	Baker Lake to Lower Kazan River	183	*Anautalik, Anautalik's husband,* 3 Inuit (2 youth, 1 adult)
7/25	All-terrain vehicle	Baker Lake to Prince River	33	3 non-Inuit
7/27	All-terrain vehicle	Baker Lake to guide's cabin	24	*Anautalik* 1 non-Inuk
11/27	Snowmobile	Baker Lake to guide's cabin	20	*Anautalik* 3 Inuit (2 youth, 1 adult)

raise questions about cultural practices different from their own, and clarify cultural norms with respect to responsibility to and for this special and changing riverscape. The same photographs were used in the Lutsel K'e workshop I described in this chapter's introduction. Implemented initially as modes of participatory interpretation, the photograph workshops evolved to play an important role in establishing new partnerships with a northern First Nation and advancing a new phase of *Picturing the Thelon River* (2013–2015).

Conventional approaches to data analysis, which would be fair to consider well removed from the direct contexts of the field, have also been incorporated into *Picturing the Thelon River*. For example, content analysis was used to organize manifest themes and interpret latent meanings associated with the qualitative and visual data generated by Thelon tourists and inhabitants (Grimwood & Doubleday, 2013a, 2013b). These analyses, however, were not performed under the guise of neutrality or meant to authorize an irrevocable truth about the Thelon's social-ecological-cultural realities. Rather, interpretation emulated what Kulchyski (2006) describes as an "ethics of reading": a critical and situated engagement with social theory and community-oriented research practice that aims to "give a sense" of cultural alternatives to the logics of totalization. It is about using iterative interpretations and writing to illuminate expressions of value, meaning—and perhaps even responsibility—that present positive possibilities for the communities we work with (Kulchyski, 2006). So, when content analysis was used to illuminate Inuit uses and relationships with the Thelon River (Grimwood & Doubleday, 2013a), we did so to prompt visions of Arctic river system governance—and northern futures more generally—based on values of collaboration, equity, democracy, and plurality of perspectives; it is a reading that challenges the singular federal vision of Canadian sovereignty fixated on securing a resource frontier. Such interpretations are in line with the action agenda of PAR insofar as they represent relevant entry points for future transformations (Khan, Bawani, & Aziz, 2013).

PAR researchers also often commit to analytical and interpretive work that, in addition to fostering research results, churns critical reflection and learning with respect to methodological processes and the structural circumstances within which they are positioned (Brydon-Miller et al., 2003). Indeed, engaging the nexus of action–reflection and theory–method lies at the heart of PAR (Kindon, Pain, & Kesby, 2007c). The methodological construct of engaged acclimatization, discussed earlier in this chapter, was the result of critically reflecting on how I negotiated the meaning and practice of responsible research during initial experiences with community-based participatory approaches in Nunavut. Fieldnotes, observations, and photographs from these early community encounters, coupled later with academic literature, served as source material for reflexive and critical engagement with the processes involved in establishing research partnerships. The analytical work was very much iterative. Ideas and illustrative moments unpinning the conceptualization were fleshed out and refined through conversations with coauthors, cycles of reading and writing, numerous revisions based on feedback from colleagues and editors, and consistent attentiveness to the possibility of being overly prescriptive or losing touch with the situated and contextual genesis of engaged acclimatization. The most significant and obvious limitation of this interpretation and writing is that voices of community research partners were largely absent. As such, we acknowledge in the paper that engaged acclimatization is derived from situated *Qablunaat* (non-Inuit) perspectives; therefore, the thinking, experiences, and merit we associate with the process should be scrutinized from other vantage points.

Clearly, interrogating the relations of power within which we are embedded as PAR researchers is imperative to advancing social transformation and more democratic forms of knowledge production. All of us assume multiple positionalities at any one time (Herr & Anderson, 2005) and are disciplined to perform in certain ways by various structural factors and forces (Foucault, 1980). As Freire (1970) observes, the focus of social change is not entirely about escaping oppressive situations; it is also about escaping that piece of the oppressor planted deep within each of us. This, of course, can never be a *final* escape, since power relations, as we know from Foucault, are ever present and only shift in terms of how, what, and whom they effect.

Considerations Related to Social Justice

Socio-political discourses that reinforce perceptions of the Arctic as empty wilderness and/or resource frontier depend on the erasure of Indigenous peoples and their histories from within a landscape. Within the colonial context of Canadian nation building, these narratives have entitled, and continue to entitle, non-Aboriginal people (mainly white settlers) to occupy and claim territory. Since 2007, for instance, Canadian Prime Minister Stephen Harper has repeated his clarion call with respect to Arctic sovereignty—"use it or lose it"—an unfortunate if not explicit denial of generations of Aboriginal occupancy and legal realities of Aboriginal title written into treaties and comprehensive land claims.

Academic research and recreational canoeing—two very different sets of practices, to be sure, but overlapping at least insofar as they both play out in my own identity performances (Grimwood, 2011b)—have abetted this dispossession and denial (for insight into the intellectual's role, see Smith [1999]; for the canoeist's, see Erickson [2013]). Indeed, my scholarly passions and leisure pursuits are inextricably linked to these egregious legacies. But instead of abandoning them outright, or clutching them steadfastly to defend against the burden of guilt, I participate in the Arctic intent on mobilizing my relative privilege as a beneficiary of colonialism in ways that might prompt things to be done differently. The orienting values and features of PAR have proven effective. They have helped create and nurture collaborative spaces (institutional, interpersonal, representational) for learning with communities, identifying with the Arctic as "homeland" of resilient societies, and critically reflecting on research praxis and its potential for enacting positive social change. Before concluding this chapter, I'd like to draw on my experiences to identify and briefly discuss five key considerations when employing PAR as an approach to social justice research.

1. Distribution of Research Benefits/Resources

The social and institutional contexts within which academic researchers are situated afford us degrees of relative privilege. We are paid to pursue research and teaching interests and are protected by academic freedoms. We travel to fieldwork sites, international conferences, or the institutions of our colleagues. We have extraordinary access to information, technology, and agencies that financially support what we do. Whether we like it or not, we are often perceived as the gatekeepers of knowledge. PAR and its affiliated approaches compel us to distribute these and other benefits and resources within the communities that we work. In Arctic communities, paying honoraria is a modest, albeit generally appreciated, way to acknowledge participants' knowledge contributions. Similarly, hiring community members to respected positions within the research team—e.g., research assistants, community liaisons, guides, and interpreters—contributes to flows of household income and honors local knowledge. Training and skill development with respect to research methodology, communication, and project management can also foster individual and community capacity, leading to new projects designed and implemented exclusively by the communities themselves. Research-related resources can also be directed to methodological processes that support participants' expression of identity and/or culture. For example, the experiential river trips noted above were a form of data collection that supported/prompted subsistence practices and connections to homeland. In the current phase of *Picturing the Thelon River*, a headwaters land camp experience will provide a context for Dene hunters and youth to exchange knowledge while working with academic researchers to plan future collaborative and land-based research. The Lutsel K'e Dene First Nation identified several benefits associated with the research land camp, including greater awareness of Dene land use, occupancy, and livelihoods within their community and beyond; improved protection of traditional lands; and increased opportunities for culturally meaningful land use and economic alternatives to resource extraction.

2. Democratization of Knowledge

PAR represents the democratization of knowledge in terms of knowledge access, ownership, and generation. Much like PAR itself, democratizing knowledge is an emergent process and—more often than not—an ideal to which researchers strive. Rarely, if ever, does a project begin with conditions of free and equal knowledge/knowledge production already in place. Nor is democracy ever fully achieved or maintained during PAR processes. Instead, PAR instructs us to be consistently attentive to opportunities for enhancing the democratic nature of research processes and outcomes. Working to improve the level of community involvement during project design, field research, and data analysis stages is important to these ends (Stewart & Draper, 2009). This requires researchers and their sponsoring institutions to accept degrees of methodological malleability (or messiness). In Baker Lake, for example, my initial consultations with community representatives and residents led to modifying the study objectives to better reflect local interests and concerns with respect to the Thelon, as well as to improve the communication of project intentions, which was especially necessary when translating between English and Inuktitut. With respect to field research, community members had a great deal of input in terms the content of data collected and analyzed, but also when, where, and how these processes were accomplished.

Democratizing knowledge goes far beyond the conventional stages of research (i.e., from design to analysis/interpretation). It also demands that researchers and community partners engage in open and ongoing dialogue about issues of ownership and dissemination. I share the view that participating communities are the rightful owners of knowledge documented via research, as well as the outcomes generated, whether tangible, conceptual, action-oriented, and so forth. For me, this translates into asking permission to copy and use participant photographs, or to document river journeys and research workshops, while ensuring that all original data sources remain in the community. It also means that participants are given the choice of being named (or not) for their knowledge contributions (Wilson, 2008). When I write, I represent a partial, albeit hopefully convincing, perspective that acknowledges and values the contributions made by Aboriginal participants. In many cases, academic researchers are collaborating with individuals (e.g., Laidler & Elee, 2008) and entire communities/First Nations (e.g., Castleden et al., 2008) as coauthors of peer-reviewed manuscripts. Of course, democratizing knowledge does not stop there. Journal editorial boards, for example, remain the terrain of disproportionately white male voices from developed nations and thus demand careful rethinking and restructuring (Brydon-Miller et al., 2003).

3. Politics of Participation

Despite its laudable potential for social justice research and spurring social change, PAR has been faced with some stinging critiques that cast doubt on its utility and legitimacy. According to Kesby, Kindon, and Pain (2007), most critiques have centred on negative power effects associated with "participation." Kesby et al. (2007) summarize these critiques as follows:

- PAR de-legitimizes research methods that are *not* participatory;
- PAR produces participants as subjects *requiring* "research"/"development";
- PAR disciplines these subjects as *participants* expected to perform appropriately within participatory processes;
- PAR allows researchers to retain control over knowledge while presenting themselves as benign arbitrators of benevolent processes;
- PAR re-authorizes researchers as experts *in* participatory approaches;
- PAR often romanticizes or marginalizes local knowledge produced through its processes;
- PAR reinforces pre-existing power hierarchies among participating communities; and
- PAR legitimizes the elite local knowledge that tends to be conveyed through its processes.

In effect, the formulaic and researcher-led application of participatory techniques has the potential to reinforce the kinds of inequalities and power relations between researchers and communities that PAR is meant to address (Kindon, 2005).

Moreover, in many situations beyond academia, participation has been co-opted as a strategy for further exploiting marginalized peoples and extracting resources, knowledge, or free labor for private interests and economic gain (Cornwall & Jewkes, 1995). While intentions of social responsibility, cultural sensitivity, or sustainability might factor into private-sector engagement with participatory approaches, these ideals must be interrogated and cautiously weighed. During my fieldwork in Baker Lake, the presence of exogenous resource extraction industries (gold, uranium) was palpable, in large part due to the participatory-related activities that they finance and perform, which include regular meetings with local consultation committees, documentation of traditional knowledge, community events, and competitions involving helicopter rides to proposed mine sites located within traditional hunting grounds. Without question, these participatory endeavors are designed to garner community support for extracting resources on Inuit-owned and/or ancestral lands.

In my view, however, politicizing participation does not automatically reduce PAR to methodological villain or render it ineffectual. Rather, it serves as an important reminder that no one narrative, methodological or otherwise, is universally virtuous or without silences, something that poststructuralists have called attention to for some time. My application of participatory methods and engagement with northern Aboriginal communities is, therefore, always cautious and responsive. Borrowing from Kindon (2005), "being open to sharing facilitation and innovating techniques in response to specific contexts can play a vital role in helping to monitor who is framing participation and how" (p. 217). These sentiments also apply to who takes responsibility for activating the change associated with a PAR project. When community representatives are placed as equal partners in research, "responsibility for action is not to be appropriated by the researchers, not to be abandoned by the researchers, but seen as a joint responsibility of the two—researchers and research-partners" (Khan et al., 2013, p. 162). To illustrate briefly, I'll point to the action of immersing Inuit youth in cultural traditions associated with the Thelon River, which occurred during some of the experiential river journeys. The local Inuk guide/research coordinator determined these trips to be opportunities for youth engagement; so together we adapted research plans and methods to accommodate their involvement. Much like Kesby et al. (2007), these and other experiences suggest to me that PAR is always a work in progress. Attuning ourselves to the multiple faces of participation and action provides important checks and balances in the process of inviting spaces for positive interaction, dialogue, transformation, and authentic partnership (Dupuis et al., 2011; Kesby et al., 2007).

4. Questioning Dominant Ideologies

One complication associated with doing PAR for social justice work arises when participants' perspectives of their community mirror— and are clearly shaped by—the kind of dominant cultural ideologies that enforce marginalization in the first place. The Thelon canoeists that I have worked with, for example, tend to reify conceptions of external and primordial nature (Muldoon, Qiu, Yudina, & Grimwood, 2013). If researchers embrace PAR as a process that values participants' views, how might dominant ideologies expressed in their voices be countered or resisted? Smith et al.'s (2010) approach to this challenge is to "strike a balance between honoring these perspectives but also facilitating a questioning of the taken-for-granted assumptions behind them" (p. 413). Although uncorroborated, I have found that sharing Inuit participant photographs with Thelon canoeists provokes this kind of introspection and questioning of norms. Photographs allowed the Other to be seen and heard. Moreover, when engaged in judgement-free, dialogical, and arts-based processes, I have found members of "outdoors subculture" to be quite keen and capable of expressing complex concerns with their own ideologies of nature (see Figure 8.2). Some of the onus I also place upon myself as a fellow canoeist. I often turn inward, reflecting and writing into my own positionality to initiate degrees of transformation that I can feel, own, persistently aspire to, and hopefully communicate (e.g., Grimwood, 2011b). In a critical commentary about the burgeoning academy of hope in tourism studies, Higgins-Desbiolles and Whyte (2013) convey the relevance of such personal scrutiny to solidarity and social justice work. They argue that the basis of dialogue with marginalized populations "rests on those in positions of privilege first acknowledging and then interrogating privilege and then reaching out to those in positions of colonized/marginalized subjectivities for developing an emancipatory praxis in *collaboration*" (Higgins-Desbiolles & Whyte, p. 431, original emphasis). Indeed, reaching out with PAR demands that we also reach in.

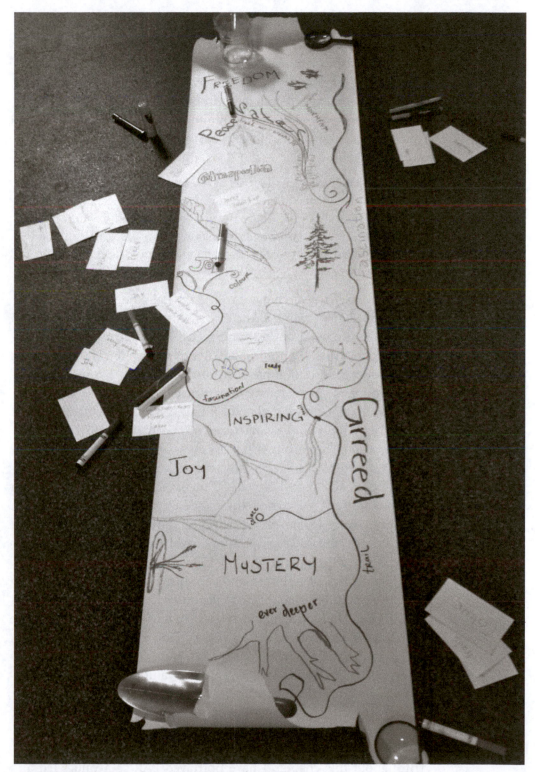

FIGURE 8.2. The complexity of nature as represented by outdoor educators in Ontario, Canada.

5. Research Ethics

PAR also demands institutional changes to champion political and personal transformations occurring during research and to accommodate researchers committed to knowledge production that is flexible, reflexive, and messy rather than linear in structure (Cornwall & Jewkes, 1995). For instance, PAR's underpinning values and features call for a fundamental reconsideration of what constitutes research ethics. According to Brydon-Miller et al. (2011), the conventional system:

> relies upon a contractual model of research ethics with an emphasis on informed consent and the academic researcher's ownership and control of data. This model reinforces the power and authority of the academic researcher.... [It] also calls into question the principles of caring and commitment that are at the heart of participatory action research by recasting these relationships as potential sites of coercion. (pp. 390–391)

In Canada, recent changes to the ethical guidelines set forth by principle federal funding agencies (CIHR et al., 2010) are helping to generate awareness that PAR and related approaches, and Aboriginal research broadly conceived, involve dynamic ethical relationships and accountabilities that are difficult to systemize. Because PAR values encounters with alternative worldviews, including what constitutes good, right, and moral behavior, research ethics will fall short if limited to written rules, abstractions, or purely rationalistic methods. In Grimwood, Doubleday et al. (2012), we prompt further discussion about the nature of research ethics by suggesting it involves embodied, affective, social, and everyday dimensions. Following Rundstrom and Deur (1999), we argue "ethics and ethical behaviour in research does not emerge from isolated reflection, but has to be negotiated as a form of...reciprocal appropriation, involving exchange of information as part of long-term relationships" (pp. 207–208). To be sure, this is an ethics of response and responsibility that is lived. Much like Brydon-Miller et al.'s (2011) vision of "community covenantal ethics" as an alternative model of research ethics for PAR, it is a stance framed by relationships, reciprocity, collaborative decision-making, and power sharing. When research, as a historical and contemporary enterprise, is laced with controversy, such values-led visions are clearly necessary for realizing research that is truly done *with* others.

Conclusion

Throughout this chapter, I have portrayed PAR as a values-led and contextually specific orientation to inquiry. From this perspective,

PAR is less a prescriptive methodological framework than it is an emergent process for enacting change, an ideal but evolving partnership between academic and community researchers who commit to engaging together in research to address locally determined and locally relevant social circumstances. Social justice is thus an inherent feature of both the process and product of PAR. Indeed, from articulating the questions, issues, and rationale driving or initiating a given project, through to the data collection and analysis procedures, the transformative actions taken, and even the way research outcomes are disseminated and reported, the promotion of social justice is and—if one agrees with Fals Borda (2006)—always has been a central concern to PAR researchers. This marks an important point of distinction for PAR relative to the methodologies discussed elsewhere in this book. Whereas well-founded disciplinary and epistemological roots of other methodologies have shifted to adopt social justice mandates, inextricable and inescapable intentions of social justice exist behind the origins, trajectories, and contemporary performances of PAR.

REFERENCES

Aporta, C. (2011). Shifting perspectives on shifting ice: Documenting and representing Inuit use of the sea ice. *The Canadian Geographer, 55*(1), 6–19.

Barnett, G. (2012). Moving north: Engaging community with place through dance. *Polar Geography, 35*(3–4), 291–307.

Bennett, N., Lemelin, R. H., Johnston, M. E., & Lutsel K'e Dene First Nation. (2010). Using the social economy in tourism: A study of National Park creation and community development in the Northwest Territories, Canada. *Journal of Rural and Community Development, 5*(1/2), 200–220.

Brydon-Miller, M., Greenwood, D., & Maguire, P. (2003). Why action research? *Action Research, 1*(1), 9–28.

Brydon-Miller, M., Kral, M., Maguire, P., Noffke, S., & Sabhlok, A. (2011). Jazz and the banyan tree: Roots and riffs on participatory action research. In N. K. Denzin & Y. S. Lincoln (Eds.), *The Sage handbook of qualitative research* (4th ed.) (pp. 387–400). Thousand Oaks, CA: Sage.

Caine, K. J., Davison, C. M., & Stewart, E. J. (2009). Preliminary fieldwork: Methodological reflections from northern Canadian research. *Qualitative Research, 9*(4), 489–513.

Castleden, H., Garvin, T., & Huu-ay-aht First Nation. (2008). Modifying photovoice for community-based participatory Indigenous research. *Social Science and Medicine, 66*, 1393–1405.

Canadian Institutes of Health Research, Natural Sciences and Engineering Research Council of Canada, & Social Sciences and Humanities Research Council of Canada (CIHR, NSERC, & SSHRC). (2010). *Tri-Council policy statement: Ethical conduct for research involving humans.* Ottawa, ON, Canada: Canadian Institutes of Health Research. Retrieved from http://www.pre.ethics.gc.ca

Cooperrider, D. L., & Whitney, D. (2005). *Appreciative inquiry: A positive revolution in change.* San Francisco, CA: Berrett-Koehler.

Cornwall, A., & Jewkes, R. (1995). What is participatory research? *Social Science and Medicine, 441*(12), 1667–1676.

Cuerrier, A., Downing, A., Johnstone, J., Hermanutz, L., Siegwart Collier, L., & Elders and Youth participants of Nain and Old Crow. (2012). Our plants, our land: Bridging aboriginal generations through cross-cultural plant workshops. *Polar Geography, 35*(3–4), 195–210.

Dick, B. (2006). Action research literature 2004–2006: Themes and trends. *Action Research, 4*(4), 439–458.

Dick, B. (2009). Action research literature 2006–2008: Themes and trends. *Action Research, 7*(4), 423–441.

Dupuis, S. L., Gillies, J., Carson, J., Whyte, C., Genoe, R., Loiselle, L., & Sadler, L. (2011). Moving beyond patient and client approaches: Mobilizing "authentic partnerships" in dementia care, support and services. *Dementia, 11*(4), 427–452.

Erickson, B. (2013). *Canoe Nation: Nature, race, and the making of a Canadian icon.* Vancouver, BC, Canada: UBC Press.

Fals Borda, O. (2006). The North-South convergence: A 30-year first-person assessment of PAR. *Action Research, 4*(3), 351–358.

Ford, J. D., & Smit, B. (2004). A framework for assessing the vulnerability of communities in the Canadian Arctic to risks associated with climate change. *Arctic, 57*(4), 389–400.

Foucault, M. (1980). *Power/knowledge: Selected interviews and other writings 1972–1977.* New York: Pantheon Books.

Freire, P. (1970). *Pedagogy of the oppressed.* New York: Seabury.

Gearheard, S., Aporta, C., Aipellee, G., & O'Keefe, K. (2011). The Igliniit project: Inuit hunters document life on the trail to map and monitor arctic change. *The Canadian Geographer, 55*(1), 42–55.

Greenwood, D., Whyte, W. F., & Harkavy, I. (1993). Participatory action research as a process and as a goal. *Human Relations, 46*(2), 175–192.

Grimwood, B. S. R. (2011a). *Picturing the Thelon: Natures, ethics, and travel within an Arctic riverscape.* Unpublished doctoral dissertation. Carleton University, Ottawa, ON, Canada.

Grimwood, B. S. R. (2011b). "Thinking outside the gunnels": Considering natures and the moral terrains of recreational canoe travel. *Leisure/Loisir, 35*(1), 49–69.

Grimwood, B. S. R., Cuerrier, A., & Doubleday, N. C. (2012). Introduction: Arctic community engagement during the 2007–2008 International Polar Year. *Polar Geography, 35*(3–4), 189–193.

Grimwood, B. S. R., & Doubleday, N. C. (2013a). From river trails to adaptive co-management: Learning and relating with Inuit inhabitants of the Thelon River, Canada. *Indigenous Policy Journal, 23*(4). Retrieved from http://www.indigenouspolicy.org/index.php/ipj/article/view/146

Grimwood, B. S. R., & Doubleday, N. C. (2013b). Illuminating traces: Enactments of responsibility in practices of Arctic river tourists and inhabitants. *Journal of Ecotourism, 12*(2), 53–74.

Grimwood, B. S. R., Doubleday, N. C., Ljubicic, G. J., Donaldson, S. G., & Blangy, S. (2012). Engaged acclimatization: Towards responsible community-based participatory research in Nunavut. *The Canadian Geographer, 56*(2), 211–230.

Harper, D. (2002). Talking about pictures: A case for photo elicitations. *Visual Studies, 17*(1), 13–26.

Herr, K., & Anderson, G. (2005). *The action research dissertation*. Thousand Oaks, CA: Sage.

Higgins-Desbiolles, F., & Powys Whyte, K. (2013). No high hopes for hopeful tourism: A critical comment. *Annals of Tourism Research, 40*, 428–433.

Ip, M., Grimwood, B. S. R., Kushwaha, A., Doubleday, N. C., & Donaldson, S. G. (2008). Photos and plants through time: Monitoring environmental change in the Canadian Arctic with implications for outdoor education. *Pathways: The Ontario Journal of Outdoor Education, 21*(1), 14–18.

ITK (Inuit Tapiriit Kanatami), & NRI (Nunavut Research Institute). (2007). *Negotiating research partnerships with Inuit communities: A guide for researchers*. S. Nickels, J. Shirley, & G. J. Laidler (Eds.). Ottawa, ON, and Iqaluit, NU, Canada: ITK & NRI.

Jensen, A. M. (2012). Culture and change: Learning from the past through community archaeology and the North Slope. *Polar Geography, 35*(3–4), 211–227.

Johnson, J. T. (2010). Place-based learning and knowing: Critical pedagogies grounded in indigeneity. *Geojournal, 77*, 829–836.

Kemmis, S., & McTaggart, R. (2000). Participatory action research. In N. K. Denzin & Y. S. Lincoln (Eds.), *Handbook of qualitative research* (2nd ed.) (pp. 567–605). Thousand Oaks, CA: Sage.

Kesby, M., & Gwanzura-Ottemoler, F. (2007). Researching sexual health: Two participatory action research projects in Zimbabwe. In S. Kindon, R. Pain & M. Kesby (Eds.), *Participatory action research approaches and methods: Connecting people, participation, and place* (pp. 71–79). New York: Routledge.

Kesby, M., Kindon, S., & Pain, R. (2007). Participation as a form of power: Retheorising empowerment and spatialising participatory action research. In S. Kindon, R. Pain & M. Kesby (Eds.), *Participatory action research approaches and methods: Connecting people, participation and place* (pp. 19–25). New York: Routledge.

Khan, K. S., Bawani, S. A. A., & Aziz, A. (2013). Bridging the gap of knowledge and action: A case for participatory action research (PAR). *Action Research, 11*(2), 157–175.

Khanlou, N., & Peter, E. (2005). Participatory action research: Considerations for ethical review. *Social Science and Medicine, 60*, 2333–2340.

Kindon, S. (2005). Participatory action research. In I. Hay (Ed.), *Qualitative methods in human geography* (pp. 207–220). Don Mills, ON, Canada: Oxford University Press.

Kindon, S., Pain, R. & Kesby, M. (2007a). Introduction: Connecting people, participation and place. In S. Kindon, R. Pain & M. Kesby (Eds.), *Participatory action research approaches and methods: Connecting people, participation and place* (pp. 1–5). New York: Routledge.

Kindon, S., Pain, R., & Kesby, M. (2007b). Participatory action research: Origins, approaches and methods. In S. Kindon, R. Pain & M. Kesby (Eds.), *Participatory action research approaches and methods: Connecting people, participation and place* (pp. 9–18). New York: Routledge.

Kindon, S., Pain, R., & Kesby, M. (Eds.). (2007c). *Participatory action research approaches and methods: Connecting people, participation and place*. New York: Routledge.

Klodawsky, F. (2007). "Choosing" participatory research: Partnerships in space–time. *Environment and Planning A, 39*, 2845–2860.

Koster, R. L. P., & Lemelin, R. H. (2009). Appreciative inquiry and rural tourism: A case study from Canada. *Tourism Geographies, 11*(2), 256–269.

Kulchyski, P. (2006). Six gestures. In P. Stern & L. Stevenson (Eds.), *Critical Inuit studies: An anthology of contemporary Arctic ethnography* (pp. 155–167). Lincoln, NE: University of Nebraska Press.

Laidler, G. J. (2007). *Ice, through Inuit eyes: Characterizing the importance of sea ice processes, use, and change around three Nunavut communities*. Unpublished doctoral dissertation. University of Toronto, Toronto, ON, Canada.

Laidler, G. J., & Elee, P. (2008). Human geographies of sea ice: Freeze/thaw processes around Cape Dorset, Nunavut, Canada. *Polar Record, 44*(2), 51–76.

Laidler, G. J., Ford, J. D., Gough, W. A., Ikummaq, T., Gagnon, A. S., Kowal, S., Qrunnut, K., & Irngaut, C. (2009). Travelling and hunting in a changing Arctic: Assessing Inuit vulnerability to sea ice change in Igloolik, Nunavut. *Climatic Change, 94*, 363–397.

Lemelin, R. H., Dawson, J., Stewart, E. J., Maher, P. T., & Lück, M. (2010). Last chance tourism: The doom, the gloom, and the boom of visiting vanishing destinations. *Current Issues in Tourism, 13*(5), 477–493.

Lemelin, R. H., Wiersma, E. C., Trapper, L., Kapashesit, R. , Beaulieu, M. S., & Dowsley, M. (2013). A dialogue and reflection on photohistory: Engaging indigenous communities in research through visual analysis. *Action Research, 11*(1), 92–107.

Louis, R. P. (2007). Can you hear us now? Voices from the margin: Using Indigenous methodologies in geographic research. *Geographical Research, 45*(2), 130–139.

Markey, S., Halseth, G., & Mason, D. (2010). Capacity, scale and place: Pragmatic lessons for doing community-based research in the rural setting. *The Canadian Geographer, 54*(2), 158–176.

Muldoon, M., Qiu, J., Yudina, O., & Grimwood, B. S. R. (2013). *A postcolonial reading of responsibility in tourism.* Paper presented at the International Critical Toursim Studies Conference V, Sarajevo, Bosnia & Herzegovina, June 25–28. Retrieved from http://cts.som.surrey.ac.uk/sample-page/tourism-and-its-potential-as-a-social-force/?wpa-paged=2

Pain, R. (2004). Social geography: Participatory research. *Progress in Human Geography, 28*(5), 652–663.

Panelli, R. (2008). Social geographies: Encounters with Indigenous and more-than-White/Anglo geographies. *Progress in Human Geography, 32*, 1–11.

Pulsifer, P., Gearheard, S., Huntington, H. P., Parson, M. A., McNeave, C., & McCann, H. S. (2012). The role of data management in engaging communities in Arctic research: Overview of the Exchange for Local Observations and Knowledge of the Arctic (ELOKA). *Polar Geography, 35*(3–4), 271–290.

Reason, P., & Bradbury, H. (2008). *The Sage handbook of action research: Participative inquiry and practice* (2nd ed.). Thousand Oaks, CA: Sage.

Reason, P., & Torbert, W. R. (2001). Toward a transformational science: A further look at the scientific merits of action research. *Concepts and Transformation, 6*(1), 1–37.

Rundstrom, R., & Deur, D. (1999). Reciprocal appropriation: Toward an ethics of cross-cultural research. In J. D. Proctor & D. M. Smith (Eds.), *Geography and ethics: Journeys in a moral terrain* (pp. 237–250). New York: Routledge.

Smith, L. T. (1999). *Decolonizing methodologies: Research and Indigenous peoples*. London, UK: Zed Books.

Smith, L., Bratini, L., Chambers, D. A., Jensen, R. V., & Romero, L. (2010). Between idealism and reality: Meeting the challenges of participatory action research. *Action Research, 8*(4), 407–425.

Stewart, E. J., & Draper, D. (2009). Reporting back research findings: A case study of community based tourism research in northern Canada. *Journal of Ecotourism, 8*(2), 128–143.

Stewart, E. J., Jacobson, D., & Draper, D. (2008). Public participation geographic information systems (PPGIS): Challenges of implementation in Churchill, Manitoba. *The Canadian Geographer, 52*(3), 351–366.

Whyte, W. F., Greenwood, D., & Lazes, P. (1989). Participatory action research: Through practice to science in social research. *American Behavioral Scientist, 32*(5), 513–551.

Wilson, S. (2008). *Research is ceremony: Indigenous research methods*. Halifax, NS, Canada: Fernwood Publishing.

Evocative Inquiry: Saving the World, One Story at a Time

Caitlin M. Mulcahy

Prologue

The night after I submitted the first draft of this chapter to the editors of this book, I had the oddest thing happen to me. All of my children fell asleep at a reasonable hour. My husband was out for the night. I was…alone.

This rarely happens to me, a mother of three young children and now a very new assistant professor; I rarely have time on my hands, and as such, I didn't know how to spend it.

It was raining out, lovely warm rain that came in through the windows that I'd propped open to get rid of some of the diaper smell, and I was sitting at my desk, beside which sits heaps of Lego and a tent full of Barbies and their furniture. I crossed my arms, leaned back in my chair, and puzzled: What was I to do? Nintendo? Netflix? Highly problematic yet satisfying romance novel? Beer and candy? I grew antsy with possibilities.

I'm not sure what caused me to deviate from this light, leisurely fare and instead turn on my laptop and start searching, but that's what I did, scrolling through folder and subfolder until I found it. The one article I'd always pretended to read, but actually never had. It had a strange, lurid feel to it. I was both attracted and repelled. I had avoided Carol Rambo Ronai's (1995) firsthand account of childhood sex abuse for as long as I'd known about it for the same reason I avoid slasher films and my own teenaged diaries: there are some things that I just can't stomach. Yet there I was, double-clicking on the icon just after I had come to the realization that evocative inquiry probably doesn't really change the world after all.

Let me back up for a second. Hours earlier I submitted to the editors of this book a chapter arguing for the social justice–promoting powers of evocative inquiry pieces like Ronai's. I wasn't thrilled with the draft. There was a lackluster feel, an absence of energy, of conviction, that I was attempting to push past to get the thing done. Truth was, I wasn't really sure evocative inquiry did what I was saying it did. I had nagging concerns about evocative inquiry's ability to create change, and what's more, what kind of change would that be, anyway? I couldn't for the life of me, even after writing forty-four pages of it, imagine what that change, brought about by evocative inquiry, would look like. But I was prepared to put those concerns aside so I could move on to the next project requiring my attention, probably Lego related.

I think the part of me that sought out and double-clicked on the article was the same part of me that imagined I could just skim the Ronai piece. Nope. Once clicked, I was immediately sucked into the vortex of Ronai's achingly painful account of the sex abuse she suffered at the hands of her father. *"If I hid from him well…"* she begins, and I began as well, to change. And by the end of the article, I was a different person.

I was physically ill for the rest of the night and had nightmares for days. I couldn't look my husband or children in the eye. I skipped an evening out with friends. I went for long runs and long showers, all in an attempt to shake this article. I wished I had never set eyes on the thing. I railed against evocative inquiry and decided I hated it. One evening while I was running and trying valiantly to distract my thoughts with *Buffy the Vampire Slayer*, a shadow of an idea formed in the back of my mind. When I turned off the treadmill and stepped onto the ground, a line from the article popped into my head: "If male supremacy and patriarchal families were eliminated, then incest and other forms of rape would be eliminated" (Ronai, 1995, p. 406). For the first time since reading the article, I felt my body calm. I knew what I had to do. I raised a fist and spoke aloud to a dingy, empty basement: "I call for a revolution."

In the following days, I staged my own tiny revolution. I "liked" feminist Facebook pages. I circulated articles to friends that might affront their politics. Instead of quietly maintaining the peace during afterschool playgroup at our suburban park, I openly expressed distaste for Tinkerbell. And at home, I bundled up the glorious set of Barbies, clothes, and furniture that had been given to my daughter and stuffed them into a black garbage bag. My revolution was neither large, nor organized, nor even perhaps detectable to anyone else but me. But I felt it. It made a difference to me.

That was five weeks ago. Now the Ronai article sits at the back of my mind (and on the front of my syllabus for a new course) as a reminder to me that feminist work is important, that systems of oppression have to go, and that I have to work to create that change in my everyday life. Ronai, in writing a piece of evocative inquiry nearly twenty years ago, is keeping me vigilant and pushing for social justice. I had been lulled into the sweet cocoon of white, suburban, dual-income life, and this piece of evocative inquiry woke my raging feminist sensibilities back up with a vengeance. Today, Barbie; tomorrow—with any hope—the world. And so as I submit this new draft, still questioning but less uncertain, I guess I don't know if evocative inquiry *does* create change, but I guess I do know that it *can*. And right now, that's enough for me. I have been *moved* by evocative inquiry. And now I'll invite you to come along for the ride.

The Move Toward Being Moved

The move toward evocative inquiry is part of a larger shift in contemporary qualitative research toward creating research that moves people. Contemporary qualitative research has, according to Denzin and Lincoln (2011), transitioned through seven periods to arrive at today's "eighth moment": the traditional period of "objective" ethnographers (1900–1950), the modernist or golden age of positivist and postpositivist social critique (1950–1970), the blurred genres period of initial migration between the arts and social sciences (1970–1986), the crisis of representation period of the emergence of reflexivity and critical theory (1986–1990), the postmodern period of "the narrative turn" (1990–1995), the postexperimental period of "the new ethnographies" (1995–2000), and the methodologically contested present (2000–2010), a period of confronting backlash and mixing methods. Qualitative research in its eighth moment has arrived in "the future" (2010–present), wherein Denzin and Lincoln (2011) urge qualitative researchers to become better at connecting personal troubles to social justice, lived experience to social policy. Here I argue what I deem "evocative inquiry" provides qualitative researchers the opportunity to rise to the challenge of the eighth moment by conducting social science research that moves people: to think, to feel, to change. To begin, I outline the historical and disciplinary roots of evocative inquiry, explore three key expressions of evocative inquiry, detail strategies for data collection and analysis, discuss considerations for social justice, and conclude with suggestions for further readings in evocative inquiry research that have moved me, and might very well move you, too.

Historical and Disciplinary Roots:
The Origins of Evocative Inquiry

Evocative inquiry, otherwise known as "experimental ethnography" (van Maanen, 1988), "creative analytic practice" (L. Richardson, 2000), "arts-based inquiry" (Finley, 2003), and "the new ethnography" (Goodall, 2008) among others, appears in many different forms, including fiction (Banks, 2000), nonfiction (Ellis, 1995), short stories (Parry, 2006), poetry (Brady, 2009), drama (Poulos, 2010), photography (Holmes, 2012), drawing (Picart, 2002), plays (Mulcahy, Parry, & Glover, 2009), dance (Cancienne & Snowber, 2003), visual arts (Minge, 2006), and so forth; however, despite the wide variety of forms this research can take, good research in this realm of study should be evocative (produces a vivid impression of reality; calls up, summons, elicits, draws forth the smells, colors, sounds and shapes of social life) and inquiring (questions, explores, seeks truth). Researchers in this tradition aim to produce research that joins "ethics, aesthetics, political praxis, and epistemology" (Denzin, 2000, p. 258), while calling into question issues of subjectivity, authority, authorship, reflexivity, and the academic research and writing process (L. Richardson, 2000). Whereas more traditionally postpositivist researchers might consider themselves reporters of data, researchers who practice evocative inquiry are more likely to consider themselves storytellers (Goodall, 2008), poets (Tillman-Healy, 1996), or artists (Finley, 2003). Though researchers have proposed a variety of different and sometimes conflicting rubrics of criteria for judging evocative inquiry (more on the specific criteria proposed to follow), it is generally agreed upon that readers of evocative inquiry should be "emotionally aroused and cognitively engaged" by this research (Ellis, 2004, p. 254).

The objective to keep readers engaged through evocative writing arose out of the crisis of representation in social science literature. Many social scientists were questioning what they were writing, how they were writing it, and for whom they wrote. Anthropologists wondered how it came to pass that the ethnographies they produced were "resolutely person-specific" but yet somehow decidedly "not personal" (Behar, 1996, p. 8). Sociologists grappled with the academic imperative to stay "invisible, our own voices mute" despite prominent sociologists such as C. Wright Mills defining the discipline as "at the intersection of biography and history" (Kolker, 1996, p. 135). A. Bochner (1997) suggests some scholars were also frustrated with the quality of social science literature; indeed, Bochner describes the bulk of social science literature as boring and poorly written:

> We pay a steep price for producing texts that sustain the illusion of disinterest and neutrality by keeping the personal voice out. Our work is underread, undergraduates find many of our publications boring, graduate students say our scholarship is dry and inaccessible, seasoned scholars confess they don't finish half of what they start reading, and the public hardly knows we exist. (p. 433)

As such, social scientists, feeling impersonal, ineffective, invisible, and boring, began to turn toward narrative.

During this "narrative turn" (Denzin & Lincoln, 2011) social scientists struggled with issues of voice, authorship, and reflexivity and searched for new ways to represent themselves and their research. The goal of this exploration was to create social science writing that "blurred text and context" (p. 3). The author would be positioned in the text, resisting the postpositivist tradition of the objective, omniscient author, and the text would be messy, uncertain, and multivocal, resisting the demand for the fact-based, incontrovertible linearity that dominated social science literature to this point. This so-called "renaissance" in qualitative research was concerned with reexamining relationships in social science research—relationships between researcher and participant, researcher and reader, and researcher and self—and with creating social science research that was rich, imaginative, creative, and compelling. In this sense, the narrative turn borrowed and benefitted from both the critical conversations about truth, objectivity, and marginalized voices happening in critical and feminist theories, and the conversations about literary tools and rhetoric devices happening in the humanities. What resulted from these crises in representation and narrative turns was nearly two decades of social science literature that both evokes (feelings, sensations, emotions, lived experience) and provokes (thoughts, questions, action, change). Evocative inquiry pieces from this time are gut-wrenching (Ellis & Bochner, 1992), soul-haunting (Ronai, 1996), mind-bending (M. Richardson, 2003), and heart-breaking (Halley, 2003). There are pieces that enrage (Fox, 1996), engage (Tillman-Healy, 1996), incite (Ronai, 1995), and instruct (Jenkins, 2010). There are also pieces that fall short, confuse, drag, and leave cold; yet the effort to create transformative qualitative research is still worthwhile. Because, as Behar (1996) puts it, an "anthropology that doesn't break your heart just isn't worth doing anymore" (p. 177).

So what kind of anthropology is worth doing anymore? What do the parameters of this new tradition of research look like? By what criteria should evocative inquiry be judged? Clough (2000) uses caution when she discusses possible criteria for judging evocative inquiry, arguing that too much emphasis on criteria can invite and encourage methodological policing, leaving less emphasis on imagination, ethics, and producing good, innovative work. Instead, she suggests asking oneself the following kinds of questions when reading evocative inquiry: Does the work have the possibility to create a better world? Does it motivate cultural criticism? Is it closely aligned with theoretical reflection, thus inspiring new sociological thought? On a more aesthetic note, Denzin (2000) offers this advice: these texts should be "poetic, performative, and narrative...hopeful, well-written, and well-plotted stories that show memorable characters and unforgettable scenes" (p. 260). A. Bochner (2000) looks for six criteria when reading evocative inquiry: concrete details, structurally complex narratives, the author's attempt to dig under the superficial to get to vulnerability and honesty, a standard of ethical self-consciousness, a moving story, and transformation, wherein the main character moves in a believable way from who she was to who she becomes. Finley (2003) maintains she does not look for craftspersonship when evaluating evocative inquiry; rather, she finds "great artistry in experiences of passion, communion, and social responsibility" (p. 294). L. Richardson (2000) lays out five criteria: substantive contribution, aesthetic merit, reflexivity, impact, and expression of reality.

At first I subscribed to Richardson's criteria, and yet upon reflection, many of the evocative inquiry pieces I admire and revere could arguably be considered weak when judged against these five specifications. For instance, one could argue Lahman's (2008) exceptionally powerful poem about postpartum depression, printed in *Qualitative Inquiry* without analysis, preamble, or epilogue, failed to make a substantive contribution, and was not explicitly reflexive. But it was incredibly moving. As such, my criteria for judging evocative inquiry have evolved as I have read and written more. As it stands, all I ask of evocative inquiry is that it moves me: moves me to feel, moves me to think, moves me to change, moves me to reflect, moves me to act, moves me into new and different positions and perspectives. This is what separates evocative inquiry from all other forms of research: evocative inquiry allows social scientists the space to focus on creating research that is moving. As I see it, this focus on moving research is what makes evocative inquiry truly powerful and distinct. The criteria set out by previous researchers (social responsibility, reflexivity, transformation) are quite obviously important, but secondary for me. If I am not moved by the research, I consider the piece not to have done its job. To demonstrate the move toward being moved in social science research, we now turn to four examples of the shape evocative inquiry can take.

Variations of Evocative Inquiry

Creating moving research is not an easy feat. It means compelling ourselves to be raw, intimate, and vulnerable. It means not only capturing the *how* and the *why* of the social experience, but also capturing what the social experience *is like*. And it means writing texts that are complex, polyvocal, and multilayered. Though by no means exhaustive of the various forms evocative inquiry can take, here I explore as examples four forms of evocative inquiry that researchers use to create moving research: autoethnography, performance, poetry, and visual arts.

Autoethnography

Autoethnography is part of the autobiographical genre of writing and researching. Perhaps the most widely used form of evocative inquiry, David Hayano (1979) coined the term *autoethnography* to refer to ethnographic work done on one's "own people." The researcher is an "insider" in the culture or experience studied, as opposed to traditional ethnography that necessarily positioned the researcher as an "outsider" studying a culture or experience that was foreign to the anthropologist. Autoethnographers write evocatively in part by writing about themselves: the researcher is a so-called walking laboratory (Ellis, 2004). The autoethnographer studies oneself, one's own lived experiences, and the lives of others connected to those experiences. In this sense, the autoethnographer is intimately embedded in the text, engaging the reader through self-revelation, vulnerability, and reflexivity, provoking empathy, reflection, and critical thought. Autoethnographic narrative is characterized by a multilayered, complex, often fragmented writing style, infused with a critical social analysis and a focus on conveying what a social experience "is like." Researchers have used autoethnography to evoke experiences of abortion (Ellis & Bochner, 1992), child abuse (Ronai, 1996), sex reassignment surgery (Dent, 2002), and eating disorders (Tillmann-Healy, 1996). I have used autoethnography in my own research on the gendered nature of family memory keeping and the impact of a mother's memory loss, during which I interviewed my family members including my mother, who suffers from dementia (Mulcahy, 2012).

Good autoethnography should connect "the teller of the tale" to their audience and should create meaning that is both imaginative and analytical (Goodall, 2008). In other words, good autoethnography should move the reader both emotionally and intellectually. My autoethnographic research dealing with my mother's dementia aimed to move the reader into new positions wherein they could come to new understandings about genetic disease, the gendered nature of family memory keeping, and the complexity of coping with a mother's memory loss. In turn, the reader might be moved to change and to act, to value and celebrate the overlooked labor women perform in the home, to use a feminist lens to critique the gendered division of labor, and to imagine better services for families coping with genetic disease and/or a mother's memory loss. This movement can be created by drawing the reader into the piece through autoethnographic vulnerability, and yet it can also be accomplished through a more polyvocal approach.

Performance Text

With more and more frequency, researchers are turning to the more polyvocal form of performance texts to move their readers to feel, think, and act differently. Denzin (2003) argues performance texts are uniquely powerful in their ability to convey complicated life experiences. These texts create the opportunity for multiple speakers, meanings, layers, realities, experiences, and interpretations (Ellis, 2004). Educational theorists have long used performance as a means of creating empathy; famed educator and activist Augustus Boal (1979) suggested that theatre created the opportunity for audience members to step into the scene (sometimes literally), to take on different roles, to experience life in another's shoes, to experiment with where to go from "here." In writing theatre, researchers are able to use that creative space to play with emotions, space, and voice. Researchers can be disorderly, autobiographical, fictional, representational, abstract, fragmented, and/or incomplete. Plays, ethnodramas, screenplays, and performance pieces have been constructed (and sometimes produced) by researchers to explore varied social experiences such as cancer (Lobel, 2008), American race relations (Denzin, 2008), spousal abuse (Tamas, 2011b), the founding of grassroots feminist organizations (Jenkins, 2010), father–son relationships (Pelias, 2002), and the tenure process (Poulos, 2010). I used a performance text to explore my father's experiences of caring for my mother over the fifteen years of her illness, as well as the gendered division of memory keeping in our home (Mulcahy, 2012).

The performance text allows us to stage the contradictory voices and interpretations present during the research and analysis process. In staging our research as a reflexive performance text, notions of absolute truth, authority, objectivity, and omniscience in research are destabilized. Instead, we are left with a messy, unresolved text and a fractured narrative voice, leaving room for multiple interpretations, movement between positions, and, ultimately, conversation. Moreover, this reflexivity enables a transparency of knowledge production that is not often seen in more traditional methods of representing research. As Tamas (2011b) describes, "the reader is aware that I have scripted everybody…at least we both know that it's a show" (p. 437). In this sense, performance text offers the possibility of both drawing the audience into the social experience by putting on an evocative show and moving the audience into new and dynamic positions emotionally and intellectually. Within these new positions, readers might be moved to think more critically about, as was the goal in my own research, gender, care work, health, illness, and family, and to act more passionately to advance justice and strategize for improved policy and services in these areas as well.

Poetry

Many researchers who practice evocative inquiry find poetry a uniquely expressive and emotional representation of social life. These researchers argue poetry "shows" rather than "tells"; evokes rather than spells out; enables image, metaphor, and freedom of form; empowers the researcher to use rich textures and vivid hues perhaps unavailable through other methods; provokes deep emotional and intellectual response; and facilitates the capturing of elusive moments of truth. Indeed, M. Richardson (1998) suggests, "Poetry wants us to see. To see what? Those instantaneous sights, when things stand so clearly before us, when truth shows its face" (pp. 453–454). Faulkner (2007) outlines a variety of labels for poetry in social science research, including ethnographic poetics, investigative poetry, research poetry, and autoethnographic poetry, but maintains all of these labels describe "a method of turning research interviews, transcripts, observations, personal experience, and reflections into poems or poetic forms" (p. 219). Poetry is used by evocative inquiry researchers in a variety of different ways: some researchers layer their poetry throughout an autoethnographic narrative (Picart, 2002); some present the poem(s) along with an extensive analysis elucidating the meaning of the poem and its relation to research findings or reflexive theorizing (Furman, Langer, Davis, Gallardo, & Kulkarni, 2007). One recent trend in evocative inquiry research is the standalone poem published in peer-reviewed journals and collections without prefacing or following the piece with interpretation (Brady, 2009).

The use of poetry in evocative inquiry attempts to draw readers into the raw, dynamic, and layered experiences of social life, "showing" terror, despair, love, rage, and ambivalence with few words rather than "telling" the experience through traditional statistics, percentages, or block quotes. Through the often tangled and elusive mode of poetry, the author is resisting using the traditional methods of social science writing that value linearity and objectivity, instead opting for writing that suggests rather than substantiates, provokes rather than proves; writing that is more labyrinth than lab. Poetry engages readers' emotional and intellectual responses by writing social research that is deeply engrossing; the hope is that the reader becomes ensnared in the experience, willed to feel empathy, compassion, identification, rejection, or revulsion, but to *feel* nevertheless. In this sense, poetry as evocative inquiry can provide researchers brief, fleeting opportunities to capture readers and refuse to let them go until, as M. Richardson (1998) describes, "truth shows its face" (pp. 453–454), and the reader is irrevocably moved.

Visual Arts

Writing has been a privileged form of evocative inquiry, and the written word has largely dominated evocative inquiry research in the past two decades (Finley, 2003). However, in recent years, many researchers have taken the "visual turn," publishing photography (Church, 2002), painting (Minge, 2006), video (Holmes, 2012), sculpture (Phoenix, 2010), and so forth, that stand alone as social science research (M. Bochner, 2002) or are layered with other forms of text and representation (Picart, 2002). Some researchers suggest visual arts are necessary when the experience they wish to convey goes beyond the written word. As Rich (2004) argues, in these cases, show *is* tell. Evocative inquiry as visual arts makes visible the researcher's findings; however, this method also draws attention to the tension between the seemingly objective (the image) and the necessarily subjective (the multiple levels of interpretation at work of participant, researcher, viewer). This once again throws into question the positivist imperative of absolute truth and objectivity in research, instead inviting multiple interpretations and ways of knowing. Visual arts enable representations of social life that are dynamic, multidimensional, and reflective of our highly graphic and sensual culture. Sighted individuals live in and through images; thus, images can be used to interpret and represent our lived experiences (Pink, 2007). Moreover, images can be particularly vivid, shocking, intriguing, eye-catching, and can provoke strong visceral, emotional, and intellectual reactions, sometimes in just a moment's glance.

In my own research, images have been used to create a layered account of the social experience of family memory keeping (Mulcahy, 2012). I used a variety of images of memory artifacts and the women who keep this memory to explore the ways in which mothers keep, maintain, and shape a family's memory and identity. These images were interspersed with theory, analysis, and reflection, creating a rich, multilayered, dynamic presentation of my findings. However, images used in evocative inquiry research are also often provocative and moving as standalone pieces in their own right, singularly capturing and evoking the researcher's questions and findings in a way that perhaps was not possible to be achieved via the written word. At the very least, the use of images in social science research can create more compelling, absorbing, and aesthetically pleasing research, engaging the reader's imagination and intellect on a variety of different levels, moving the reader to new meanings and understandings.

These four examples of evocative inquiry—autoethnography, performance text, poetry, and visual arts—are by no means exhaustive, nor are they exclusive of one another. Often, researchers will use any or all of these methods of expression within a single piece of evocative inquiry (compare Denzin, 2008). Despite some attempts to claim one method as better than the others, most researchers agree that none of these methodologies/methods hold the key to best understanding or representing the social world. Rather, each should be considered as useful and potentially powerful tools for moving readers to think, act, and change. I now consider how to use those tools by looking more specifically at data collection.

Data Collection Strategies

Collecting data for a research project that uses evocative inquiry can be done in a variety of ways. Some researchers follow more traditional qualitative data collection methods such as participant observation (Johnson & Samdahl, 2005) or interviews with participants previously unknown to them (Banks, 2000). Some interview unknown participants, but participants who share membership in the same culture or experience as the researcher (Doloriert & Sambrook, 2009). Others specifically interview only those within their family or circle of friends (Goodall, 2005). Some researchers interview both known and unknown individuals (Jago, 2006). And some researchers do not do any interviews at all, drawing data instead from physical artifacts, literature, text, music, photographs, video, or their own recollections, dreams, reflections, experiences, observations, and interpretations to create their work (Denzin, 2008). Some researchers, of course, sample from each of these methods, creating the complex, multilayered pieces we have come to anticipate from evocative inquiry research (Holmes, 2012). Here I explore several examples of these multiple strategies for data collection from my own research.

Several of the pieces that later became published performance texts began as relatively traditional semistructured, qualitative interviews with twenty-two to twenty-four individuals who we initially did not know (Mulcahy & Parry, 2011; Mulcahy, Parry, & Glover, 2009). In these cases, it was only upon data analysis that a narrative turn, as it were, was taken (more on this analysis to follow). However, for my research on family memory, genetic disease, and the loss of a mother's memory, data was collected with an autoethnographic research design—I always intended to produce an evocative inquiry piece—and as such, specific interview techniques and data collection strategies were used. As I have discussed, in an autoethnography, the researcher necessarily recruits herself as a participant (Ellis, 2004). I also chose to recruit twenty-three participants from my family and friends. I conducted seven individual interviews and seven group interviews. For the individual interviews, I employed a "reflexive, dyadic" interview approach (Ellis, 2004), for the group interviews, I conducted relatively traditional focus group interviews (Lindelof & Taylor, 2002), and one "interactive interview" (Ellis, 2004); for all interviews I made use of elicitation methods (Loizos, 2000) through what I call *memory artifacts*. Here I explore these strategies in depth, and discuss the benefits and challenges of interviewing family and friends in evocative inquiry research.

Reflexive, Dyadic Interviews

The reflexive, dyadic interview is characterized by an inclusion of the interviewer's thoughts, feelings, and perceptions, alongside the interviewee's words, stories, and interpretations. This means that although the focus remained on my participant's story, I also included my own reflections on the interview to create a more reflexive, layered account of the experience. The reflexive, dyadic interview is also characterized by a conversational style fostered by the interviewer, and the presence of mutual disclosure; in my research on family memory, I was always open with my participants about what drew me to the project, sharing my own experiences as both a mother and a daughter grappling with her mother's dementia. However, these interviews are not merely a conversation between two friends; participants still looked to me to direct the interview, and I still referred to an interview guide during the process. Yet I allowed the conversation to deviate from the specific questions frequently, which can lead the interview into different and unexpected areas.

I used this style of interviewing during my individual interviews with family, friends, and friends of friends. After the interview I journaled my thoughts and impressions about the conversation, and returned to these notes when transcribing. These notes and subsequent thoughts were then typed into the transcript using italics for my recollections and reflections, and regular font for the verbatim conversation. Though these interviews were similar in technique to the "active interviews" I had conducted in previous research (compare Mulcahy, Parry, & Glover, 2012), I value this method for the explicit emphasis on reflexivity and the specific positioning of the researcher within the research. This process was deeply helpful in both maintaining a sense of reflexivity and laying the groundwork for future analysis.

Interactive Interviews

For this study I also used interactive interviewing (Ellis, 2004). In interactive interviewing there are usually more than two individuals (though two might work if appropriate), and all those participating act as both researcher and participant. As opposed to the more reflexive, one-on-one style of the dyadic interviews, this style of interviewing is more collaborative, focused on the story that evolves out of the interaction amid this particular group of people. And as opposed to other group interviewing techniques, this style actively attempts to minimize the researcher's authority and control over the direction of the conversation. There is no interview guide, just the announcement of the topic of conversation. I used this technique when interviewing my three siblings in our family home. I began the conversation by simply stating, "Let's talk about Mum's role in our lives as family memory-keeper." This is a topic that my siblings and I have already discussed (albeit much more informally and for far more brief periods of time), so I was confident that the conversation would flow somewhat easily from there. Ellis (2004) posits this technique is most useful when "all participants have had personal experience with the topic under discussion.... [T]his strategy is particularly useful when researching personal and/or emotional topics" (p. 64).

This style of interviewing recognizes each player as an expert and as an equal contributor to the content and direction of the conversation; however, I have not always been entirely successful in this regard. For instance, in my interactive interview with my siblings, though the conversation flowed easily and organically, helped along by the practiced dynamic between the four of us, my siblings understandably returned to me at regular intervals to ask for direction and/or clarification. Incidentally, these were always important interruptions that allowed us to return to the more raw, emotional conversations we were often attempting to circumvent with surface-level digressions. Thus, while interactive interviews can be successful in terms of collaborative storytelling among a group of experts in a particular experience, a guiding voice is sometimes still necessary (and perhaps welcomed), and the sense of a researcher's authority may never be completely vanquished.

Focus Group Interviews

I have also used focus groups in evocative inquiry when interviewing groups of individuals known to each other—and to me—in my life. This included specific groups of friends, couples, and parents and children. I used focus groups in these instances rather than interactive interviewing because I wanted to remain a facilitator and a guide in these discussions instead of relinquishing control through the more collaborative interactive interview. As such, I use an interview guide, though again, conversation often deviates from that guide into new and interesting territories. During group interviews, I find participants seem at ease, insofar as those individuals can be listeners and/or speakers, drawing inspiration from what others have said about the topic at hand (Ellis, 2004). I also find focus groups allow for participants to disagree, to challenge each other, to affirm the others' experiences; in doing so, an interactive picture of the experience begins to form. As Lindlof and Taylor (2002) describe:

> Group discussion produces data and insights that would be less accessible without interaction found in a group setting—listening to others' verbalized experiences stimulates memories, ideas, and experiences in participants. This is also known as the group effect where group members engage in a kind of "chaining" or "cascading" effect; talk links to, or tumbles out of, the topics and expressions preceding it. (p. 182)

Finally, I find focus group interviews helpful in the comfort they appear to bring to participants. Many of my focus group interviews were created at the request of individual participants who suggested a friend or family member come along. Thus, while focus groups can certainly result in less in-depth information, excluded voices, and "group think" (Lindlof & Taylor, 2002), these interviews can be successful insofar as they put participants at ease, enable the interviewer to bear witness to fascinating dynamics between friends and family members, and provide a level of comfort the participants might have found necessary to partake in the discussion. This level of comfort was often essential in my motherhood, memory, and loss research, given the sensitive, multilayered, dynamic, and complicated nature of the interviews I conducted; however, this often meant that data were created that, in turn, were sensitive, multilayered, dynamic, and complicated.

Elicitation Methods

During these interviews, I invited all participants to bring with them a family memory artifact that was meaningful to them in some way. I described this artifact as something their mother collected for them, something they collected as mothers, or any other family memory artifact of choice. This is referred to as an "elicitation method," wherein the participant might find their memories easier to recall by having a memory artifact on hand (Loizos, 2000). As Loizos (2000) suggests:

> Images are resonant with submerged memories and can help interviewees focus, free up their memory, and create a piece of "shared business" in which the researcher and the interviewee can talk together, perhaps in a more relaxed manner than without such a stimulus. (p. 98)

I find the elicitation method effective for participants, often simply as a starting point for conversation, and a focal point to return to as well that is significant, evocative, and meaningful for the participant. If the participant is nervous or anxious, or unable to connect with my explanations of the study or my interview questions, she can look down at her artifact, touch it, smell it, to bring herself back to the meaning of our interview. And as an interviewer, we can observe how the artifact is held and being handled, giving us cues to the artifact's meaning that might not be expressed by the participant verbally.

Before the interviews, I ask participants if I might take a photograph of their artifact to include anonymously in my research, and in any publications that might follow. This agreement is documented in writing on a separate informed consent form. The photographs create rich data for the interviewer, again enabling data that is complex, dynamic, and multilayered. However, ethically the interviewer must be attuned to the significance of this artifact, and handle even a photograph of the artifact with ethical care. Indeed, a blessing and a curse of autoethnographic research is that "self-revelations always involve revelations about others" (Ellis, 2007, p. 25). To protect my participants and myself as a researcher, I made clear prior to our interview that I could not completely guarantee their anonymity and before each interview, I discuss these issues of anonymity—including the ethical issues surrounding the photographs—at length.

The Benefits and Challenges of Autoethnographic Interviews

There is much an interviewer must handle with ethical care when collecting autoethnographic data, and these complications can be both beneficial and challenging in evocative inquiry research. Interviews with family and friends, so-called "insider interviews," are touted for their advantages, including personal knowledge of the experience at hand (Crossley, 2009), expediency of rapport-building (Jenks, 2002), and the easy detection of nonverbal gestures (Chavez, 2008). My experience with autoethnographic interviews confirms these advantages. Quite frequently, I felt my personal knowledge of the experience at hand enabled a more comfortable interview environment. For instance, I could easily draw upon my experience as a mother and as a daughter of a mother losing her memory. Because my participants had prior knowledge of our shared experiences, there was a level of depth to our interviews that was more easily accessed than if the participant had viewed me as an "outsider." Likewise, because of this preexisting relationship, rapport was very naturally established and an intimate interview quickly developed. I was also particularly attuned to nearly every participant's nonverbal gestures, given the preexisting familiarity between us. This enabled me to navigate the interview carefully and sensitively, and with great attention paid to underlying meanings and responses that were going unsaid. Each of these advantages to the autoethnographic interview allowed me to collect data that were rich, dynamic, and multilayered.

However, this form of interviewing is not without its disadvantages. Many of the reported advantages of "insider" interviews also can create significant challenges during interviews. Personal knowledge of the experience at hand can lead to incomplete exchanges wherein, without realizing it, the participant and interviewer fail to completely flesh out the discussion, relying instead on shorthand, or the shared understanding they have of the experience. For example, during one interview I conducted, the following dialogue occurred: "Well, it was like that time when he wouldn't save that card you sent, and I was so...remember?" "Yeah, I remember, that's exactly what I mean." "So, you know, it's important." As I transcribed the interview, I was left wondering: "*What* time? *What* happened? *Who* was there? What does it *mean*? *Why* was it important?" Likewise, the expediency of rapport building is incredibly useful in gaining access to participants with relative ease; however, this easy rapport is necessarily accompanied by an already established relationship between interviewer and the interviewee. The existent dynamic can guide and shape the interview and the data collected from the interview, meaning I often felt restrained by my need to remain polite and respectful of boundaries and conscious of leaving the interview with the relationships firmly intact. As Ellis (2004) notes, "With autoethnography, the context you're representing is yourself and your life, which is messier than ethnographies of people who live apart from you; here you're writing about individuals you talk to on birthdays and holidays" (p. 324). This often prevented me from asking questions that were more direct or probing in nature. Finally, existing relationships with participants enables easy detection of the meaning of verbal cues and nonverbal gestures; however, this knowledge can also result in the failure to probe for more information or emotional depth during an interview. For example, because I was familiar with certain participants, I easily recognized signs that we were approaching sensitive topics and would redirect the conversation. In many instances, I wondered if this redirection was helpful and ultimately wished I had asked the question and left the decision to speak about it up to the participant.

As such, I have several suggestions for preparing for insider interviews whether they be reflexive, dyadic interviews, interactive interviews, focus groups, and/or make use of elicitation methods. First, prepare for intense emotional connections and extremely personal conversations, but properly prepare as well to emotionally detach during the interview. The researcher should remind herself of the larger intentions of the interview: to collect data for a particular project. I recommend preparing a more structured, practiced interview when interviewing family and close friends that acts to consistently remind the interviewer to oscillate between insider and outsider perspectives. Though this seems counterintuitive given the intimate and informal nature of the autoethnographic interview, such structure could guard against the difficulty focusing that comes with being too deep "inside" an interview. Second, a useful strategy is to prepare a statement, perhaps even written on an interview guide, reminding the interviewer to collect data that are fleshed out with as little shorthand as possible. Phrases such as, "Pretend we don't know each other," "I know we've spoken about this before, but," and "Imagine you're describing this to a stranger" could be helpful in creating richer data. Finally, prepare beforehand by journaling about the boundaries of each specific relationship. Describe the relationship in detail, outlining the boundaries and weighing the possible risks and benefits associated with crossing those boundaries. Researchers should write about questions they fear asking and workshop a variety of ways they could ask those questions in a manner sensitive to a particular relationship. As Chavez (2008) maintains, "Traditional training begins with 'getting to know the field'; understanding participants, gaining access, and developing rapport. Insider scholars, on the other hand, need to be trained in a reverse manner: They need to get into their own heads first before getting into those of participants" (p. 491). Researchers must be confident they are prepared "in their own heads" so they can be successful in connecting and reconnecting with those they already know.

Strategies of Data Analysis and Representation

Whether the data collected result in interview transcripts, fieldnotes, photographs, reflexive recollections, diary entries, or dreams, the first step of data analysis for many evocative inquiry researchers is determining what kind of story a researcher wants to tell. Many researchers begin the process through traditional qualitative analysis methods such as narrative analysis, phenomenology, or grounded theory: researchers work inductively with their data and "write up" their findings in the form of traditional themes and categories. While ruminating on the meaning of these themes and categories, a researcher might move from the more traditional analysis to experiment with "writing up" their findings in a variety of ways, trying poetry, reader's theatre, screenplays, sketching, and so forth. Further, in evocative inquiry, processes of data collection, data analysis, and creating the final product are often intertwined, sometimes occurring simultaneously and certainly not linearly; thus, each shift in form might also enable a shift in analysis, tone, and meaning (Ellis, 2004). For instance, Banks (2000) turned to fiction when he felt that his traditional approach to analyzing and representing the findings from his study on holiday letters "failed to evoke" the emotional layers he felt were present in his data (p. 400). Berbary and Johnson (2012) noted they initially "played around" with their data within the structure of a screenplay—the form the manuscript eventually took—because they felt their analysis needed polyvocality, movement, and space (p. 250). As researchers experiment with these different forms of writing, they simultaneously reanalyze the data; each new form lends new meaning, and the researcher makes new choices about how to craft that meaning. And as the piece of evocative inquiry takes shape, the researcher might choose to pull from new data, new stories, new recollections, in an attempt to create a stronger final product. For examples of this complex process of data collection, analysis, and representation, I now draw upon several of my own complicated journeys in evocative inquiry.

The Journey to "Between Diagnosis and Death"

"Between Diagnosis and Death: A Performance Text about Cancer, Shadows, and the Ghosts We Cannot Escape" (Mulcahy, Parry, & Glover, 2009) began as a traditional, constant comparative analysis (Glaser & Strauss, 1967) of twenty-six transcripts of interviews with survivors of cancer and members of Gilda's Club, an organization that supports cancer survivors and their families. Through open and axial coding, themes were emerging about the notion of cancer as a journey. For instance, many participants spoke of "getting thrown off course," "trying to get my bearings," and "looking down the road ahead" on their "journey." The narratives also tended to follow a particular pattern or sequence of events, beginning with the experience of symptoms, followed by often frustrating and upsetting diagnosis processes, and then a subsequent period of feeling lost. The discovery of Gilda's Club was often presented as a turning point in the narrative. At this point, the narrator reflected upon how far they have come and attempted to map the road ahead. At the same time as these themes were emerging, however, I was also grappling with reading through transcripts that were so reminiscent of my own experiences as an adolescent living with my father as he endured cancer treatments. Given the narrative themes that were emerging, and my experience being haunted by the "ghosts" (Doucet, 2008) of my father's cancer while analyzing the transcripts, I began writing the data as a narrative, a father telling his seemingly disaffected teenaged daughter his "cancer story" as they trek to Gilda's Club on a cold winter's day.

When I submitted this story and the accompanying analysis to the *International Review of Qualitative Research*, I was confident the piece was creative, expressive, and made use of my own experience to explore the complexity of the cancer journey. I felt it was reflexive, powerful, and analytical; held aesthetic merit; and made a substantive contribution to the literature. However, the editor responded by suggesting the manuscript was too superficial; he was not moved enough. He pressed me to include more voices, to reflect more deeply and critically on both the data and my experiences, and to try performance text, with the assertion that this form of writing will "open up a range of meanings." And so I turned to performance text, creating multiple speaking parts (a narrator, a daughter, a father, and a "ghost"). In doing so, I mined the data anew for inspiration, pieces of dialogue, and rich descriptors, and I mined new data as well, delving back into my own memory to record and critically reflect upon my own experiences as the daughter of a cancer patient. These data were then analyzed and worked into what was becoming "Between Diagnosis and Death," a far more raw, vulnerable, and—in my opinion—moving story about cancer, shadows, and the ghosts that haunt our research.

In this sense, as the research went from traditional qualitative coding to narrative to performance text, the data were continuously collected and recollected, analyzed and reanalyzed, and the focus of the manuscript shifted slightly as new meanings took the spotlight. As the performance text built and became the bulk of the manuscript, the academic analyses were condensed into a brief abstract and epilogue bookending the dramatic piece. Thus, in evocative inquiry, the research process is not linear, as the postpositivist paradigm would insist upon; nor perhaps should it be, for what can result from this lack of linearity is a rich and complicated representation of one interpretation of multiple levels of experience at a particular time in the participants' and author's lives, a representation that also reveals the necessarily uncertain, multilayered, *human* nature of social research.

The Journey to "Awakenings"

Similarly, in our project on grassroots mothers' groups (Mulcahy & Parry, 2011), the transcripts from twenty-four interviews with new mothers were originally analyzed using the phenomenological method, insofar as we were interested in the meaning of grassroots mothers' groups within the lived experience of new motherhood. We developed five descriptive themes that we felt emerged from the data: exhausted, overwhelmed, bored, housebound, and lonely. However, as I struggled to attempt rewrites while caring for my infant son, the stories of the young mothers and my story as a young mother began to blend together until the parity could no longer be denied; I, too, was exhausted, overwhelmed, bored, housebound, and lonely, and I decided to use that experience once again as data to reflect upon. And so we turned again to performance text to explore these multiple levels of data and analysis. I wrote reflexively about my own experience as a new mother and my relationship to the data, as well as my relationship to my supervisor (herself a new mother), drawing upon emails sent between us when our children were infants. I revisited the data from the study to craft the transcripts into a conversation between five women. The result, "Awakenings: A Performance Text about First Time Mothers Making Connections" (Mulcahy & Parry, 2011) set three scenes of motherhood: me and my infant son downstage left, my supervisor and coauthor (also a mother of young children) upstage right, and the voices of the twenty-four research participants represented in verbatim quotes by five mothers sitting with babies and coffee, downstage right. We staged these experiences of new motherhood and watched how they paralleled and diverged. Only when the separate circles of motherhood interact, when the mothers reach out to each other and connect, do the mothers experience an "awakening." For me, the awakening I received as a result of my interactions with these other women was felt as both a researcher and a mother.

This manuscript became about more than just five themes offering one analysis regarding new mothers making connections. Instead, the performance text enabled us to tell the story of making connections on multiple levels: the importance of connecting first-time parents through our proposed programming for first-time parents in Canada, the importance of illustrating how we as researchers make connections in our data that then connect back to our lives in meaningful ways, and the importance of connecting academically, emotionally, and viscerally with the experience of first-time motherhood. We wanted our readers to be moved into the position of a mother for a moment: to see the empty bottles in the sink, to hear the child's sharp wail, to fight the heavy weight of drooping eyelids, and, perhaps most of all, to experience the pangs of loneliness and the yearning for something more. We also wanted our readers to be moved into the position of a social critic: to raise questions about authorship, reflexivity, and the transparency of knowledge production. And we wanted our readers to be moved into the position of a feminist: to feel the need for improved postpartum services, stronger social safety nets for mothers, and better academic representations of the overwhelming transition to motherhood. We found that in this case, the performance text allowed us the space to be in all these positions at once.

The Journey to "Shaking up the Family Tree"

Unlike the previous two examples, "Homing of the Home" (Mulcahy, 2012), or what I jokingly call "Shaking up the Family Tree," was always intended as a piece of evocative inquiry. However, when I embarked on my autoethnographic study of my family's experiences with family memory keeping, genetic disease, and our mother's memory loss to Huntington's disease, I imagined I would write a narrative out of the data. I analyzed interview transcripts with my mother, father, sisters, and brother, and began to write what I thought would be a poignant and provocative personal narrative of family memory keeping in the cleverly apropos form of a memoir. Specifically, I used narrative analysis and thematic analysis of narrative, which is similar in approach to grounded theory (Ellis, 2004). The difference is that grounded theory tends to be presented in theoretical groups and categories, whereas narrative analysis uses the storytelling form to express findings. I paid particular attention to the narrative structure of the stories, including recurring symbols, metaphors, figures of speech, and sequences of events. I then looked for overarching themes that brought these stories together. I also took reflexive, retrospective fieldnotes on my experiences with family memory keeping. This included every detail I could remember about why I was interested in the topic, what had drawn me to the project, and what life experiences I had with family memory keeping. Next I turned to the interviews, journaling about the tone, setting, and atmosphere of each interview. I concentrated on emotions and dialogue, place, colors, smells, sounds, and movements. As Ellis (2004) suggests, I wrote about the interviews when my feelings were intense, and then returned to them when I felt more emotionally removed. I reread the transcripts, inserting notes on what went unsaid during particular exchanges. At times, I found this process supremely boring and time consuming. Initially, I used none of this information in crafting my story and resented having to adhere to the process. Yet as I continued to rewrite drafts, I found I returned to these notes to layer the text with meaning, sound, atmosphere, character, tension, movement, and setting.

However, my first draft of the memoir was terrible. I attempted to write as Ellis (2004) writes, in first-person narrative form with an emphasis on realism rather than abstract prose. I wrote with "thick description" (Geertz, 1973) and used participants' own words as often as possible, as Ellis (2004) suggests. Unfortunately for my participants' words, my writing was cloying and forced, resulting in a dull piece with very little to offer theoretically. The narrative I constructed was far too neat, linear, and clean for the complex data it was supposedly representing. My voice was far too dominant and thus the story had the sense of being too confident, too in control. I began revisions, only to find I was unhappy with the entire structure of the piece. I considered starting again, for as Ellis (2004) maintains, "One of the values of this approach is its flexibility.... [Y]ou must be aware of possible dynamics and open to improvisation and changing strategies along the way to better match the constraints and needs of the project" (p. 68). I opened a new document and began to write a fresh performance text that turned out to be far superior to my first narrative. Through the performance text, I could quite literally stage my struggle and see how it played out. Thus, I created a character sitting at a desk listening to the recordings of her interviews with her family and attempting to write something about those interviews, just as I was. I staged my struggles with the research, and watched as the characters interacted and ultimately came to insights and realizations, seemingly on their own.

I had to be "permanently vigilant" about the ethics of this research (Ellis, 2009, p. 19). In a discussion that resonated strongly with my experience, Ellis (2007) describes the fear she felt when working on a project about her ill mother, fearing her representation of her mother's body, smells, noises, movements, and so forth would hurt or embarrass her. Autoethnographic work such as the performance text I wrote about my mother's illness requires considerable attention to the "relational ethics" of the stories we tell, and I had to constantly ask myself, "Do the benefits of writing and sharing these stories outweigh the risks?" (Ellis, 2009, p. 19). I sought feedback from my family on most drafts of the research, though I have yet to feel completely comfortable with representing my mother in the throes of her illness. Part of the process of analyzing and representing data through evocative research is this constant cycle of ethical questioning; as Tamas (2011a) suggests, "We are never ethically home free" (p. 262). However, part of the process, too, is accepting responsibility for those representational choices we make.

With each of these examples of evocative inquiry, the data analysis process was anything but linear. Every rewrite almost necessarily means a reanalysis, and in many instances requires a recollection of data, whether that means mining existing data for inspiration or mining one's own experiences, memories, or dreams for new insight. With every rewrite, reanalysis, and recollection, a reexamination of ethics also is required. Whether the analysis is performed through more traditional qualitative methods such as narrative analysis, phenomenology, or grounded theory, or whether the researcher explicitly sets out to use creative means of expressing the findings, data analysis in evocative inquiry research is ultimately about deciding what story to tell, and embarking on the (far-from-linear) journey of telling it.

Evocative Inquiry and the Move Toward Change

Within this move toward evocative inquiry research, Denzin (2003) argues, is the possibility of hope, revolution, freedom, justice, and change. Evocative inquiry shares theoretical underpinnings with queer theory (a shared interest in disrupting notions of linearity, fixity, and firmness and problematizing that which was traditional, normal, and true), feminist theory (a shared concern with power, perspective, and lived experience), and critical theory (a shared questioning of marginalized voices, intersecting identities, and representations of the Other). However, evocative inquiry research is not necessarily political: our research can just as easily reproduce positivist notions of objectivity and linearity, or oppressive ideologies such as racism, homophobia, or misogyny. Rather, there lies within evocative inquiry the *opportunity* to enact social justice through research that moves people (Cheek, 2010). Indeed, researchers have used the space opened up by moving, evocative inquiry to promote social change surrounding academic life and writing (Doty, 2010), misogyny in gay male culture (Johnson & Samdahl, 2005), disability rights and prenatal screening (Neville-Jan, 2005), the medicalization of women's bodies (Parry, 2006), poverty and child protection (Krumer-Nevo, 2009), and calls for black women's anger (Griffin, 2012). This space is provided via evocative inquiry's methodological focus on moving people: moving us to feel, moving us to think, moving us to change.

Evocative inquiry has the potential to move readers by drawing us into the experience with rich, emotional, "thick" descriptions of what social life "is like," told from a position of vulnerability wherein the researcher demonstrates "an unflinching commitment to write close to the bone" (Tamas, 2011a, p. 262), and a faithfulness to complex, multilayered, *human* storytelling. We then become connected to the social experience; the piece moves us into different perspectives and positions, requiring us to think *with* the story rather than simply about the story. We are then moved to care: about the characters, the experiences, and the issues with which we are engaged. As we are moved to feel, to think, to care, we are changed, sometimes without even realizing it. And that change, occurring because we have been *moved* rather than bored by social science research, prompts us to ask, as invested, engaged, *feeling* citizens, where we can go from here.

Change can mean a number of different things within the context of evocative inquiry. Doty (2010) argues evocative inquiry creates change insofar as this method challenges the status quo, creates space for revolutionary conversations about the nature and goals of social science research, and makes possible change in individual academics. Similarly, Ellis (2004) imagines evocative inquiry has the capacity to "move inward toward social change.... Increased self-understanding can sometimes provide a quicker and more successful route to social change than changing laws or other macropolitical structures" (p.

254). Jones and Adams (2010) maintain the importance of bearing witness through evocative inquiry to the stories of others. And Tamas (2011a) adds that telling our stories of trauma or the traumatic stories of our participants can work therapeutically toward the process of healing. Finley (2003) presses for a more specific, more politicized change through evocative inquiry, citing a responsibility to create research that is locally useable and takes a stand against social injustice: "research efforts that examine how things are but also imagine how they could be otherwise" (p. 293). Perhaps fittingly, the concept of change in evocative inquiry research is as multilayered, messy, and dynamic as its content.

I still have the Barbies. They are bundled in the black garbage bag in my closet. In the spirit of telling reflexive, *human* stories, I couldn't end the chapter without admitting their whereabouts. The evocative inquiry piece that moved me moved the Barbies as well, not to a garbage truck, but on to a better place. I took those Barbies, and their clothes, accessories, and furniture, to my new office, where they act every day as pieces of evocative inquiry themselves, moving students to engage, perform, critique, change (at the very least, their outfits), and begin to play at moving others into new and different positions as well.

REFERENCES

Banks, S. P. (2000). Five holiday letters: A fiction. *Qualitative Inquiry,* 6(3), 392–405.

Behar, R. (1996). *The vulnerable observer: Anthropology that breaks your heart.* Boston: Beacon Press.

Berbary, L., & Johnson, C. W. (2012). The American sorority girl recast: an ethnographic screenplay of leisure *in context. Leisure/Loisir,* 36(3-4), 243–268.

Boal, A. (1979). *Theatre of the oppressed.* London, UK: Pluto Press.

Bochner, A. (1997). It's about time: Narrative and the divided self. *Qualitative Inquiry,* 3(4), 418–438.

Bochner, A. (2000). Criteria against ourselves. *Qualitative Inquiry,* 6(2), 266–272.

Bochner, M. (2002). "If the color changes": (1996–1997). In A. Bochner & C. Ellis (Eds.), *Ethnographically speaking: Autoethnography, literature, and aesthetics* (pp. 295–296). Walnut Creek, CA: AltaMira Press.

Brady, I. (2009). How to die in the desert. *International Review of Qualitative Research,* 2(1), 155–161.

Cancienne, M. B., & Snowber, C. N. (2003). Writing rhythm: Movement as method. *Qualitative Inquiry, 9*(2), 237–253.

Chavez, C. (2008). Conceptualizing from the inside: Advantages, complications, and demands on insider positionality. *The Qualitative Report, 13*(3), 474–494.

Cheek, J. (2010). Human rights, social justice, and qualitative research: Questions and hesitations about what we say about what we do. In N. K. Denzin & M. D. Giardina (Eds.), *Qualitative inquiry and human rights* (pp. 100–111). Walnut Creek, CA: Left Coast Press.

Church, K. (2002). The hard road home: Toward a polyphonic narrative of the mother–daughter relationship. In A. Bochner & C. Ellis (Eds.), *Ethnographically speaking: Autoethnography, literature, and aesthetics* (pp. 234–257). Walnut Creek, CA: AltaMira Press.

Clough, P. (2000). Comments on setting criteria for experimental writing. *Qualitative Inquiry, 6*(2), 278–291.

Crossley, M. L. (2009). Breastfeeding as a moral imperative: An autoethnographic study. *Feminism & Psychology, 19*(1), 71–87.

Dent, B. (2002). Border crossings: A story of sexual identity transformation. In A. Bochner & C. Ellis (Eds.), *Ethnographically speaking: Autoethnography, literature, and aesthetics* (pp. 191–200). Walnut Creek, CA: AltaMira Press.

Denzin, N. K. (2000). Aesthetics and qualitative inquiry. *Qualitative Inquiry, 6* (2), 256–265.

Denzin, N. K. (2003). Performing [auto]ethnography politically. *The Review of Education, Pedagogy, and Cultural Studies, 25*, 257–278.

Denzin, N. K. (2008). *Searching for Yellowstone: Race, gender, family, and memory in the postmodern West.* Walnut Creek, CA: Left Coast Press.

Denzin, N. K., & Lincoln, Y. S. (2011). Introduction: The discipline and practice of qualitative research. In N. K. Denzin & Y. S. Lincoln (Eds.), *Handbook of qualitative research* (4th Ed.) (pp. 1–20). Thousand Oaks, CA: Sage.

Doloriert, C., & Sambrook, S. (2009). Ethical confessions of the "I" of autoethnography: The student's dilemma. *Qualitative Research in Organizations and Management: An International Journal, 4*(1), 27–45.

Doucet, A. (2008). "From her side of the gossamer wall(s)": Reflexivity and relational knowing. *Qualitative Sociology, 31*, 73–87.

Doty, R. L. (2010). Autoethnography—Making human connections. *Review of International Studies, 36*, 1047–1050.

Ellis, C. (1995). *Final negotiations: A story of love, loss, and chronic illness.* Philadelphia: Temple University Press.

Ellis, C. (2004). *The ethnographic I: A methodological novel about autoethnography.* New York: AltaMira Press.

Ellis, C. (2007). Telling secrets, revealing lives: Relational ethics in research with intimate others. *Qualitative Inquiry, 13*(1), 3–29.

Ellis, C. (2009). Telling tales on neighbors: Ethics in two voices. *International Review of Qualitative Research, 2*(1), 3–27.

Ellis, C., & Bochner, A. (1992). Telling and performing personal stories: The constraints of choice in abortion. In C. Ellis & M. Flaherty (Eds.), *Investigating subjectivity: Research on lived experience* (pp. 79–101). Newbury Park, CA: Sage.

Faulkner, S. (2007). Concern with craft: Using Ars Poetica as criteria for reading research poetry. *Qualitative Inquiry, 13*(2), 218–234.

Finley, S. (2003). Arts-based inquiry in QI: Seven years—From crisis to guerrilla warfare. *Qualitative Inquiry, 9*(2), 281–296.

Fox, K. (1996). Silent voices: A subversive reading of child sexual abuse. In C. Ellis & A. Bochner (Eds.), *Composing ethnography: Alternative forms of qualitative writing* (pp. 330–356). Walnut Creek, CA: AltaMira Press.

Furman, R., Langer, C. L., Davis, C., Gallardo, H. P., & Kulkarni, S. (2007). Expressive research and reflective poetry as qualitative inquiry: A study of adolescent identity. *Qualitative Research, 7*(3), 301–315.

Geertz, C. (1973). *The interpretation of cultures.* New York: Basic Books.

Glaser, B., & Strauss A. (1967). *Discovery of grounded theory: Strategies for qualitative research.* Mill Valley, CA: Sociology Press.

Goodall, Jr., H. L. (2005). Narrative inheritance: A nuclear family with toxic secrets. *Qualitative Inquiry, 11*(4), 492–513.

Goodall Jr., H. L. (2008). *Writing qualitative inquiry: Self, stories, and academic life.* Walnut Creek, CA: Left Coast Press.

Griffin, R. A. (2012). I AM an angry Black woman: Black feminist autoethnography, voice, and resistance. *Women's Studies in Communication, 35*, 138–157.

Halley, J. (2003). To speak of my mother. *Qualitative Inquiry, 9*(1), 49–56.

Hayano, D. (1979). Auto-ethnography: Paradigms, problems and prospects. *Human Organization, 38*(1), 99–104.

Holmes, R. (2012). A fantastic decomposition: Unsettling the fury of having to wait. *Qualitative Inquiry 18*(7), 544–556.

Jago, B. J. (2006). A primary act of imagination: An autoethnography of father-absence. *Qualitative Inquiry, 12*(2), 398–426.

Jenkins, M. M. (2010). The personal is the political: Capturing a social movement on stage. *International Review of Qualitative Research, 3*(1), 125–148.

Jenks, E. (2002). Searching for autoethnographic credibility. In A. Bochner & C. Ellis (Eds.), *Ethnographically speaking: Autoethnography, literature, and aesthetics* (pp. 170–186). Walnut Creek, CA: AltaMira Press.

Johnson, C. W., & Samdahl, D. (2005). "The night they took over":

Misogyny in a country-western gay bar. *Leisure Sciences, 27*(4), 331–348.

Jones, S. H., & Adams, T. E. (2010). Autoethnography and queer theory: Making possibilities. In N. K. Denzin & M. D. Giardina (Eds.), *Qualitative inquiry and human rights* (pp. 136–157). Walnut Creek, CA: Left Coast Press.

Kolker, A. (1996). Thrown overboard: The human costs of health care rationing. In C. Ellis & A. Bochner (Eds.), *Composing ethnography: Alternative forms of qualitative writing* (pp. 132–159). Walnut Creek, CA: AltaMira Press.

Krumer-Nevo, M. (2009). Four scenes and an epilogue: Autoethnography of a critical social work agenda regarding poverty. *Qualitative Social Work, 8*(3), 305–320.

Lahman, M. K. E. (2008). The blue period. *Qualitative Inquiry, 14*(8), 1540–1542.

Lindlof, T. R., & Taylor, B. C. (2002). *Qualitative communication research methods* (2nd ed.). Thousand Oaks, CA: Sage.

Lobel, B. (2008). BALL: The script. *Text and Performance Quarterly, 28*(12), 160–177.

Loizos, P. (2000). Video, film and photographs as research documents. In M. W. Bauer & G. Gaskell (Eds.), *Qualitative researching with text, image and sound* (pp. 93–107). London, UK: Sage.

Minge, J. M. (2006). Painting a landscape of abortion: The fusion of embodied art. *Qualitative Inquiry, 12*(1), 118–145.

Mulcahy, C. M. (2012). The homing of the home: Exploring gendered work, leisure, social construction, and loss through women's family memory keeping. Doctoral dissertation, University of Waterloo, Canada. Retrieved from http://hdl.handle.net/10012/7104

Mulcahy, C. M., & Parry, D. C. (2011). Awakenings: A performance text about first time mothers making connections. *International Review of Qualitative Research, 4*(4), 335-352.

Mulcahy, C. M., Parry, D. C., & Glover, T. D. (2009). Between diagnosis and death: A performance text about cancer, shadows, and the ghosts we cannot escape. *International Review of Qualitative Research, 2*(1), 29–42.

Mulcahy, C. M., Parry, D. C., & Glover, T. D. (2012). *From mothering without a net to mothering on the Net: The impact of an online social networking site on experiences of postpartum depression.* Paper presented at the Institute for Gender and Health Advancing Excellence in Gender, Sex and Health Research conference, Montréal, QC, Canada, October 29–31.

Neville-Jan, A. (2005). The problem with prevention: The case of spina bifida. *American Journal of Occupational Therapy, 59*, 527–539.

Parry, D. C. (2006). Women's lived experiences with pregnancy and midwifery in a medicalized and fetocentric context: Six short stories. *Qualitative Inquiry, 12*(3), 459–471.

Pelias, R. J. (2002). For father and son: An ethnodrama with no catharsis. In A. Bochner & C. Ellis (Eds.), *Ethnographically speaking: Autoethnography, literature, and aesthetics* (pp. 35–43). Walnut Creek, CA: AltaMira Press.

Phoenix, C. (2010). Seeing the world of physical culture: The potential of visual methods for qualitative research in sport and exercise. *Qualitative Research in Sport and Exercise, 2*(2), 93–108.

Picart, C. (2002). Living the hyphenated edge: Autoethnography, hybridity, and aesthetics. In A. Bochner & C. Ellis (Eds.), *Ethnographically speaking: Autoethnography, literature, and aesthetics* (pp. 258–273). Walnut Creek, CA: AltaMira Press.

Pink, S. (2007). *Doing visual ethnography.* Thousand Oaks, CA: Sage.

Poulos, C. N. (2010). Transgressions. *International Review of Qualitative Research, 3*(1), 67–88.

Rich, M. (2004). Show is tell. In M. Bamberg & M. Andrews (Eds.), *Considering counter-narratives: Narrating, resisting, making sense* (pp. 151–158). Philadelphia: John Benjamins.

Richardson, L. (2000). Evaluating ethnography. *Qualitative Inquiry, 6*(2), 253–255.

Richardson, M. (1998). Poetics in the field and on the page. *Qualitative Inquiry, 4*(4), 451–462.

Richardson, M. (2003). Mamma lied: I discovered death, became an anthropologist, and found you. *Qualitative Inquiry, 9*(2), 303–311.

Ronai, C. R. (1995). Multiple reflections of child abuse: An argument for a layered account. *Journal of Contemporary Ethnography, 23*(4), 395–426.

Ronai, C. R. (1996). My mother is mentally retarded. In C. Ellis & A. P. Bochner (Eds.), *Composing ethnography: Alternative forms of qualitative writing* (pp. 109–131). Walnut Creek, CA: AltaMira Press.

Tamas, S. (2011a). Autoethnography, ethics, and making your baby cry. *Cultural Studies, Critical Methodologies, 11*(3), 258–264.

Tamas, S. (2011b). Biting the hand that speaks you: (Re)writing survivor narratives. *International Review of Qualitative Research, 4*(4), 431–460.

Tillman-Healy, L. (1996). A secret life in a culture of thinness: Reflections on body, food, and bulimia. In C. Ellis & A. Bochner (Eds.), *Composing ethnography: Alternative forms of qualitative writing.* Walnut Creek, CA: AltaMira Press.

van Maanen, J. (1988). *Tales of the field: On writing ethnography.* Chicago, IL: University of Chicago Press.

The Future of Social Justice: Paradigm Proliferation

Diana C. Parry & Corey W. Johnson

> At the beginning of the second decade of the 21st century, it is time to move forward. It is time to explore new discourses. We need to find new ways of connecting persons and their personal troubles with social justice methodologies. We need to become better accomplished in linking these interventions to those institutional sites where troubles are turned into public issues and public issues transformed into social policy. (Denzin & Lincoln, 2011, p. ix)

We hope the seven methodological approaches presented here outline the possibility for change when a social justice paradigm is combined with qualitative inquiry. One of our underlying goals is to illustrate that social inequities can be addressed in productive ways and that change can come from anywhere, especially from the bottom up. As a result, we ALL are capable of, and therefore responsible for, making our world a better place. Qualitative inquiry is an important part of change as it enables us to connect "to the hopes, needs, goals, and promises of a free democratic society" (Denzin & Lincoln, 2011, p. 3). Although the role for qualitative inquiry in creating positive social change has not always been clear, today "qualitative researchers [are] able to understand the connection between social science writ broadly and the quest for better policy, for a more just and democratic society, for a more egalitarian distribution of goods and services" (Lincoln & Denzin, 2011, p. 716). Whereas in the past critical perspectives were in some cases simply a companion, today that has changed, and qualitative inquiry and social justice are a conjoined voice (Lincoln & Denzin, 2011).

There is a vast and ever-growing group of qualitative scholars who embrace a social justice paradigm. As a field of inquiry, social justice researchers should be proud of the broad scope of substantive topics and critical paradigmatic approaches published in a large range of journals. This reflects what Denzin and Lincoln (2011) refer to as "paradigm proliferation" and includes "a rainbow coalition of racialized and queered post-ism, from feminism, to structuralism, ... post-scientism, Marxism, and postconstructivism" (p. ix) across various fields and disciplines. Indeed, scholars in sociology, cultural studies, anthropology, literary studies, marketing, geography, women's studies, various ethnic studies, education, and nursing are all using qualitative inquiry as a means to enact social justice (Kincheloe, McLaren & Steinberg, 2011, p. 168).

As a result of this proliferation, we are inundated with a variety of qualitative research strategies, methods of data collection, analysis, and representation. The number of options might seem paralyzing, especially to novice researchers. Looking forward, paradigmatic choices will only continue to grow as scholars blur boundaries and *define and redefine themselves* as researchers. These are exciting times for qualitative researchers as we discover multiple entry points into the complexities of social experiences within a global context. A multitude of lenses and strategies for social justice is critical as qualitative researchers engage with people from across the world—thinking, feeling, living human beings—who encounter constraint, discrimination, marginalization, oppression, and violence in their everyday lives and creatively reposition themselves. These injustices and responses demand our attention. In this way, a social justice paradigm reflects the eighth moment of qualitative inquiry, which "asks that the social sciences and the humanities become sites for critical conversations about democracy, race, gender, class, nation-states, globalization, freedom and community" (Denzin & Lincoln, 2011, p. 3).

Such changes in society will simultaneously bring about parallel changes in our research practices (Plummer, 2011). Plummer (2011) explains, "As the social world changes, so we may start to sense new approaches to making inquiries" (p. 196). Reflecting an iterative process inherent to qualitative inquiry, it is clear that as research changes the world, so too will the world change its research practices. Thus, we aim in this last chapter to outline the considerations we think are critical to the future of a social justice paradigm given the theoretical and methodological tools collected in this book. We begin with the need to embrace a deep interdisciplinarity.

Embrace Deep Interdisciplinarity

> Research—like life—is a contradictory, messy affair.
> (Plummer, 2011, p. 195)

It is increasingly apparent that to get at the complicated, messy affairs that create and are created by social inequities, research acts also need to be complex affairs. Such complexity can be achieved through inter-disciplinarity, which Kincheloe (2001) describes as "a process where disciplinary boundaries are crossed and the analytical frames of more than one discipline are employed by the researcher" (p. 685). Inter-disciplinarity enables researchers to adopt different theoretical per-spectives and methodological approaches to address dynamic issues, problems, and inequities through various lenses. In addition, inter-disciplinarity enables researchers from different backgrounds and traditions to work together under an umbrella of respect for various approaches. Such diversity is important "as parts of complex systems and intricate processes, objects of inquiry are far too mercurial to be viewed by a single way of seeing or as a snapshot of a particular phe-nomenon at a specific moment in time" (Kincheloe et al., 2011, p. 170). Yet, interdisciplinarity itself is no longer enough to achieve so-cial justice aims. We need to go *deep* (Kincheloe et al., 2011)!

Whereas interdisciplinarity enables researchers to adopt various lenses/approaches and respects a multiplicity of perspectives, *deep* interdisciplinarity creates *new* levels of awareness and *new* modes of research. Deep interdisciplinarity seeks to "modify disciplines and the view of research each person brings to the table; everyone leaves the table informed by the dialogue in a way that idiosyncratically influ-ences the research methods they subsequently employ. The point of interaction is not standardized agreement…but awareness of the di-verse tools in the researcher's toolbox" (Kincheloe et al., 2011, p.170).

Part of deep interdisciplinarity is what Newbury (2011) calls *theoretical inconsistency*. Newbury explains:

> If I am committed to the ideals of social justice…then I must realize that not everyone will share my view of what this looks like. I must accept the fact that there will be readers who view my research from a drastically different theoretical orientation than my own. And if I wish to dialogue across the expanse that lies between our world-views, then my work must hold some relevance to their own lives and work…. And this may in turn create space for important genera-tive dialogues and collaborations that previously did not take place, contributing to the potential of positive social change (p. 340).

Theoretical inconsistency creates the forum for critical discussions that Denzin and Lincoln (2011) argue are vital in the eighth moment. Such discussion can spark questions between researchers, but also within individual researchers as scholars think through who they are, what they stand for, and why. For example, Plummer (2011) finds himself pondering: "So here am I, like many others, a bit of a humanist, a bit post-gay, a sort of feminist, a little queer, a kind of liberal…. Who am I? How can I live with these tensions?" (p. 197). If you are doing this work well, you will likely encounter similar tensions. Reconciling such tensions, however, is likely not possible, nor desirable (Newbury, 2011; Plummer, 2011). We must *live* the tensions to learn and grow, even when they are painful (Johnson, 2009, 2014).

Rather than viewing paradigmatic advances through a polarizing lens of one or two paradigms (such as postpositivism or interpretivism), we encourage an exploration of the multitude of social justice approaches and accompanying theories and related hybrids—those embodied in Marxism, LGBT theory, critical race theory, feminist theory, queer theory, postscientism, and participatory action research, to name a few—that would enable researchers to most effectively enhance social justice within their communities of concern. With a growing group of researchers embracing social justice as the goal of the research (both in the process and the products of research), we look forward to a "proliferation, intermingling, and confluence of paradigms" that will underpin future social justice paradigms (Denzin & Giardina, 2009, p. 34).

We must take care, however, as we embark on paradigm proliferation to avoid the "Oppression Olympics" (Davis & Martinez, 1998; Johnson, 2014) wherein one equity-seeking group competes with another similarly oppressed group for attention and resources. The goal in deep interdisciplinarity is to gain a deeper, more nuanced appreciation for the pain felt and strategies used by various groups so that we might learn from one another, develop new models of research, and work together to advance a more just society for *all* groups. The desired outcome of deep interdisciplinarity is recognizing the conditions operating in society that continue to exploit and dehumanize people and the development of strategies for change.

Engage in Risky Reflexivity and Radical Research

Writers/researchers make a space of analysis in which the motives, consciousness, politics, and stances of informants and researchers/writes are rendered contradictory, problematic, and filled with transgressive possibilities. (Fine, 1994, p. 75)

Deep interdisciplinarity requires researchers to recognize when tensions develop in the research process, to be willing to move in unanticipated directions, and to be open to surprises along the way (Newbury, 2011). Deep interdisciplinarity requires a self-reflexive researcher. According to Johnson (2014), self-reflexivity is one of the most important considerations for those involved in social justice research. It involves the interest and willingness to "privately and publicly unpack the very real, but constructed dichotomies between our personal and professional lives" (p. 7). Unpacking these issues is risky, both personally and professionally. Consider for a moment, the risk of being a white, male, gay scholar revealing a racist upbringing (Johnson, 2009), or a female feminist scholar who struggles to deal with her transprejudice. Risk is a critical component of self-reflexivity, and qualitative researchers must confront it "if they are to work for social justice/change. In that uncomfortable place is where a space imbued with official academic discourses meets a space of testimony and witness where one of the dilemmas of reflexive inquiry lies" (Johnson, 2009, p. 488).

The reward of risky reflexivity is the ability to conduct radical research. Whereas much research is "about keeping the lid on the dustbin" (Schostak, 2012, p. 4), radical research is about blowing the lid off. Radical research is a collective endeavor that aims to create conditions in which *all* people can make a difference in their own lives (Schostak, 2012). To make a difference in the lives of others, however, we must be able to interrogate our own landscape. Researchers who engage in risky reflexivity are able to question the conditions in which she/he is part of the problem of social inequities (vis-à-vis various forms of privilege) and are willing to own those mistakes as well as give up resources to begin to become part of the solution (Johnson, 2009).

Radical should not imply, however, that the sole focus of research is the large, macro-level inequities that create major inequities (such as pay inequities). On the contrary, radical research appreciates that it is often the conditions of *everyday life* that require attention as ordinariness can conceal systematic constraints that create social inequities (Parry, 2014). One means by which radical research facilitates the sharing of voices to be equally heard and made effective is through texts that involve and speak to the everyday experiences of people.

Create Evocative Texts that Enact an Ethical Experience

We change the world by the way we make it visible.
(Denzin, 2000, p. 266)

Radical researchers want to bring experiences to life and avoid representational strategies in which the voices of participants are "buried beneath layers of analysis" (Denison, 1996, p. 352) or co-opted for the purposes of academic reward. Instead, radical researchers want to represent research in a manner that honors people (Richardson, 2000). As a result, radical researchers create texts that "move from the personal to the political, from the local to the historical and the cultural. These are dialogic texts and presume an active audience, which create spaces for give-and-take between reader and writer. They do more than turn the Other into the object of the social science gaze" (Denzin & Lincoln, 2011, p. 5).

Creative analytic practice (CAP) is one effective way to create texts that enact an ethical experience while being engaging and accessible to a wide audience, including those outside of academia (Richardson, 2000). CAP involves expressing what one has learned in research through evocative and creative writing techniques including artistic and literary genres such as stories, poems, plays, vignettes, and other performance pieces (Parry & Johnson, 2007). Using CAP, radical researchers are able to integrate their voice with those of their participants to show the author is always present in research, which stands in sharp contrast to traditional social scientific work wherein researchers are taught to suppress the "I" in their write-ups (Richardson, 1997). CAP challenges the political and interpretative authority and legitimacy of a text (Schwandt, 2001). As a result, "these works constitute the next set of critical conversations among qualitative social researchers, eroding fixed categories and provoking possibilities for qualitative research that is designed *against* Othering, *for* social justice" (Fine, 1994, p. 81, original emphasis).

Richardson (1997) suggests five criteria for creating and judging texts that attempt to convey what is learned in research for social justice. The first criterion is the substantive contribution of the text. For a text to succeed substantively, it must contribute to a deeper understanding of social life, including being grounded or embedded in a human perspective. The human perspective must then inform the ways in which the text itself is constructed. For example, in Diana's dragon boat study, women made sense of their experiences with breast cancer through stories (Parry, 2007), and were thus presented as short vignettes. The second criterion for judging social justice research is its aesthetic merit. Aesthetically, radical researchers want to draw the audience in and enable readers to empathetically identify with the people in their studies and/or challenge the reader's perception of the represented group. Either way, as Mulcahy (chapter 9) articulates, to enact a social justice agenda, a text needs to be complex, interesting, and engaging: in other words, not boring! Reflexivity, as discussed above, is the third criterion to judge texts. When writing up the dragon boat study, Diana was clear about how the text was created, including her role as the researcher. She held herself accountable for the knowledge she put forth and disclosed ethical issues surrounding the creation of the text. The goals were to illustrate an adequate self-awareness/ self-exposure so that readers were able to judge her position, relation, and articulation of the experience. Richardson suggests asking how the text would affect the reader on an emotional and intellectual level. Diana hoped her dragon boat text would generate new questions, motivate others to write, and/or to try new research practices. Ultimately, Diana hoped her text would inspire readers to take social action, broadly defined, regarding women's experiences with breast cancer. The final criterion involves an expression of a reality. A text needs to convey an embodied sense of lived experience. The text needs to be believable and convey a credible account of a cultural, social, individual, or communal sense of the "real" (Richardson, 2000, p. 254).

The turn toward nontraditional and creative forms of representation enables researchers to think broadly about the audience of their research and write in a manner accessible to people besides academics (Parry & Johnson, 2007). CAP resists esoteric language that prevents scholars from putting their research to use, or a specialized lexicon that serves as barriers for non-experts to understand. Reid (2004) explains that esotericism keeps the knowledge constructed by scholars out of the hands of participants, activists, and practitioners while also preventing scholars from understanding one another. In its process and representation, CAP facilitates a higher propensity for social justice, placing participant stories in the public domain to influence change. For example, when Corey (Johnson, Singh, Gonzalez, 2014) asked the LGBTQ youth in their PAR study on bullying in high school how their data could really make a difference to create change, they said, "Our teachers and counselors don't read journals; you should make a documentary." And so they did. Although they had no previous experience with filmmaking, they gave it a shot, and the experimentation paid off. The resulting documentary films have now been shown in more than 1,000 schools in the state of Georgia; they live on the Web for anyone to access; they mobilized a movement for enumerated bullying policies in most of the state; and they launched the Georgia Safe Schools Coalition and sustain organizations taking up the issue of LGBTQ youth empowerment statewide.

So as we look to the future of social justice, it is clear "we are in a new age where messy, uncertain, multivoiced texts, cultural criticism, and new experimental works will become more common, as will more re-flexive forms of fieldwork, analysis, and intertextual representations" (Denzin & Lincoln, 2011, p. 26).

Develop Communities of Friendly/Critical Participants

We were advocating for a new performative cultural politics, a radical democratic imagination that redefined the concept of civic participation and public citizenship (especially within the academy)…. [T]his imagination dialogically inserts itself into the world, provoking conflict, curiosity, criticism, and reflection, and contributes to a public conversation. (Giardina & Denzin, 2011, p. 324)

Texts that create and enact moral meaning require researchers to work *with*, rather than *for*, a community or group (Angrosino & Rosenberg, 2011; Denzin, 1997). Working for a community or group (a value of postpositivism) implies a philosophically distant stance between the researcher and the researched with objectivism as a goal of the research process (Lincoln, Lynham & Guba, 2011). Working *with* a community or group dictates that the researcher have a deep kinship (political and emotional) with research participants based upon membership or social ties (Angrosino & Rosenberg, 2011). Within a social justice research agenda, participants are not distant objects of study, but rather neighbors, lovers, friends, family members, and/or allies in the goals of emancipation. Such transparency in relationships creates a community of critical informants (Dupuis, 1999) where knowledge can be built from the lived experiences of people.

Understanding the lived experience of people is essential because social justice researchers frequently become spokespersons or advocates for causes and issues; they can help people articulate enduring and emergent problems and bring together key stakeholders for community discussions/actions (Angrosino & Rosenberg, 2011). Social justice research reflects an emancipatory vision that involves the researcher who is part of and working with the community to create a different world (Charmaz, 2011) for that community. Horsfall and Titchen (2009) have found:

Working this way promotes different understandings and outcomes of whose and what knowledge gets to count, and of what types of knowing or researching are worth more than others…disrupting edges and opening up research spaces in these ways and creating the conditions for human flourishing can be more inclusive and accessible for people, cultures, environments not trained in, or using, research or academic-speak. (p. 158)

One place to begin creating communities of friendly, but critical informants is through our pedagogy.

Link Social Justice Research to Critical Pedagogy

Education either functions as an instrument which is used to facilitate integration…or it becomes the practice of freedom, the means by which men and women deal critically and creatively with reality and discover how to participate in the transformation of their world. (Freire, 2000, p. 34)

Many academics ask themselves, "How can I ensure that my research and teaching make a positive impact on societal and educational transformation?" (Wood, 2010, p. 108). The future of social justice demands a shift in which everyone can be a radical researcher, if that is their desire. To accomplish this aim, we must energize and engage students with social justice issues that are important to them so they are empowered to change the world. The goal is for all educators to ask, "How can teaching for social justice be conceptualized so that every individual may locate his or her position within it?" (Sonu, 2012, p. 177). In other words, how can we teach students to confront social inequities and use research "as a transformative endeavour with an emancipatory consciousness" (Kincheloe et al., 2011, p. 164)? Students must learn the process of investigation, examination, criticism, and re-investigation so that they see and think more critically and recognize the forces that subtly shape their lives (Freire, 2000; Kincheloe et al., 2011). To accomplish this, we must teach students to "read" differently. We use *reading* here to note multiple forms of literacy, from reading a book or play to websites or graphic novels. Reading needs to move beyond comprehension of words on a page to a deeper understanding and engagement with the "unstated dominant ideologies hidden between the sentences" (Kincheloe et al., 2011, p. 165). In short, we must teach students to read the world differently, including texts, social situations, language, and the actions of people (Freire, 2000).

However, before we adopt a critical pedagogy, we must pause and examine the process of teaching (and learning) our research methods. This pause, or what Kincheloe, McLaren, and Steinberg (2011) refer to as a "step back…allows us a conceptual distance that produces critical consciousness…[refusing] the passive acceptance of externally imposed research that tacitly certify modes of justifying knowledges that are decontextualized, reductionistic, and inscribed by dominant modes of power" (p. 169). We believe we need a "reimagination" of qualitative inquiry that is radical, unconventional, and exciting (St. Pierre, 2011, p. 613). Giardina and Denzin (2011) argue four important pedagogical outcomes of a new, imaginative social science:

> First, as a form of instruction, it helps persons think critically, historically, and sociologically. Second, as critical pedagogy, it exposes the pedagogies of oppression that produce and reproduce oppression and injustice (see Freire, 2000, p. 54). Third, it contributes to an ethical self-consciousness that is critical and reflexive. It gives people a language and a set of pedagogical practices that endeavors to turn oppression into freedom, despair into hope, hatred into love, doubt into trust. Fourth, in turn, this self-consciousness shapes a critical racial self-awareness. This awareness contributes to utopian dreams of racial equality and racial justice. (Giardina & Denzin, 2011, p. 324)

A new critical pedagogy enables us to imagine the possibilities of all people linked to a social justice paradigm in which we all have stories that frame a larger, grander story where we take action against injustices (Sonu et al., 2012). In applying a critical pedagogical lens, "we create an empowering qualitative research, which expands, contracts, grows, and questions itself within the theory and practice examined" (Kincheloe et al., 2011, p. 167). Such an approach is critical to the future of a social justice paradigm.

Conclusion

As we see it, these are the five key areas that shape the future of a social justice paradigm. Part of that future includes you, the reader. Our aim in writing this book is to provide the methodological processes for qualitative inquiry so that others are able to move forward and enact social justice. While we hope the historical evolution of a social justice paradigm and its key considerations provide a necessary context, the crux of the book are the seven methodological approaches that serve as guidance as you embrace a social justice paradigm through qualitative inquiry. When considering *your* particular methodological approach to a social justice paradigm for each given project, remember that

> the process of becoming a social justice researcher includes the discovery of a new set of lenses, emerging tools, and new pathways while maintaining a critical and post perspective rooted in anti-oppressive praxis. Research becomes an extension of one's own identity

as a human/animal/environment rights activists, which requires leveraging the skills and capacities of research as a strategy to move to a more socially just world. (Lorenzetti, 2013, p. 451)

Whatever lenses you adopt, we hope this book inspires you and gives you the tools to take on the "thorny issues" (Rossman & Rallis, 2010, p. 381) of society by using your subjectivity, experience, creativity, and research design skills to transform the world by championing dignity for all people, reducing suffering, and promoting wellbeing (Plummer, 2011). Such research advances are what Denzin and Lincoln (2011) have called a "civic social science….committed up front to issues of social justice, equity, nonviolence, peace, and universal human rights" (p. 613).

With this call to action in mind, we position this book within a "politics of possibility" (Giardina & Denzin, 2011, p. 319). Such a politics demands a focus on "how far we can 'push' the boundaries of qualitative research into new fields, strategies, and political/moral awareness" for a more just society (Plummer, 2011, p. 198). Our own social justice goal in writing this book is to provide a pathway for conducting research that not only gets "heads" but also "hearts" working for social justice (Horsfall & Titchen, 2009, p. 148).

We agree with Lincoln and Denzin (2011) that "we have work to do, important work, and we must do it fast and well" (p. 718). Our hope is that this book provides you with what you need to begin *your* important work. Start with a politics of hope (Denzin, 2000). As Freire (2000) argues, hope underpins the desire/dream for improving human existence. In his words, "Hope is ethical. Hope is moral. Hope is peaceful and nonviolent. Hope seeks the truth of life's sufferings. Hope gives meaning to the struggles to change the world. Hope is grounded in concrete performative" (p. 8). Embrace hope and move forward to create the type of world you see and think is just. We wish you all the best as you embrace a social justice paradigm and look forward to learning about the ways you have made the world a better place for everyone.

REFERENCES

Angrosino, M., & Rosenberg, J. (2011). Observations on observation: Continuities and challenges. In N. K. Denzin, & Y. S. Lincoln (Eds.), *The Sage handbook of qualitative research* (4th ed.) (pp. 467–478). Thousand Oaks, CA: Sage.

Charmaz, K. (2011). Grounded theory methods in social justice research. In N. K. Denzin, & Y. E. Lincoln (Eds.), *The Sage handbook of qualitative research* (4th ed.), (pp. 359–380). Thousand Oaks, CA: Sage.

Davis, A. Y., & Martinez, E. (1998, May). *Coalition building among people of color.* Paper presented at the University of California, San Diego. Retrieved from http://culturalstudies.ucsc.edu/PUBS/Inscriptions/vol_7/Davis.html

Denison, J. (1996). Sport narratives. *Qualitative Inquiry, 2*(3), 351–362.

Denzin, N. K. (1997). *Reading the crisis: Interpretive ethnography.* Thousand Oaks, CA: Sage.

Denzin, N. K. (2000). Aesthetics and the practices of qualitative inquiry. *Qualitative Inquiry, 6* (2), 256–265.

Denzin, N. K., & Giardina, M. D. (Eds.). (2009). *Qualitative inquiry and social justice.* Walnut Creek, CA: Left Coast Press.

Denzin, N. K., & Lincoln, Y. S. (Eds.). (2011). *The Sage handbook of qualitative research* (4th ed.). Thousand Oaks, CA: Sage.

Dupuis, S. (1999). Naked truths: Towards a reflexive methodology in leisure research. *Leisure Sciences, 21,* 43–64.

Fine, M. (1994). Working the hyphens: Reinventing self and others in qualitative research. In N. K Denzin & Y. S Lincoln (Eds.), *Handbook of qualitative research* (pp. 70–82). Thousand Oaks, CA: Sage.

Freire, P. (2000). *Pedagogy of the oppressed.* London, UK: Continuum.

Giardina, M. D., & Denzin, N. K. (2011). Acts of activism Politics of possibility toward a new performative cultural politics. *Cultural Studies Critical Methodologies, 11*(4), 319–327.

Horsfall, D., & Titchen, A. (2009). Disrupting edges–opening spaces: Pursuing democracy and human flourishing through creative methodologies. *International Journal of Social Research Methodology, 12*(2), 147–160.

Johnson, C. W. (2009). Writing ourselves at risk: Using self-narrative in working for social justice. *Leisure Sciences, 31*(5), 483–489.

Johnson, C. W. (2014). All you need is love: Considerations for social justice leisure research. *Leisure Sciences, 36*(8), 388–399.

Johnson, C. W., Singh, A. A., & Gonzalez, M. (2014). "It's complicated": Collective memories of LGBTQQ youth. *Journal of Homosexuality, 61*(3), 419–434.

Kincheloe, J. L. (2001). Describing the bricolage: Conceptualizing a new rigor in qualitative research. *Qualitative Inquiry, 7*(6), 679–692.

Kincheloe, J. L., McLaren, P., & Steinberg, S. R. (2011). Critical pedagogy, and qualitative research: Moving to the bricolage. In N. K. Denzin, & Y. S. Lincoln (Eds.), *The Sage handbook of qualitative research* (4th ed.) (pp. 163–178). Thousand Oaks, CA: Sage.

Lincoln, Y. S., & Denzin, N. K. (2011). Epilogue: Toward a "refunctioned ethnography." In N. K. Denzin, & Y. S. Lincoln (Eds.), *The Sage handbook of qualitative research* (4th ed.) (pp. 715–718). Thousand Oaks, CA: Sage.

Lincoln, Y. S., Lynham, S. A., & Guba, E. G. (2011). Paradigmatic controversies, contradictions, and emerging confluences, revisited. In N. K. Denzin, & Y. S. Lincoln (Eds.), *The Sage handbook of qualitative research* (4th ed.) (pp. 97–128). Thousand Oaks, CA: Sage.

Lorenzetti, L. (2013). Research as a social justice tool: An activist's perspective. *Affilia, 28*(4), 451–457.

Newbury, J. (2011). A place for theoretical inconsistency. *International Journal of Qualitative Methods, 10*(4), 335–347.

Parry, D. C. (2007). "There is life after breast cancer": Nine vignettes exploring dragon boat racing for breast cancer survivors. *Leisure Sciences, 29*(1), 53–69.

Parry, D. C. (2014). My transformative desires: Enacting feminist social justice leisure research. *Leisure Sciences, 36*(4), 1–16.

Parry, D. C., & Johnson, C. W. (2007). Contextualizing leisure research and encompassing complexity in lived leisure experience: The need for creative analytic practice. *Leisure Sciences, 29*(2), 119–130.

Plummer, K. (2011). Critical humanism and queer theory: Living with the tensions. In N. K. Denzin, & Y. S. Lincoln (Eds.), *The Sage handbook of qualitative research* (4th ed.) (pp. 195–212). Thousand Oaks, CA: Sage.

Reid, C. (2004). Advancing women's social justice agenda: A feminist action research framework. *International Journal of Qualitative Methods, 3*(3), 1–15.

Richardson, L. (1997). *Fields of play: Constructing an academic life*. New Brunswick, NJ: Rutgers University Press.

Richardson, L. (2000). Writing: A method of inquiry. In N. K. Denzin, & Y. S. Lincoln (Eds.), *Handbook of qualitative research* (2nd ed.) (pp. 923–948). Thousand Oaks, CA: Sage.

Rossman, G. B., & Rallis, S. F. (2010). Everyday ethics: Reflections on practice. *International Journal of Qualitative Studies in Education, 23*(4), 379–391.

Schostak, J. (2012). *Social justice, education and the politics of research methodology*. Paper presented at University of East London, London, UK, April 2012. Retrieved from http://www.academia.edu/5275076/Social_Justice_Education_and_the_Politics_of_Research_Methodology

Schwandt, T. A. (2001). *Dictionary of qualitative inquiry*. Thousand Oaks, CA: Sage.

Sonu, D. (2012). Illusions of compliance: Performing the public and hidden transcripts of social justice education in neoliberal times. *Curriculum Inquiry, 42*(2), 240–259.

Sonu, D., Oppenheim, R., Epstein, S. E., & Agarwal, R. (2012). Taking responsibility: The multiple and shifting positions of social justice educators. *Education, Citizenship and Social Justice, 7*(2), 175–189.

St. Pierre, E. A. (2011). Post qualitative research: The critique and the coming after. In N. K. Denzin, & Y. S. Lincoln (Eds.), *The Sage handbook of qualitative research* (4th ed.) (pp. 611–626). Thousand Oaks, CA: Sage.

Wood, L. (2010). The transformative potential of living theory educational research. *Educational Journal of Living Theories*, *3*(1), 105–118.

APPENDIX ||||||||||||||||||||||||||||||||||||||||||||||||||||||||||||||||||||||||||||||||||||

Dig Deeper into Additional Readings

MARXIST THEORY

Marx, K., & Engels, F. (2002). *The communist manifesto* (S. Moore, Trans.), G. S. Jones (Ed.). New York: Penguin Putnam Inc. (original work published 1848).

It is here that Marx makes his well-known statement that all history is that of class struggle. This short but profound text is an elaboration of this basic proposition. By tracing the struggles between the bourgeois and proletarians, the proletariats and communists, and by exploring the relation between his socialist moment and those of previous generations, Marx arrives at his revolutionary call to communists and other opposition parties to move against the existing social and political order. This clarion, though dated and troubled by the failings of the many movements his work inspired, is still worthy of consideration for scholars working with issues of social class. With the intensification of many of the struggles Marx details, and their proliferation within late capitalist societies, his thought is such that change can scarcely be conceived without it.

Marx, K. (1979). *A contribution to the critique of the political economy* (N. I. Stone, Trans., from the second German edition). Chicago, IL: Charles H. Kerr & Company (original work published 1859).

Many of the ideas Marx develops in this contribution were elaborated in *Capital, Volume 1*; however, this earlier text retains its value and importance as it focuses on the underpinnings of the capitalist system as well as the theory of historical materialism that Marx developed to explain human history. Both aspects of the text reveal the complexity of Marx's thought in relation to his extensive project of socialist revolution. Though dense and a challenging read, this text is indispensible for grappling with the nuance of Marxist theory.

Marx, K. (2011). *Capital, volume 1: A critique of political economy* (S. Moore & E. Aveling, Trans.), F. Engels (Ed.). Mineola, NY: Dover Publications (original work published 1867).

Involving more than 30 years of deliberation, and ultimately unfinished prior to his death, this work is often considered Marx's masterpiece. The analysis yields a passionate denouncement of the brutality of nineteenth-century capitalism, constructed by close examination of its inner workings. This text establishes the foundations for most of Marx's theories, and provides the groundwork for his conclusion that capitalism cannot be reformed but only overthrown by a revolution led by the working class.

CRITICAL RACE THEORY

Bell, D. A. (1992). *Faces at the bottom of the well: The permanence of racism.* New York: Basic Books.

Within the so-called "post-racial" epoch of the Obama administration, this relatively early work by Derrick Bell reasserts itself to debunk the myth of racial equality. Moreover, this text discredits any notion of a progressive, step-by-step movement toward an inevitable racial equity. Bell reveals how even the occasional judicial, political, and legislative changes in the discourse of race operate to obscure the harsh reality that racism is permanent. Yet, the permanence of racism is matched with a hopeful political and economic struggle, which is to make meaning in the face of absurdity. This book is invaluable in striking down and shattering the whitewashed imagination of social justice, building in its place a permanence of political struggle full of meaning.

Delgado, R., & Stefancic, J. (Eds.) (2005). *The Derrick Bell reader.* New York: New York University Press.

Delgado and Stefancic's edited collection brings together some of the most influential works of Critical Race Theory founder Derrick Bell. Of interest are both Bell's analytical methods and their effective disruption of majoritarian tropes in legal and sociological discourse. The presumed orthodoxy behind much racial thought is critiqued with equal provocation and inspiration. Though this text dispenses with versions of social change that "feel good," this collection does provide many intimations of change that can become the fuel for less placid and domesticated movements toward racial justice.

Delgado, R., & Stefancic, J. (Eds.). (2001). *Critical race theory: An introduction.* New York: New York University Press.

This reader edited by Delgado and Stefancic provides an accessible collection of essays that outlines the undergirding principles, tenets, and commitments of Critical Race Theory. The volume is not only accessible as an overview, but it is also equally provocative, demonstrating the underlying racial oppression permeating legal, sociological, and political life. Though much of the essays included in this volume may appeal more directly to the question of law, its terminology and concepts articulate profound ideas ready for application in the broader social sciences and humanities.

Crenshaw, K., Gotanda, N., Peller, G., & Thomas, K. (Eds.). (1996). *Critical race theory: The key writings that formed the movement*. New York: The New Press.

This volume of essays edited and compiled by Crenshaw, Gotanda, Peller, and Thomas provides a great service to the field of Critical Race Theory by delineating the theoretical structure and critical features of the movement. The movement is nothing less then the critical examination of contemporary legal thought and doctrine and the dismantling of its reification of social dominance and subordination of people of color.

FEMINISM

Irigaray, L. (1985). *Speculum of the other woman* (G. C. Gill, Trans.). Ithaca, NY: Cornell University Press (original work published 1974).

Luce Irigaray's text is one of the most important works of 1970s feminist theory. The text offers critical readings of both Freud and Plato, which remain relevant a generation later. The readings attack the masculine ideology inherent in psychoanalysis and Western discourse, as well as the origins in philosophical metaphors that work to exclude women from the production of discourse. Between these critiques of Freud and Plato are 10 essays that attend to far-ranging aspects of history and philosophy as they relate to women, which explores what Irigaray is most widely known for celebrating: the sexual difference of women.

de Beauvoir, S. (2011). *The second sex* (C. Borde & S. Malovany-Chevallier, Trans.). New York: Vintage Books (original work published 1949).

Primarily known as an existential philosopher, de Beauvoir gained an additional reputation as a radical when this text was originally published in 1949. *The Second Sex* was placed on the Vatican's list of forbidden books, and as such it speaks to the vehement and—at the time—controversial tones of her writing. Yet, this text was highly influential to the development of subsequent works by Friedan (*Feminine Mystique*) and Millett (*Sexual Politics*), equally considered critical sources for feminist theory. In addition to the text offering a continental perspective within an historical context of the late 1940s, its enduring strength lies in de Beauvoir's rigorous review of data from biology, physiology, ethnology, anthropology, mythology, folklore, philosophy, economics, and literary criticism to support her arguments against the forced relegation of women to a secondary position to men in Western society. The book stands as an early feminist text of merit for its many profound insights into women's lives, struggles, and politics, and helps one to understand what it means to be a woman.

hooks, b. (1999). *Ain't I a woman: Black women and feminism*. Brooklyn, NY: South End Press (original work published 1981).

Considered by many to be a seminal work in black feminism, bell hooks offers a thorough critique of white male patriarchal oppression, the failings of various historical freedom movements intended to include black women, and the tendency in feminism to treat sex and race as separate social categories. Leveling her argument that these identities are inseparable through a broad historical reading of black women's oppression by both black and white male patriarchy, she provides a detailed chronology of feminism within a broad historical context. This text is one that must be read and read again, especially by feminist scholars who want to work for emancipatory politics that counters the historical exclusion of women of color.

McCann, C. R., & Kim, S. (Eds.). (2013). *Feminist theory reader* (3rd ed.). New York: Routledge.

This collection of essays edited by McCann and Kim provides a thorough reading of feminist theory. Global and third-world texts are incorporated throughout the volume, which provides a significant contribution of a broad survey of feminist theory. In addition, it emphasizes intersectionality between theories, topics, and authors by bringing their historical context to the fore. The volume provides a quality overview of feminist theory while also examining the fluidity and intersectionality of gender discourses.

LGBT THEORY

Rubin, G. S. (1993). Thinking sex: Notes for a radical theory of the politics of sexuality. In H. Abelove, M. A. Barale, & D. M. Halperin (Eds.), *The Lesbian and gay studies reader* (pp. 3–44). New York: Routledge (original work published 1984).

Rubin's essay is a provocative critique of the limitations of feminist theory and supposed innocence of children, which she intended to cast as a myth. This essay, originally published in 1984, was groundbreaking at the time, but requires further analysis. As such, it is a good launching point for scholars interested in determining critical avenues for contemporary critique of sexual politics and the history of sexual persecution.

Sedgwick, E. K. (1990). *Epistemology of the closet*. Oakland, CA: University of California Press.

Eve Kosofsky Sedgwick is considered one of the founders of LGBT studies. This text's critical argument is that every aspect of Western culture is intimately touched, affected, and implicated in the gender and sexual binary distinctions undergirding its structure. Equal parts literary, historical, and critical analysis, she attacks these binaries, revealing several contradictions valuable for conceiving sexuality and gender differently. This text also provides a thoughtful and provocative analysis of the first-wave AIDS epidemic. Frequently interweaving diverse sources such as Nietzsche, Foucault, Melville, Wilde, and Proust, the introduction and first chapter provide an excellent overview of her theoretical stance and the trajectory it sets for the then-burgeoning project of her scholarship.

Halberstam, J. (1998). *Female masculinity*. Durham, NC: Duke University Press.

With the growing body of literature exploring issues of masculinity coming at the expense of women, Judith Halberstam's text works to disrupt this problematic by focusing specifically on the complex and multiple masculinities females embody. Her text argues that granting ownership of masculinity to white men enables the condemnation of female masculinities embodied by both straight and lesbian feminists. Ultimately, this text works towards an acknowledgment of gender indeterminacy as a valid and celebrated identity.

Stryker, S., & Whittle, S. (Eds.) (2006). *The transgender studies reader*. New York: Routledge.

Susan Stryker's and Stephen Whittle's edited collection of essays from a wide range of scholars are drawn together to demonstrate the developing scholarly and popular discourses related to transgender theory, in particular how notions of gender, sexuality, agency, and identity evolve and transform with its development. Including work from before the 1990s, the medicalization and psychologization of transgender identities and bodies is discussed in conjunction with its subsequent displacement by a 1990s-and-beyond line of scholarship dedicated to activism. The linguistic determination of transgender persons is discussed in relation to postmodern deconstruction whereby possibilities for reconstructive, reinventive, and recuperative processes of understanding the gendered self in its thorough disordered-ness is highlighted. Essay by essay, the editors of this volume engender a political struggle against inherited meanings of gender and sex, and in the process offer a poignant overview of construction of transgender studies.

QUEER THEORY

Foucault, M. (1990). *The history of sexuality: Volume 1: An introduction* (R. Hurley, Trans.). New York: Vintage Books (original work published 1976).

This book by Michel Foucault begins from a very different perspective of sex and sexuality than hypotheses that suppose their repression in discourse; instead, he argues that sex and sexuality have proliferated and intensified in discourse, and questions how sex and sexuality are considered the essential definition of a human being. Far from a repressive force deployed in a law-like structure, Foucault sees power in relations and circulating in all directions. Sexuality is seen as a conduit for the circulation and movement of such power. The technologies deployed to discipline and control sexuality and sex deemed deviant is considered a means to normalize and regulate the population. Instead of sex/sexuality being the defining essence of human being, it is posited as a social construct enabling population control.

Butler, J. (1990). *Gender trouble: Feminism and the subversion of identity*. New York: Routledge.

Judith Butler is a philosopher perhaps most recognized for this book, in which she critiques the assumed stable and fixed categories of gender and the presupposition that these extend from nature and a necessary heterosexuality. Her arguments trouble the fictions as well as their supporting regulatory, hierarchical structures. Her troubling lends to her theorization of gender performativity. Understanding gender performativity requires more than a superficial engagement with this groundbreaking text; it is the primer for any subsequent work on the performance of gender, its construction, reification, and destabilization.

Jagose, A. (1996). *Queer theory: An introduction*. New York: New York University Press.

Annamarie Jagose's book provides a particularly valuable historical overview of the diverse theories and movements that are commonly grouped under the rubric of "queer theory" as if it had no antecedents. Equally valuable is her unflinching interrogation of supposedly essential categories of *gay, lesbian,* and *bisexuality,* along with the essential notions of *man, woman, sex,* and *gender,* which she sees as the challenge of queer theorists proper, to disrupt the essentialism undergirding such concepts.

Vaid, U. (1995). *Virtual equality: The mainstreaming of gay & lesbian liberation*. New York: Anchor Books.

As an activist and critical voice in the discourses of sexuality and gender, Urvashi Vaid wrestles with the difficult questions of what unites and divides us. In this book, she posits that there can be no coming together, consensus, or unity among the issues that divide.

In the quest for liberation and legitimacy, she argues that gay and lesbian issues have become coopted in their mainstreaming, resulting in disappointment, disillusion, envy, and only an appearance of acceptance. Vaid appeals for caution in how legitimacy and liberation is sought, noting the problems and tensions between action and rhetoric that often ring hollow, superficial, and inconsiderate of race and class. For Vaid, the mainstream attention given to the movement for legitimatization and liberation is paradoxical insofar as these goals are only achieved to the degree that marginalization is maintained. Vaid's is a call for more than rhetoric, more than lip service, and more than one movement, as the battle to assert rights and have them legally guaranteed has not ended but widened.

POSTSTRUCTURALISM

Derrida, J. (1978). Structure, sign and play in the discourse of the human sciences (Alan Bass, Trans.). In *Jacques Derrida, writing and difference* (pp. 278–293). Chicago, IL: The University of Chicago Press (lecture delivered 1966).

Jacque Derrida is undoubtedly one of the most profound figures in poststructuralism, and this lecture is considered by many to mark the beginnings of that theoretical premise. What Derrida presents in the lecture is an analysis of structuralism, primarily as pertains to linguistics, the hallmark of "centering." Centering is the fixing of a structure on a privileged term, whether man, God, presence, or being, to locking it in to an established mode that can no longer "play" or move along to other modes of thought. This text is one of two particularly relevant for the pragmatic work of affirmative deconstruction, for which Derrida is most widely known. Derrida's text is complex and dense, but equally beautiful in its composition. As a primary text for poststructuralist theory, Derrida is indispensible reading.

Derrida, J. (1998) *Of Grammatology* (G. Spivak, Trans.). Baltimore, MD: Johns Hopkins University Press (original work published 1967).

The second text that establishes Derrida's theory of affirmative deconstruction and critiques of phenomenology, psychoanalysis, and structuralism is *Of Grammatology*. It is indispensible for understanding the basic response to the problems of structuralism, particularly in relation to linguistics, which accounts for much of the association with Derrida's version of poststructuralism to the linguistic turn and its affinity amongst critical literature studies. This text provides extensive forays into Derrida's philosophical oeuvre, and the translator's introduction captures much of its impetus as a pragmatic, ethical urgency to live and act in the midst of decentered uncertainty.

Foucault, M. (1970). *The order of things: An archaeology of the human sciences*. New York: Vintage Books (original work published 1966).

Although Foucault is perhaps most often known for his work on the genealogy of sexuality, this text deploys his archaeological method to establish a distinction between his attempt to understand the organizing and structuring models of human perception and knowledge, their shifts and alterations, between the Renaissance and the end of the nineteenth century from the projects of phenomenology and history. The models Foucault examines are biology, linguistics, and economics as the disciplines of the human science par excellence. Through his analyses, the idioms and presuppositions of these sciences are leveraged to disrupt the Western structure of human being and reality. Though this text is perhaps more difficult, verbose, and obscure than his later works, it is provides many significant insights into his philosophical preoccupations, giving a certain shape to many later critical polemics.

Deleuze, G. & Guattari, F. (1987). *A thousand plateaus: Capitalism and schizophrenia* (B. Massumi, Trans.). Minneapolis, MN: University of Minnesota Press (original work published 1980).

Though Deleuze wrote several monographs and theoretical texts on his own, this is a second book in a series on capitalism and schizophrenia, and stands as a rich culmination of much of the previous and subsequent work. Taking Spinoza, Nietzsche, and Bergson as their antecedents, Deleuze and Guattari develop many concepts that are increasingly finding traction in critical discourses. Though it is impossible to encapsulate the diverse range of topics and concepts they espouse in their text, it is perhaps not too simplistic to characterize their overarching project as the subversion and uprooting of the arborescent structures of linguistics, phallogocentrism, and the supremacy of the interiority of human being. As such they celebrate—and exemplify in each plateau of the text—the many ways that these structures not only undo themselves, but necessarily must. Social change for Deleuze and Guattari is not simply a matter of replacing one structure for another, one majority for another, but necessarily a becoming-molecular of bodies that generates micropolitical movements capable of subverting molar regimes. The text is intended to be taken up and applied, even without full understanding, to social projects. It is this reason we offer this text as suggested reading alongside those of Foucault and Derrida. The translator's introduction provides a thoughtful and equally polemic overview of the text.

POSTCOLONIALISM

Young, R. J. C. (2001). *Postcolonialism: An historical introduction.* Malden, MA: Blackwell Publishers Inc.

Robert Young is recognized as a leading exponent of postcolonial theory. This reader is suggested as much for its historical depth as its comprehensive breadth. As an introductory text, scholars approaching postcolonialism for the first time will benefit from its clear and accessible language, thorough explanation of key concepts and terminology, exposition of historical antecedents, and interpretation of many early postcolonial works.

Said, E. W. (1979). *Orientalism.* New York: Vintage Books.

This book by Edward Said is considered by many to be among the founding texts of postcolonial theory. He deploys the term "orientalism" as both an epistemological and ontological style of thought necessary to distinguish between "the Orient" (principally referring to what the West calls the Middle East) and "the Occident." From this onto-epistemological orientation, Said discusses institutionalized, historical-cultural disparities between East and West. With a blend of Foucauldian and Marxist theory, he probes these power relations, noting how even Western scholarship inscribes a supposed inferiority upon the regions and people of the East, shaping subjectivities, knowledges, and languages with colonial discourses and colonial rule structured by an assumed "superiority" of the West.

Spivak, G. C. (1999). *A critique of postcolonial reason: Toward a history of the vanishing present.* Cambridge, MA: Harvard University Press.

Gayatri Spivak is among the most widely recognized scholars of postcolonial and third-world feminist theory for the complexity and nuance of her thought as well as her provocative writing style. This relatively recent text may be read as a challenge to, and a distancing from, the field of postcolonialism she has long been associated with, by offering powerful critiques of many lines of thought currently circulating as orthodox within its purview. In so doing, she focuses attention on the reach of global power, the cultural forces that enable destruction of people and the environment, yet presses equally hard against the limits of postcolonial theory by reasserting the value of feminism, Marxism, and even the philosophy of Kant. Of particular interest is a revision of her most influential essay, "Can the Subaltern Speak?", which in many ways encompasses the major themes of her critique.

INDEX ||||||||||||||||||||||||||||||||||||||||||||||||||||||||||||||||||||||||||||||||||||||||||||||||||||||||||||||||||||||||

ABOUT THE AUTHORS ||||||||||||||||||||||||||||||||||||||||||||||||||||||||||||||||||

ABOUT THE EDITORS

Corey W. Johnson is a professor and program chair of the Qualitative Research Program in the Department of Leadership, Education Administration at The University of Georgia (UGA). He teaches courses on social justice, gender and sexuality, qualitative data collection, ethnography, and philosophy of science. His scholarship focuses on the power relations between dominant and nondominant populations in the cultural contexts of leisure. This examination provides important insight into both the privileging and discriminatory practices that occur in contemporary settings. In 2012, he received the UGA President's MLK Jr. Achieving the Dream award for his efforts to make society more just.

Diana C. Parry is an associate professor in the Department of Recreation and Leisure Studies at the University of Waterloo in Canada. Using a feminist lens, Diana's research privileges women's standpoints and aims to create social change and enact social justice by challenging the medical model of scholarship. In particular, Diana's research explores the personal and political links between women's leisure and women's health, broadly defined. Diana serves as a special advisor to President Barack Obama on women's and gender issues.

ABOUT THE CONTRIBUTORS

Bryan S. R. Grimwood is an assistant professor in the Department of Recreation and Leisure Studies at the University of Waterloo, Canada. His research explores nature–society relationships in contexts of leisure/tourism, learning, and livelihoods and is informed by principles of community-based participatory research, qualitative inquiry, and geographical notions of nature, ethics, and mobility. As a parent and outdoor educator, Bryan is also interested in the "nature stories" we tell ourselves and live, and what these stories say about our being human and the extent to which they foster resilient children, communities, and ecologies.

Brett D. Lashua is a senior lecturer in the Carnegie Faculty at Leeds Beckett University, United Kingdom. His scholarship is concerned primarily with the ways that young people make sense of their lives through arts, leisure, and cultural practices such as popular music. He is coeditor of *Sounds and the City: Popular Music, Place and Globalization* with Karl Spracklen and Stephen Wagg.

Denise L. Levy is an associate professor of social work and director of the Master in Social Work (MSW) program at Appalachian State University (ASU), where she teaches courses on cultural competence, family therapy, field/internship, and spirituality and religion in social work practice. Social justice is a common theme in her courses as well as her research. Using qualitative methods, specifically grounded theory, Denise's research focuses on how GLBTQ individuals with a Christian upbringing resolve conflict between sexual/gender identity and religious beliefs. She has received several grants/stipends and has published articles in social work, religion, and interdisciplinary journals. Prior to her time in academia, Denise, a licensed clinical social worker (LCSW), worked as an in-home family therapist and program director. A lifelong learner, she recently earned a graduate certificate in expressive arts therapy.

Caitlin M. Mulcahy is an assistant professor in the Department of Sexuality, Marriage, and Family Studies at St. Jerome's University in the University of Waterloo. Caitlin's research focuses on a sociology of the intimate through a feminist lens, connecting private experiences of friendship and family back to the dominant gender discourses that shape everyday life and the impact of these intimate experiences on social justice. Her research has explored intimate contexts such as women's diary-keeping, friendships between cancer patients, connections made between new mothers, and the intimate context of family memory keeping and the loss of a mother's memory to dementia.

Tracy Penny Light is executive director of the Centre for Student Engagement and Learning Innovation at Thompson Rivers University in Canada. She was previously director of women's studies and associate professor in the Departments of Sexuality, Marriage, and Family Studies and History at the University of Waterloo. Her disciplinary research explores the medical discourse on gender and sexuality in Canada and the United States in the twentieth century. She has two coedited books forthcoming: *Bodily Subjects: Essays on Gender and Health, 1800–2000* (with Wendy Mitchinson and Barbara Brookes), and *Feminist Pedagogy in Higher Education: Critical Theory and Practice* (with Jane Nicholas and Renée Bondy).

Jeff Rose is currently a visiting assistant professor in the Environmental Studies Department at Davidson College. His research interests pursue a diverse set of questions that critically examine issues of public space, productions of nature, connection to place, and nonnormative behaviors. Outside of academia, Jeff remains active as an instructor for Outward Bound and enjoys a variety of backcountry activities, including rock and ice climbing, backpacking, skiing, and canyoneering.

Anneliese A. Singh is an associate professor at The University of Georgia in the Department of Counseling and Human Development Services. Her research, practice, and advocacy focus on the resilience of historically marginalized populations. She is a cofounder of the Georgia Safe Schools Coalition and the Trans Resilience Project. She passionately believes in liberation, justice, and qualitative research.